Progress in Surgery — 2

Progress in Surgery
VOLUME TWO

EDITED BY

I. Taylor MD ChM FRCS
Professor of Surgery,
Southampton University Medical School,
Southampton, UK

CHURCHILL LIVINGSTONE
EDINBURGH LONDON MELBOURNE AND NEW YORK 1987

CHURCHILL LIVINGSTONE
Medical Division of Longman Group UK Limited

Distributed in the United States of America by
Churchill Livingstone Inc., 1560 Broadway, New
York, N.Y. 10036, and by associated companies,
branches and representatives throughout the world.

First published 1987

ISBN 0-443-03515-6
ISSN 0267-0399

British Library Cataloguing in Publication Data
Progress in surgery.
  Vol. 2
  1. Surgery
  I. Taylor, I.
  617   RD31

Produced by Longman Singapore Publishers (Pte) Ltd.
Printed in Singapore

Preface

In this second volume, surgical conditions in which there has been recent progress either in our overall understanding or in management have been reviewed. In the main the subjects chosen are ones which are frequently encountered either by the general surgeon or within specialist units, and accordingly any progress related to them becomes of importance. The specialist topics relate to prognosis in head and neck cancer (P. M. Stell, M. S. McCormick), the management of neonatal surgical emergencies (L. Spitz), carotid endarterectomy (A. O. Mansfield) and aspects of brain tumours (H. B. Coakham).

There has been some progress in our understanding of several depressing topics which general surgeons will undoubtedly encounter from time to time. These include the management of liver metastases (A. Flowerdew, I. Taylor), gastric cancer (W. H. Allum, J. W. L. Fielding), anal incontinence (H. L. Duthie), and radiation damage to the bowel (P. F. Schofield).

Controversies abound in surgical practice and none more so than in the role of surgery in pancreatitis (C. W. Imrie), the management of lower gastrointestinal haemorrhage (P. A. Farrands), gastro-oesophageal reflux and strictures (C. J. Stoddard), the management of stones in the common bile duct (B. J. Britton), and the role of adjuvant systemic therapy in breast cancer (T. Cooke). There has been progress in each of these five topics which has helped to clarify the guidelines for both diagnosis and treatment.

Finally, two topics which have expanded enormously in recent years are reviewed. In the case of parenteral nutrition (G. T. Royle) this is now an established and important therapeutic modality. However, the use and eventual value of monoclonal antibody and oncogene technology (I. Taylor) is still in its infancy and has yet to be incorporated into surgical practice.

Each author has been asked to review the progress which has occurred in their subject. It is hoped that the detailed analysis of these topics will be of value not only to surgical trainees during the approach of the Final Fellowship examinations, but also to surgeons-in-training and established consultants.

I would like to thank all the contributors for giving of their time in writing the reviews, my secretaries June and Lynne Daniels, and the staff of Churchill Livingstone for their co-operation. Finally, I happily acknowledge once again the support and encouragement of my wife and family.

Southampton, 1987   I. T.

Contributors

W. H. Allum BSc FRCS
Lecturer in Surgery, Queen Elizabeth Hospital, Birmingham, UK

B J. Britton FRCS
Consultant Surgeon, John Radcliffe Hospital, Oxford, UK

H. B. Coakham MRCP FRCS
Consultant Neurosurgeon, Frenchay Hospital, Bristol, UK

T. Cooke MD FRCS
Senior Lecturer in Surgery, Department of Surgery, University of Liverpool, UK

H. L. Duthie MD ChM FRCS
Provost, University of Wales College of Medicine, Cardiff, UK

P. A. Farrands MD FRCS
Lecturer in Surgery, University Surgical Unit, Southampton, UK

J. W. L. Fielding MD FRCS
Senior Lecturer in Surgery, Queen Elizabeth Hospital, Birmingham, UK

A. Flowerdew FRCS
Cancer Research Campaign Fellow, University Surgical Unit, Southampton, UK

C. W. Imrie ChM FRCS
Consultant Surgeon, Royal Infirmary, Glasgow, UK

A. O. Mansfield ChM FRCS
Consultant Surgeon, St Mary's Hospital, London, UK

M. S. McCormick FRCS
Lecturer, Royal Liverpool Hospital, Liverpool, UK

G. T. Royle MS FRCS
Senior Lecturer in Surgery, University Surgical Unit, Southampton, UK

Philip F. Schofield MD FRCS
Consultant Surgeon, Christie & Withington Hospitals, Manchester, UK

L. Spitz PhD FRCS
Nuffield Professor of Paediatric Surgery, The Hospital for Sick Children, Great Ormond Street, London, UK

P. M. Stell ChM FRCS
Professor of Otorhinolaryngology, Royal Liverpool Hospital, Liverpool, UK

C. J. Stoddard MD FRCS
Consultant Surgeon, Royal Hallamshire Hospital, Sheffield, UK

I. Taylor MD ChM FRCS
Professor of Surgery, University Surgical Unit, Southampton, UK

Contents

1   *P. M. Stell   M. S. McCormick*

Prognosis in cancer of the head and neck

INTRODUCTION

Cancer of the head and neck constitutes 5–10% of all human cancers. There are 3 main groups:

— Squamous carcinoma of the mucosal surfaces of the mouth, pharynx, etc,
— Non-Hodgkin's lymphomas
— Salivary tumours.

90% of head and neck tumours are malignant as can be seen from Table 1.1: this table is based on a series of almost 4000 patients seen personally in the past 25 years. The data on these patients have been stored prospectively, initially on cards, and for the past 10 years on a microprocessor. This chapter will be based partly on analysis of this data bank, and partly on a review of the literature. Most previous articles have looked at one factor in isolation, but we have subjected our data to multivariate analysis to identify factors which predict survival to 5 years. The advantage of this method is that it dissects out confounding factors. For instance, it is well known that survival falls with increasing size of the tumour. But the chance of developing a lymph node metastasis also increases with increasing size of

Table 1.1   Relative incidence of different tumours of the head and neck

Squamous carcinoma		75%
Lymphomas		2.5%
Non-Hodgkin's	2.2%	
Hodgkin's	0.3%	
Salivary tumours		7.5%
Benign	4%	
Malignant	3.5%	
Miscellaneous		15%
Benign	4%	
Malignant	11%	

Table 1.2   Squamous carcinoma — prognostic factors

	t	P
Age	−5.80	<0.00001
Sex (female)	+0.57	N.S.
General condition (Compared to GC 0)		
GC 1	−3.83	<0.001
GC 2–4	−4.20	<0.0001
Lymph node metastases (compared to N_0)		
N_1	−3.19	<0.01
N_2	−4.07	<0.0001
N_3	−5.10	<0.00001
T stage (compared to T_1)		
T_2	−1.14	N.S.
T_3	−2.29	<0.05
T_4	−2.28	<0.05
Histological grade (compared to SCC)		
Well differentiated	−1.97	N.S.
Mod. differentiated	−2.12	<0.05
Poorly differentiated	−1.39	N.S.
Site (Compared to tumours of the nose, sinuses, nasopharynx and ear)		
Hypopharynx	−4.49	<0.00001
Larynx	+4.18	<0.0001
Mouth	+0.42	N.S.
Year of initial treatment	−0.34	N.S.

the tumour, and this event has a marked effect on prognosis. If the effect of lymph node metastases is allowed for, the size of the primary tumour is not a very strong predictor of survival.

The significance of various prognostic factors for squamous carcinoma in our series is shown in Table 1.2. Even after identifying all the known prognostic factors, 85% of the variance in our own population remained unexplained. Clearly, we therefore know as yet little or nothing about the basic biological behaviour of this common tumour.

SQUAMOUS CARCINOMA

This is much the commonest tumour of the head and neck, a slightly surprising fact, given that large parts of the upper respiratory tract are lined by respiratory epithelium. Presumably the development of a squamous carcinoma is preceded by squamous metaplasia.

Assessment of prognostic factors would scarcely be possible without the TNM classification schemes. These began to be developed in the 1950's in Europe, and in the 1960's in North America (Smith et al, 1961). There are now 2 schemes: the American Joint Committee (AJC, 1983) and the Union

International Contre le Cancer (UICC, 1978). After a period during which the classification of these bodies grew together, their definitions are now sadly diverging again.

Age, sex and general condition

It used to be thought that cancer progressed more slowly in the elderly, but a progressive fall in survival with increasing age has been demonstrated by several authors (Cachin, 1975; Easson & Palmer, 1976). Some of these data are difficult to analyse because it is not clear whether intercurrent deaths are allowed for. Furthermore, cancer presents later in the elderly (Easson & Palmer, 1976) and this fact must be taken into account. Analysis of our own data shows that survival still deteriorates markedly with age even when deaths from intercurrent disease and differences in TNM stage are allowed for: in other words the older the patient the less able he is to resist his cancer. Indeed, age was the most significant predictor of all in our series (Table 1.2). Our results for laryngeal cancer are shown in Table 1.3.

Table 1.3 Laryngeal carcinoma — 5-year survival related to age

Age	Crude survival	Actuarial survival
0–39	65%	70%
40–49	78%	83%
50–59	57%	66%
60–69	48%	56%
70–79	34%	52%
80+	30%	45%

Many authors who have considered sex have found it to be a significant factor. Again it is not clear whether this difference is due to a different pattern of cancer in women: it is possible that women are more health conscious, and present earlier. In our series sex was completely insignificant when other factors were allowed for.

General condition

Attempts to measure the patient's general condition were initiated by Karnofsky in (1948) but have only recently been incorporated in the AJC Classification and not yet by the UICC.

Those authors (Oreggia et al, 1983) who have considered performance status have usually found it a good predictor of survival: indeed it was the most significant prognostic indicator for carcinoma of the tonsil in one series (Petrovich et al, 1980).

Karnofsky's index of performance status is now widely used, particularly in chemotherapy trials, but it is a measure of the effect of the patient's cancer on his general health, rather than an assessment of his general health per se. We have used the ECOG scale (AJC, 1983) as follows:

Grade

0 Fully active, able to carry on all predisease activities without restriction (Karnofsky 90–100)

1 Restricted in physically strenuous activity but ambulatory and able to carry out work of a light or sedentary nature, for example, light housework, office work (Karnofsky 70–80)

2 Ambulatory and capable of all self-care but unable to carry out any work activities. Up and about more than 50% of waking hours (Karnofsky 50–60)

3 Capable of only limited self-care, confined to bed or chair 50% or more of waking hours (Karnofsky 30–40)

4 Completely disabled. Cannot carry on any self-care. Totally confined to bed or chair (Karnofsky 10–20)

This classification, too, is a significant predictor of survival, grade 1 being worse than 0, and 2–4 (lumped together) worse than 1.

Size of the primary tumour (T stage)

Attempts to relate prognosis to the extent of the primary tumour began in 1961, when the American Joint Committee proposed a T staging system for laryngeal cancer. The various stages were shown to relate to survival, based on a retrospective analysis of 600 patients. Since then it has been universally accepted that T stage correlates with survival for all sites. The staging for mouth cancer is shown as a typical example in Table 1.4. However, the AJC did not consider confounding factors: it has already been mentioned that the incidence of lymph node metastases rises with advancing T stage. Such a metastasis seriously reduces survival, but if this confounding effect is allowed for, the effect of T stage becomes much less marked: indeed in our own material (Table 1.2) stage T_2 could not be distinguished from T_1.

Table 1.4 AJC system for T staging a tumour of the mouth

TX	Tumour that cannot be assessed.
TO	No evidence of primary tumour.
TI	Tumour 0–2 cm in diameter, solitary, freely mobile, facial nerve intact*
T2	Tumour 2–4 cm in diameter, solitary, freely mobile or reduced mobility or skin fixation, and facial nerve intact*
T3	Tumour 4–6 cm in diameter, or multiple nodes, skin ulceration, deep fixation, or facial nerve dysfunction*
T4	Tumour> 6 cm in diameter and/or involving mandible and adjacent bones

 * applicable to parotid tumours only.

Many of the T stages defined by the UICC and the AJC appear to be based more on administrative tidiness, than on pathological factors known to affect survival. A good example of this is pharyngeal cancer: much the most important indicators of survival are the length of the tumour (as is also true of cancer of the oesophagus) and vocal cord paralysis (Stell et al, 1986). Neither of these factors is included in the TNM scheme, and most of the factors which are included are irrelevant. Given, furthermore, that there are wide inter- and intra-observer errors in assigning a patient's tumour to a T stage, it is tempting to make the heretical suggestion that two T stages would suffice: firstly small localised tumours, and secondly large tumours causing fixation and invading neighbouring organs or tissues, e.g. the mandible. A relatively weak effect of T stage compared to N stage has been found by others (Lam et al, 1980; Hibbert et al, 1983).

Lymph node metastases (N stage)

One of the distinctive characteristics of head and neck cancer is the behaviour of the lymph nodes in the neck. This closed system forms a protective barrier which resists the spread of the cancer for many months. Resection of invaded nodes by radical neck dissection is thus a very worthwhile procedure. The 2 systems for staging nodal metastases are shown in Tables 1.5 and 1.6. As can be seen from the tables several factors are, or are thought to be, important. These include: the number of nodes, their size, and whether they are bilateral or fixed. The very worst prognosis is for patients with nodes which are bilateral and fixed (Stell, 1983), but no category is available in either staging system for these patients. Analysis of our data showed all three stages (N_1–N_3) to be good separate indicators of survival, and that the prognosis decreased with advancing stage.

Table 1.5 AJC system for staging lymph node metastases

NX	Minimum requirements to assess the regional nodes cannot be met
N0	No clinically positive node
N1	Single clinically positive homolateral node 3 cm or less in diameter
N2	Single clinically positive homolateral node more than 3 but not more than 6 cm in diameter or multiple clinically positive homolateral nodes none mere than 6 cm in diameter
N2a	Single clinically positive homolateral node more than 3 cm but not more than 6 cm in diameter
N3	Massive homolateral nodes(s), bilateral nodes or contralateral node(s)
N3a	Clinically positive homolateral node(s), one more than 6 cm in diameter
N3b	Bilateral clinically positive nodes (in this situation, each side of the neck should be staged separately; i.e. N3b: right, N2a; left, N1)
N3c	Contralateral clinically positive nodes(s) only

Table 1.6 UICC system for staging lymph node metastases

N	Regional lymph nodes
N0	No evidence of regional lymph node involvement
N1	Evidence of involvement of movable homolateral regional lymph nodes
N2	Evidence of involvement of movable contralateral or bilateral regional lymph nodes
N3	Evidence of involvement of fixed regional lymph nodes
NX	The minimum requirements to asses the regional lymph nodes can not be met

Table 1.7 Survival related to histological lymph node status (Batsakis, 1979)

	5-year 'cure' rate	
	Roswell Park Hospital	Memorial Hospital
Histologically negative	60%	60%
Histologically positive		
1. Single	31%	30%
2. Two	25%	—
3. Three or more	11%	24%
4. Contralateral	—	25%
5. Bilateral	—	5%

Histological factors such as the number of nodes of involved, and particularly capsular rupture are even more important predictors than clinical assessment of size, etc. (Snow et al, 1982). The influence of histologically positive nodes is very marked: the decreasing survival with increasing number of nodes invaded is shown in Table 1.7 (Batsakis, 1979).

The level of the node in the neck is also thought to be important. A common scheme is shown in Figure 1.1: using this scheme, analysis of our data showed survival for level I to be better than for level II (the upper deep cervical) but survival for levels III and IV did not differ from Level II.

Histological differentiation

Attempts to classify squamous carcinoma into 3 types (well, moderately and poorly differentiated) go back half a century or more to Broders, but there are many difficulties inherent in this system, including wide inter-and intra-observer error by the histopathologist, variations between different parts of the same tumour and at different times. Furthermore, at any one site most tumours are of one specific type, for example most lip tumours are well differentiated whereas most tonsillar tumours are poorly differentiated. Nonetheless, careful assessment of histological grading has been shown to

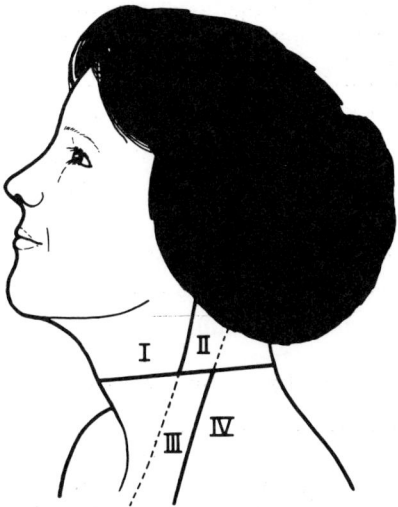

Fig. 1.1 Lymph node levels

correlate with recurrence, metastases and mortality (Lund et al, 1975). Complicated studies have been carried out of laryngeal carcinoma taking into account various histological characteristics (Batsakis, 1979). These factors correlate with survival, but are only relevant in a research environment. Our own material is based on reports made by numerous pathologists over many years; many confined themselves to a diagnosis of 'squamous cell carcinoma' without specifying the grade. Analysis showed that these haphazard gradings did not correlate with survival.

Site

The site of the tumour has long been known to have a bearing on prognosis. This is clearly shown by our data: tumours of the larynx have a relatively better prognosis, and those of the hypopharynx a relatively worse prognosis, compared to tumours of the mouth and to those of the skull base (i.e. the nose and sinuses, nasopharynx and ear) which occupy the middle ground. This is not due to a difference in biological behaviour of the tumour itself but to a combination of several local factors. Firstly, the size at presentation varies between sites — for example laryngeal tumours cause hoarseness early, whereas a tumour must grow to considerable size in the bulky piriform fossa before it causes dysphagia. Secondly, there are wide variations in lymphatic drainage of individual organs, ranging from the vocal cord which has no external drainage to the clinically silent piriform fossa which has a rich drainage. Thirdly, natural barriers such as cartilage, are present in some organs such as the larynx, but not in others. An example of the latter is the posterior part of the floor of the mouth: a carcinoma here has virtually no barrier to prevent its spread into the soft tissues of the neck. Finally, there is the question of accessibility: tumours of the middle ear, for instance, are amenable to only the most heroic surgery.

Second malignancy

One curious aspect of head and neck cancer is the propensity for a second primary squamous carcinoma to appear later in another part of the upper respiratory tract, or in the lungs. Indeed a second primary tumour in the lung is commoner than a secondary tumour at that site. Such events are thought to be more common for tumours of the mouth, and for patients who continue to smoke after treatment of their first primary. Treatment of a second primary tumour is often worthwhile, but clearly the prognosis is worsened by such an event.

Metastases

Distant metastases at the time of presentation are rare: they are found in only 1% or patients, almost always in the lungs. They are, of course, a universally bad prognostic sign.

Year of initial treatment

Some believe that the results of treatment are improving: the Director of the American National Cancer Institute is quoted as saying 'We're saving thousands of lives today that weren't saved 20 years ago'. Others disagree

Table 1.8   Advances in treatment of head and neck cancer (1960–1985)

Diagnosis
  TNM staging
  Microlaryngoscopy
  CAT scans

Reconstructive surgery
  Axial flaps
  Musculocutaneous flaps
  Revascularised flaps
  Gastric and colonic transpositions for pharyngeal cancer

Excisional surgery
  Partial laryngectomy
  Prophylactic neck dissection

Radiotherapy
  Linear accelerator
  Isotopes

Adjuvant treatment
  Radiotherapy plus surgery
  Chemotherapy plus radiotherapy

forcibly with this view. Certainly, many changes have been made in the treatment of head and neck cancer since the early 1960's (Table 1.8). Analysis of our data bank does not show increasing survival over the past 25 years. This is not really surprising: newer methods of reconstruction, for example, have improved the cosmetic and functional end result of major excisions, and shortened the time the patient spends in hospital. But the biological behaviour of the tumour and the methods of excising it remain the same. Numerous supposed advances, for example adjuvant radiotherapy and chemotherapy, have been greeted with great enthusiasm but all so far have proven to be false dawns.

Delay in diagnosis and treatment

Very little work has been done on the three phases of delay (patient, G.P. and hospital). Certainly it is known that 70% of medical and dental GP's cannot recognise a carcinoma in the mouth when they see one. Given the high intellectual capability of present day medical students this must indicate a serious deficiency in training. Also the delay in hospital is probably 2–3 months at least. Squamous carcinoma of the head and neck is an orderly disease, for example the probability of developing lymph node metastases increases with time. Delay is therefore very important. It is known that tongue tumours 1.5 cm or less in diameter can virtually always be cured. Assuming that all tumours are small at one phase in their development (which may not be true) a huge increase in survival could be achieved by greater public awareness and willingness to be treated, by greater medical suspicion and by an improved, i.e. accelerated, hospital service.

Sadly, our material does not suggest that patients are being diagnosed earlier (Table 1.9): indeed advanced tumours (T_3 and T_4) constituted only 15% of the sample in the 1960's, but 28% in the 1980's. This may partly be explained by changing referral patterns.

Table 1.9 T stage at presentation by decades

	T_1	T_2	T_3	T_4
1962–1969	22%	14%	11%	4%
1970–1979	24%	13%	19%	8%
1980–1985	21%	14%	15%	13%

MALIGNANT SALIVARY TUMOURS

Salivary tissue is traditionally divided into the major and minor glands. The former include the parotid and submandibular glands occasionally the sublingual glands, and the latter the minor salivary glands. These are scattered throughout the upper aerodigestive tract but the commonest site is the hard palate. 60% of parotid tumours are benign whereas 60% of minor gland tumours are malignant.

The most important histological types of salivary tumours are shown in Table 1.10: benign tumours will not of course be considered here. It can be seen that much the commonest tumour is the adenoid cystic carcinoma, but it must be emphasised that the relative frequency of the different tumours varies between sites: for example fewer than 5% of parotid tumours are adenoid cystic carcinomas.

Table 1.10   Histological types of salivary tumours

Adenoid cystic carcinoma	60%
Mucoepidermoid carcinoma	15%
Carcinoma ex-pleomorphic adenoma	10%
Others	15%
Squamous carcinoma	5%

Prognosis and follow-up

One thing which must be emphasised for salivary malignancies is the very long period of follow-up required before the end result can be assessed. This is particularly true of adenoid cystic carcinoma: whereas squamous cell carcinoma, if it recurs does so within 2 years, adenoid cystic carcinoma may remain dormant for 10–15 years before a recurrence is manifest.

Histological types

The most important prognostic factor in salivary tumours is thought to be the histological type. Furthermore, several tumours can be divided into a high grade and a low grade sub-group. This is particularly true of mucoepidermoid carcinoma, and may also be true of adenoid cystic carcinoma. Salivary tumours can be divided on the basis of histology into 4 groups

Table 1.11   Prognostic groups of salivary tumours (Seifert et al, 1984)

I	Well differentiated acinic cell tumour Well differentiated mucoepidermoid tumour Tubular adenoid cystic carcinoma
II	Solid and cribriform adenoid cystic carcinoma Poorly differentiated acinic cell tumour Duct carcinoma
III	Adenocarcinoma Poorly differentiated mucoepidermoid tumour Squamous cell carcinoma
IV	Carcinoma ex-pleomorphic adenoid Undifferentiated carcinoma

(Table 1.11) (Seifert et al, 1984). Specific important points about some of the commoner tumours will now be discussed.

Adenoid cystic carcinoma

One of the most important characteristics of this tumour is its tendency to spread along nerve sheaths. This tumour is very indolent, but tends to be fatal after 15 years or more. There is some evidence that its propensity for multiple recurrences may be due to inadequate initial treatment and that the prognosis can be improved by radical initial therapy.

Adenoid cystic carcinoma has well recognised different histological patterns, but whether they have prognostic significance is a matter of dispute (Batsakis, 1979).

Mucoepidermoid carcinoma

It is generally accepted that low grade mucoepidermoid carcinomas have a very much better prognosis than high grade. Intermediate and high grade carcinomas have a high rate (about 50%) of lymph mode metastasis, and their survival is stage dependant: 100% for stage 1,65% for stage II and 10% for stage III (Spiro et al, 1975). On the other hand low grade tumours have almost a 100% five-year survival irrespective of their stage, and they seldom metastasise.

Site of the tumour

The influence of site is controversial. Some authors state that tumours of the minor salivary glands are more lethal than those of the major glands because the minor glands are relatively inaccessible to the surgeon, and spread can also occur early. Other surgeons claim the reverse relationship to be true. In our material the best prognosis was for oral tumours: the prognosis for tumours in the major glands and for those at other minor sites, e.g. the nose and sinuses, was similar.

TNM staging of the tumour

The AJC has proposed a staging system based on size of the tumour, and the presence of a facial paralysis in parotid tumours. The UICC has not so far developed a system. It is generally acknowledged that T stage of the primary tumour is not a very significant predictor in salivary malignancy, and this finding is borne out by analysis of our material.

Unlike squamous carcinoma of the head and neck lymph node metastases, at presentation or later, are uncommon. When they do occur they are usually rapidly fatal.

Distant metastases, notably to the chest, again behave in an entirely different manner to those from squamous carcinoma. They may remain indolent and symptomless for many years, particularly when they arise from an adenoid cystic carcinoma: a solitary pulmonary metastasis from the latter tumour is well worthwhile resecting.

Clinical features: cranial nerve paralyses

The most marked characteristics of adenoid cystic carcinoma is its propensity to spread along nerve sheaths. It is this property which confers its uncertain long term behaviour and poor prognosis. A cranial nerve paralysis at the time of presentation, particularly a facial nerve paralysis in a parotid tumour, is a very ominous sign: 100% were dead at 10 years in one series (Eneroth, 1972).

Demographic factors

In our series age and sex were very important factors. Prognosis decreased with increasing age, but was better for women than men. Unlike squamous carcinoma general condition was not important. This might be related to the causative factor of squamous carcinoma: commonly quoted aetiological agents include heavy smoking and drinking, which are also associated with the development of chronic bronchitis, heart disease, etc. Salivary carcinomas are not thought to be due to these factors. (Fig. 1.2).

LYMPHOMA

Hodgkin's lymphoma is common in the lymph nodes in the neck. In contrast, it rarely arises within the upper respiratory tract, 95% of lymphomas at the latter site being non-Hodgkin's in type. Naturally the vast majority of the latter arise from Waldeyer's ring, that is the tonsil and adenoid. Only non-Hodgkin's lymphoma will be considered here.

The important factors influencing survival in non-Hodgkin's lymphoma are the cytological classification, the histological patterns (nodular or diffuse) and the stage of the disease.

Cytological classification

The application of recently developed immunological techniques to the study of lymphomas has resulted in numerous new classifications of the cytological type of the tumour.

In the earlier part of this century, an attempt was made to explain the diverse types of lymphoma upon the existence of a putative multipotent progenitor — the reticulum cell. The histological classification embraced the terms 'reticulum cell sarcoma', 'lymphosarcoma', and 'giant follicular

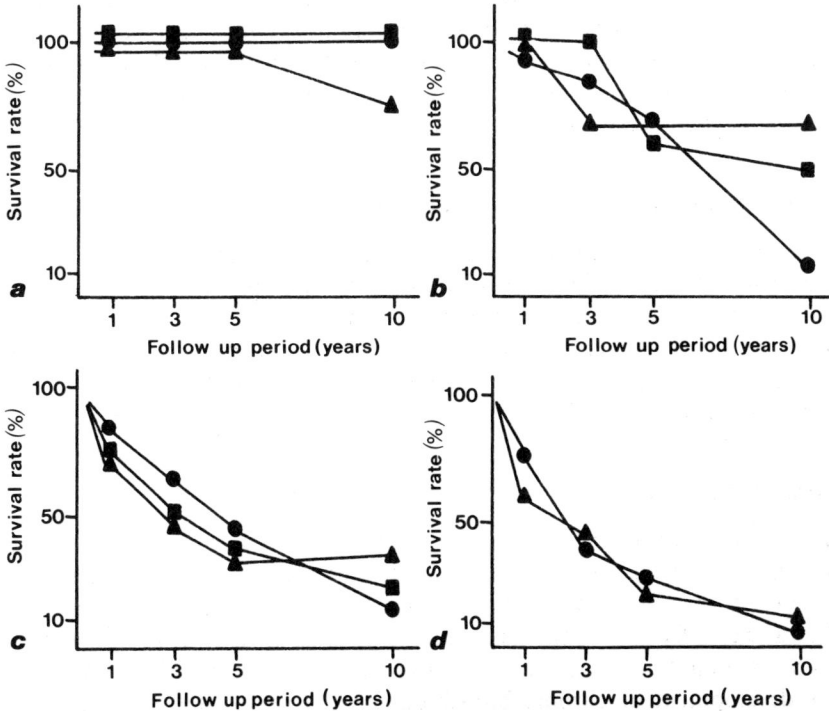

Fig. 1.2 Survival rates of different types of salivary malignancy. (a) Group I: ● = Adenoid cystic carcinoma (tubular); ■ = Acinic cell tumour (highly differentiated); ▲ = Mucoepidermoid tumour (highly differentiated). (b) Group II: ● = Adenoid cystic carcinoma (cribriform, solid); ■ = Duct carcinoma; ▲ = Acinic cell tumour (poorly differentiated). (c) Group III: ● = Adenocarcinoma; ■ = Squamous cell carcinoma; ▲ = Mucoepidermoid tumour (poorly differentiated). (d) Group IV: ● = Carcinoma or pleomorphic adenoma; ▲ = Undifferentiated carcinoma

(nodular) lymphoma' and depended primarily on cell size. Small cells were equated with lymphosarcoma, and large cells with reticulum cell sarcoma. But, these subcategories correlated poorly with prognosis.

In 1956, Rappaport proposed a morphologic classification of the non-Hodgkin's lymphomas based on 1. the resemblance of the malignant cells of various lymphomas to what was then thought to be their benign or normal tissue counterpart, and 2. the degree of supposed cellular differentiation of these cells. Thus, the 'malignant histiocyte' replaced the 'malignant reticulum cell' in those tumours in which the cells were large and resembled histiocytes. Well-differentiated lymphocytic lymphoma replaced lymphocytic lymphosarcoma, lymphomas composed of cells that were larger with more variability in size or nuclear configuration were deemed poorly differentiated lymphocytic lymphomas and further categories were created to encompass lesions with more than one cell type (mixed lymphocytic-histiocytic lymphoma) and those that appeared specially primitive or 'undifferentiated'. A nodular (follicular) pattern within any given subgroup had a favourable prognostic significance.

Clinicopathologic studies showed that this histopathologic classification was a useful guide to the management and prognosis of the non-Hodgkin's lymphomas. Simply stated, the larger or 'less-differentiated' the cell type, the worse the prognosis.

Recent advances in immunology have redefined the malignant lymphomas as neoplasms of the immune system. The Rappaport classification was a morphologic one and was proposed before recognition of the T and B cell systems, and the phenomenon of lymphocyte transformation. Lymphocytes which differentiate under the influence of the thymus are called T cells and those which differentiate in the bursal equivalent or bone marrow are called B cells. Each arm of the immune system has its own functional and anatomical characteristics as well as characteristic surface receptors and antigens. In brief, T cells control cell mediated immunity and B cells control humoral (antibody) mediated immunity.

In the early 1970's Lukes and Collins related the malignant lymphomas to the T lymphocytic and B lymphocytic systems. Normal T and B lymphocytes, after exposure to antigens or plant mitogens, transform in vitro from small inactive cells to large metabolically active dividing forms. The in vivo counterpart of this process for B cells occurs in the follicular centres of lymph nodes, hence the term follicular centre cell lymphoma. T cell transformation occurs outside the follicles. According to this new reasoning the larger cells are not 'poorly differentiated', but instead reflect the point along the continuum of lymphoid transformation at which malignant change occurs. Thus, histiocytic lymphomas are not composed of histiocytes but rather are the neoplastic counterpart of the large transformed lymphocyte. Surface membrane marker studies and other techniques have confirmed these observations. (The above is condensed from an essay by Howard & Batakis, 1985).

The Lukes and Collins system is widely used in North America. The alternative immunological method of classification used in Europe is the Kiel classification laid down by Lennert and his colleagues (1975). The 2 systems are compared in Table 1.12.

Clinicopathologic studies are said to have established the prognostic value of the new immunologic classifications, but this was not borne out by analysis of our data. It is also possible that there is confounding between staging and histology: the high grade tumours tended to present at a more advanced stage, and this fact may explain their apparently worse prognosis.

Histological classification

In the Lukes and Collins system each tumour is subdivided into a diffuse and a nodular type.

In general, improved survival is seen for each cell type with the nodular

Table 1.12 Comparison of Kiel and Rappaport classification (Lennert et al, 1975)

Kiel classification	Rappaport equivalent		
Low grade malignancy			
Lymphocytic (CLL and Others)	Well differentiated lymphocytic, diffuse		
Lymphoplasmacytoid (immunocytic)	Lymphocytic type with dysproteinemia Lymphoproliferative diseases with dysproteinemia		
Centrocytic	Well	differentiated	nodular
	Poorly	lymphocytic	diffuse
Centroblastic/centrocytic*	Well and poorly		
Follicular	differentiated; mixed cell;		nodular
Follicular and diffuse	histiocytic-lymphocytic;		diffuse
Diffuse	histiocytic		
High grade malignancy			
Centroblastic	Histiocytic, nodular or diffuse Undifferentiated, nodular or diffuse		
Lymphoblastic	Undifferentiated		
Burkitt type	Poorly differentiated lymphocytic diffuse		
Convoluted-cell type			
Others			
Immunoblastic	Histiocytic, diffuse		

* with or without sclerosis.

rather than the diffuse pattern. The well differentiated lymphocytic lymphomas, even in their widespread leukemic stage (chronic lymphocytic leukemia) and the nodular, poorly differentiated lymphocytic lymphomas even with involvement of the bone marrow (stage IV) have a good prognosis. This distinction into two types does not apply to the Kiel system.

Staging of non-Hodgkin's lymphoma

Staging of malignant lymphomas is important to define the extent of the disease and to determine the best course of treatment. Clinical and pathological staging classifications (the Ann Arbor Staging Classification) were established for Hodgkin's disease in 1971. The staging classifications take into account the presence of both nodal as well as extranodal involvement by the lymphoma.

Extranodal involvement is common in non-Hodgkin's lymphomas at the time of the initial diagnosis, whereas in Hodgkin's disease the process is usually limited to lymph nodes. The AJC staging system is shown in Table 1.13. The UICC has not yet developed a system for this tumour.

Although several studies have shown that staging laparotomy may disclose occult sites of disease in non-Hodgkin's lymphomas this has not led to a change of treatment, and this procedure laparotomy is thus thought

Table 1.13 Non-Hodgkin's lymphoma

staging classification (AJC)	
Stage 1	Involvement of a single lymph node region (I) or of a single extralymphatic organ or site (I_E)
Stage II	Involvement of two or more lymph node regions (number to be stated) on the same side of the diaphragm (II); or, localized involvement of an extralymphatic organ or site of one or more lymph node regions on the same side of the diaphragm (II_E)
Stage III	Involvement of lymph node regions on both sides of the diaphragm (III) which may also be accompanied by local involvement of extralymphatic organ site (III_E), by involvement of the spleen (III_s), or both ($III_E + S$)
Stage IV	Diffuse or disseminated involvement of one or more extralymphatic organ tisues with or without associated lymph node enlargement

to be unhelpful in non-Hodgkin's lymphoma. The presence of disseminated non-Hodgkin's lymphoma can be detected in most patients by lymphangiography and routine biochemical tests. Efficient CAT scans are now rapidly displacing invasive methods of assessment.

SUMMARY

90% of head and neck tumours are malignant and 90% of these are squamous carcinomas. Most of the rest are non-Hodgkin's lymphomas and malignant salivary tumours.

In brief, the most important factors determining prognosis in squamous carcinoma are the age of patient, his general condition, the development of lymph node metastases and the site of the primary tumour. The size of the primary tumour and its histological differentiation are less important.

Salivary carcinomas behave in an entirely different way to squamous carcinomas. The most important prognostic factors include the histological type of the tumour, its site, and the age and sex of the patient.

For non-Hodgkin's lymphoma the staging system is the most significant predictor: demographic factors (age, sex, etc) are not significant, nor was there any significant difference in survival between nodal and extranodal sites. The bad prognosis of the high grade lymphomas may be due to the fact that they usually present at an advanced stage.

REFERENCES

American Joint Committee on Cancer. 1983 Manual of Staging of Cancer, 2nd Edition. J B Lippincott Company, Philadelphia
Batsakis J G. 1979 Tumors of the Head and Neck. Clinical and Pathological Considerations, 2nd ed. Williams and Wilkins, Baltimore

Batsakis J G. 1979 Tumors of the Head and Neck. Clinical and Pathological
    Considerations, 2nd ed. Williams and Wilkins, Baltimore, p 204
Batsakis J G. 1979 Tumors of the Head and Neck. Clinical and Pathological
    Considerations, 2nd ed. Williams and Wilkins, Baltimore, p 147
Cachin Y. 1975 Cancers of the head and neck: prognostic factors and criteria of response to
    treatment. In: Staquet M J (ed) Cancer Therapy: Prognostic Factors and Criteria of
    Response. Raven Press, New York, pp 353–366
Easson E C, Palmer M K. 1976 Prognostic factors in oral cancer. Clinical Oncology
    2: 191–202
Eneroth C M. 1972 Facial nerve paralysis: a criterion of malignancy in parotid tumors.
    Archives of Otolaryngology 95: 300–304
Hibbert J, Marks N J, Winter P J, Shaheen O H. 1983 Prognostic factors in oral squamous
    carcinoma and their relation on clinical staging. Clinical Otolaryngology 8: 197–203.
Howard D R, Batsakis J G. 1985 Non-Hodgkin's lymphomas: contemporary classification
    and correlates. Annals of Otology, Rhinology and Laryngology 94: 326–328
Karnofsky, D A, Abelmann W H, Craver L F, Burchenal J H. 1948 The use of the
    nitrogen mustards in the palliative treatment of carcinoma. Cancer 1: 634–656
Lam K H, Wong J, Lim S T K, Ong G B. 1980 Carcinoma of the tongue: factors affecting
    the results of surgical treatment. British Journal of Surgery 67: 101–105
Lennert K, Mohri N, Stein H, Kaiserling E. 1975 The histopathology of malignant
    lymphoma. British Journal of Haematology 31 (Suppl):193–203
Lund C, Sogaard H, Elbrond O, Jorgensen K, Andersen A P. 1975 Epidermoid carcinoma
    of the lip. Histologic grading in the clinical evaluation. Acta Radiologica 14:465
Oreggia F, De Stefani E, Denoe-Pellegrini H. 1983 Carcinoma of the tonsil. Archives of
    Otolaryngology 109: 305–309
Petrovich A, Kuisk H, Jose L, Barton R, Rice D. 1980 Advanced carcinoma of the tonsil.
    Acta Radiologica (Therapy) 19: 425–431
Seifert G, Miehlke A, Haubrich H, Chilla R. 1984 Speicheldrusen — krankheiten. Georg
    Thieme Verlag, Stuttgart, p 299
Smith H R, Caulk R M, Russell W O, Jackson C L. 1961 End results in 600 laryngeal
    cancers using the American Joint Committee's proposed method of stage classification and
    end reporting. Surgery, Gynecology and Obstetrics October: 435–444
Snow G B, Annyas A A, Van Slooten, E A, Bartelink, H, Hart A A M. 1982 Prognostic
    factors of neck node metastasis. Clinical Otolaryngology 7: 185–192
Spiro R H, Huvos A G, Strong E Q. 1975 Cancers of the parotid gland. A clinicopathologic
    study of 288 primary cases. American Journal of Surgery 137: 452–459
Stell P M, McCormick M S, Jackson S. 1986 Prognostic factors in postcricoid carcinoma.
    (In press.)
Stell P M. 1983 Fixed, bilateral, cervical nodes. The Journal of Laryngology and Otology
    9: 851–856
UICC. 1978 TNM Classification of Malignant Tumours, 3rd edition. Geneva

The management of neonatal surgical emergencies

The neonatal period is defined as the first 28 days of extrauterine life. Surgery during this period consists largely of the treatment of congenital abnormalities. Under ideal circumstances, neonatal surgery should be concentrated in large centres and should only be undertaken by surgeons who have undergone specific training in paediatric surgery. The reasons for claiming a monopoly of neonatal surgery for the paediatric surgeon are as follows:

1. It is only the paediatric surgeon who is likely to acquire the necessary experience and expertise to be able to deal with the full range of neonatal surgical conditions.

2. By concentrating neonatal surgery in large units, the essential support services of anaesthesiology, pathology, radiology are more likely to be available.

3. The nursing care of the neonate demands specific knowledge and expertise.

4. The non-operative aspects of surgical management requires an understanding of the physiological differences between the newborn infant and older children and adults.

It is incumbant upon the general surgeon to have the ability to recognise those conditions which require prompt referral to a specialist centre.

PHYSIOLOGICAL ASPECTS OF THE NEONATAL SURGICAL PATIENT

The average full-term infant weighs 3500 g and has a surface area of 0.19 m^2. The ratio of surface area to weight is twice that of an adult and this imposes a genuine risk of excessive heat and insensible fluid loss. The neonatal kidney is immature and can only function within a narrow homeostatic range. During this period the diuretic response to a water load is poor and fluid restriction is generally better tolerated. Many hepatic enzyme systems are immature with the result that drugs and anaesthetic agents are slowly detoxified. The newborn infant's resistance to infection is limited by a combination of low immunoglobulin levels and reduced leukocyte activity. Body size itself does not present any great problems. The results of surgery in very low birth weight infants are determined more by the medical complications of prematurity than the technical limitations of surgery. The association of additional anomalies which are often multiple presents very real problems.

Intravenous fluid and electrolyte requirements

The basic solution for neonates consists of a combination of 10% dextrose in 0.18% saline. Maintenance fluid requirements vary according to age:

$$
\begin{array}{ll}
<1500 \text{ g} & - \text{ 180 ml/kg/24 hours} \\
1500\text{--}2500 \text{ g} & - \text{ 150 ml/kg/24 hours} \\
>2500 \text{ g} & - \text{ 120 ml/kg/24 hours.}
\end{array}
$$

Postoperatively, intravenous fluids are restricted to one-third of maintenance requirements for the first 48 hours and two-thirds for the subsequent 48 hours. Full requirements are only administered on the fifth and subsequent days.

Abnormal losses, e.g. nasogastric aspirate, enteric fistula output and other extracellular fluid losses, should be carefully recorded and replaced volume for volume with normal saline (0.9%) with the addition of 10 mmol potassium chloride per 500 ml of saline solution. The replacement should take place on an hourly basis and the entire fluid requirements reassessed every 6–12 hours until stability has been achieved.

The normal sodium requirement is 3 mmol/kg/day. Provided abnormal losses are accurately replaced, it is not normally necessary to calculate sodium balance on a formal basis. A plasma value of sodium of less than 130 mmol/1 requires correction. The normal potassium requirement is 2 mmol/kg/day. Provided the urine output exceeds 2 ml/kg/hours, potassium in a concentration of 20 mmol/litre should be added to the intravenous fluid solution.

The blood volume of the neonate is 80 ml per kilogram body weight. Acute blood loss should be replaced volume for volume with whole blood. An initial rate of 20 ml/kg/hour is appropriate but should be modified according to clinical response, pulse, blood pressure, and central venous pressures if available. Plasma is an excellent volume expander and in acute situations a rate of 20 ml/kg/hour is suitable. Blood should *always* be available in the operating theatre for any neonatal surgical procedure and losses in excess of 10% of the blood volume should be promptly replaced (i.e. >8 ml/kg).

RECOGNITION OF THE PRESENCE OF CONGENITAL MALFORMATION

External deformities

A thorough physical examination soon after birth will reveal externally obvious anomalies such as cleft lip, myelomeningocoele, exomphalos, imperforate anus, ectopia vesicae, limb deformities, etc.

Concealed anomalies

The recognition of the significance of specific clinical features should raise suspicions of an abnormality affecting one of the internal viscera.

1. Respiratory distress, i.e. tachycardia >160/min, tachypnoea >60/min and expiratory grunting. Surgical conditions account for approximately 15% of the pathological processes which cause respiratory distress. The major causes are idiopathic respiratory distress syndrome, meconium aspiration and cardiac failure. Surgical causes include diaphragmatic hernia, congenital lobar emphysema, pneumothorax, and oesophageal atresia when the diagnosis has been delayed and aspiration pneumonitis has developed.

2. Bile-stained vomiting. The presence of green bile in the vomitus is an indication of mechanical intestinal obstruction. Septicaemia from a whole range of sources, e.g. urinary tract infection, meningitis, pneumonia, etc., may cause a temporary ileus which will mimic mechanical obstruction. The degree of abdominal distension in mechanical obstruction varies according to the level of the obstruction. Erythema or oedema of the anterior wall signifies peritonitis and/or ischaemic intestine.

3. Delayed passage of meconium. Failure to pass meconium within the first 24 hours of life in an otherwise healthy infant should alert the clinician to the possibility of Hirschsprung's disease. A suction rectal biopsy will provide histological evidence for or against the diagnosis.

4. Failure to pass urine within the first 24 hours of life in an infant who is well hydrated indicates the need for full investigation of the urinary system.

5. Rectal bleeding. The passage of blood and mucus in the stool, especially when associated with abdominal distension and bilious vomiting, is highly suspicious of necrotising enterocolitis. The diagnostic feature on plain abdominal X-ray is pneumatosis intestinalis.

6. Abdominal masses. The more common causes of a palpable intra-abdominal mass in infancy are benign cystic lesions of the kidney such as hydronephrosis or multicystic kidneys. Tumours are rare in this age range. Mesenteric and duplication cysts invariably cause mechanical obstruction to the adjacent intestine.

TRANSPORT OF THE SURGICAL NEONATE

The newborn infant can be safely transported over long distances provided precautions are taken to maintain body temperature and the accompanying personnel are fully experienced and adequately equipped to deal with cardiorespiratory emergencies (Spitz et al, 1984). In the event of shock, hypothermia, respiratory failure, gross disturbances of fluid and electrolyte homeostasis, therapeutic measures should commence at the base hospital and continue en route during transportation. A nasogastric tube on free drainage with regular aspiration is essential in all surgical neonates to prevent vomiting and inhalation pneumonia. A specimen of maternal serum and a valid consent form should accompany the baby.

Special precautions are necessary for the transfer of infants with oesophageal atresia, diaphragmatic hernia and exomphalos. They will be elaborated in their specific sections.

SPECIFIC NEONATAL SURGICAL PROBLEMS

Congenital diaphragmatic hernia

The herniation occurs through the foramen of Bochdalek in the posterolateral portion of the diaphragm. The left side is affected 10 times more frequently than the right.

The contents of the hernia consist of a combination of small and large intestine, stomach, spleen and left kidney. The earlier the clinical presentation the more severe the pulmonary hypoplasia due to intrauterine compression of the developing lung.

Clinical features on presentation consist of respiratory distress, apparent dextrocardia, audible borborygmi in the left hemithorax and a scaphoid abdomen. The diagnosis is confirmed on straight X-ray of the chest and abdomen (Fig. 2.1).

Emergency treatment consists of placing the infant in a high oxygen atmosphere and passing a large bore (No. 8 or 10) nasogastric tube to evacuate all air from the stomach. Ventilation by face mask must be avoided as air entering the stomach and intestines is likely to increase the respiratory distress and pulmonary compression. If a stable situation cannot be achieved by placing the infant in 100% oxygen, endotracheal intubation and mechanical ventilation should be instituted. Sudden unexplained clinical deterioration should lead one to suspect a tension pneumothorax. The infant should be transferred accompanied by an experienced nurse and doctor continuing the emergency resuscitative measures.

Definitive treatment consists of reduction of the hernial contents via an abdominal approach. The defect in the diaphragm can usually be repaired by direct suturing and the associated malrotation corrected by a standard Ladd's procedure.

The prognosis is directly related to the time of presentation and the degree of pulmonary hypoplasia. Infants exhibiting symptoms within the first 6 hours of life have a 50% mortality, while virtually all infants presenting after this time should survive. Improvement in survival is due

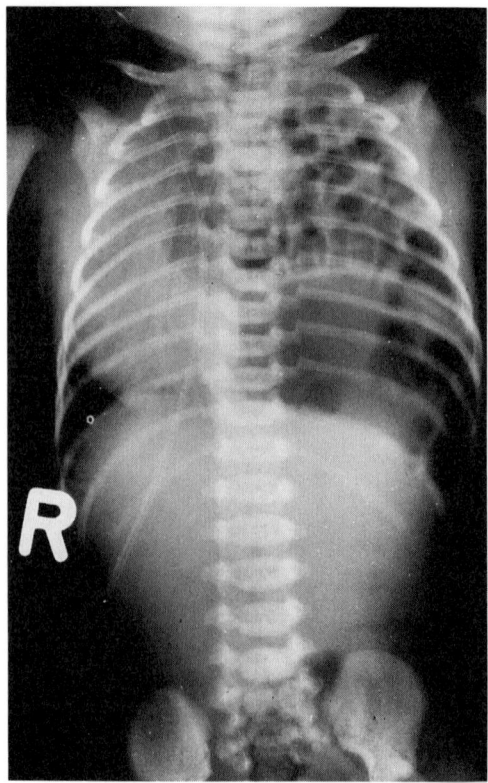

Fig. 2.1 Left diaphragmatic hernia. Plain X-ray of chest and abdomen showing a shift of the cardiac shadow to the right with bowel occupying the left hemi-thorax. There are no bowel gas shadows in the abdomen.

to improved postoperative management including elective mechanical ventilation and the administration of pulmonary vasodilators to counteract the effects of persistent foetal circulation (Brereton et al, 1985).

Oesophageal atresia

In 90% of cases the oesophageal atresia is associated with a distal tracheo-oesophageal fistula (Holder et al, 1964). The presence of polyhydramnios during the third trimester of pregnancy should alert the clinician to the possibility of either an oesophageal atresia or another form of high intestinal obstruction.

Due to the inability to swallow saliva, the infant is excessively mucusy at birth. The diagnosis is confirmed by failure to be able to pass a large bore (No. 10–12) nasogastric tube into the stomach. The level of the atresia should be confirmed on straight X-ray of the chest. Gas in the stomach and intestine is indicative of a distal tracheooesophageal fistula.

During transfer it is essential to prevent aspiration pneumonia by keeping the blind upper oesophageal pouch empty by frequent suction to an indwelling catheter (the double lumen Replogel tube is most appropriate). Treatment consists of ligation and division of the tracheo-oesophageal fistula and end-to-end anastomosis of the oesophageal segments. This can be achieved in the majority of cases. The prognosis is directly related to the presence and severity of associated anomalies and the degree of prematurity (Rickham et al, 1977). An overall survival rate of over 80% should be expected for this condition.

Intestinal obstruction

The main causes of intestinal obstruction in the neonatal period may be classified as follows:

1. Mechanical

(a) intraluminal — meconium ileus
                  — meconium plug syndrome
(b) intramural — atresia or stenosis
                  — Hirschsprung's disease
                  — anorectal anomalies
(c) extrinsic — malrotation ± volvulus
                  — irreducible inguinal hernia
                  — duplication cysts

2. Ileus

(a) septicaemia
(b) necrotising enterocolitis

The plain erect and supine abdominal X-ray are diagnostic in the majority of cases. Contrast studies may be necessary in selected cases.

Meconium ileus. Fifteen per cent of infants with fibrocystic disease present with meconium ileus (Park & Grand, 1981). The obstruction is due to thick tenacious meconium impacting within the lumen of the distal small bowel. Gross abdominal distension is usually present from birth. Bilious vomiting occurs shortly afterwards. Small amounts of greyish mucus may be passed per rectum. The meconium-filled loops of intestine may be palpable on abdominal examination. A positive family history of cystic fibrosis may be obtained.

In uncomplicated cases, the plain abdominal X-ray reveals distended loops of intestine of varying calibre, an absence of air-fluid levels and a ground-glass appearance due to the admixture of gas and meconium (Fig. 2.2). A contrast enema will show a microcolon filled with inspissated

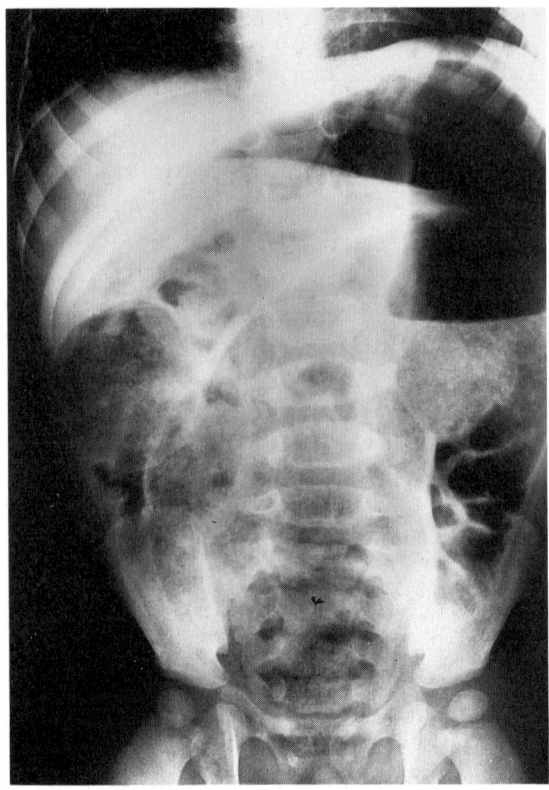

Fig. 2.2 Meconium ileus. Plain erect abdominal X-ray showing dilated loops of intestine of varying calibre with 'ground-glass' appearance of a mixture of meconium and air in the right iliac fossa.

mucus pellets. Confirmation of the diagnosis depends on the demonstration of high levels (>70 mmol/l) of sodium and chloride in the sweat. A positive sweat test can rarely be recorded in infants under one month of age.

For uncomplicated cases of meconium ileus, the gastrografin enema may be therapeutic as well as diagnostic. The emulsifying and hydrophilic properties of gastrografin assist in liquifying the inspissated meconium which can then be evacuated. It is vitally important for the gastrografin to enter the dilated intestine and for complete relief of the obstruction to have occurred at the end of the procedure (Noblett, 1961). Operative treatment is indicated in the presence of a mechanical obstruction (atresia or volvulus), peritonitis and when gastrografin enema is unsuccessful in relieving the obstruction (Bishop & Koop, 1957). Recently we have had considerable success with resection and primary anastomosis after complete intraoperative evacuation of the inspissated material.

'*Meconium plug syndrome*'. This syndrome is characterised by failure of the infant to pass meconium during the first 24 hours of life. A digital rectal examination or a saline washout produces a large greyish plug of mucus followed by a large amount of sticky meconium. There may be abdominal distension and bilious vomiting which promptly resolve on the evacuation of meconium. The syndrome is common in the stressed premature infant and in infants of diabetic mothers, but in the otherwise full-term infant, the diagnosis of Hirschsprung's disease should be considered.

Intestinal atresias and stenosis. Duodenal atresia and stenosis is a developmental anomaly which is frequently associated with additional malformations such as Down's syndrome, congenital cardiac deformities, oesophageal atresia and anorectal anomalies. The diagnosis is made on the presence of a 'double-bubble' on the plain erect abdominal X-ray (Fig. 2.3).

Treatment is by side-to-side duodenoduodenostomy. A transanastomotic feeding tube provides an invaluable means of enteral feeding in the early postoperative period (Girvan & Stephens, 1974).

Atresias of the intestine develop as a consequence of an intrauterine ischaemic process such as volvulus, intussusception, strangulated hernia or a vascular embolus (Barnard & Louw, 1956). Bile-stained vomiting is

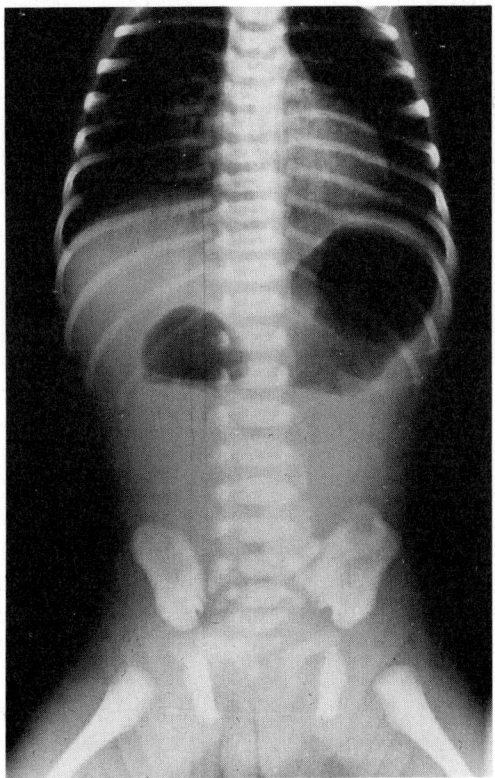

Fig. 2.3 Duodenal atresia. Plain abdominal X-ray showing classical 'double-bubble' appearance of air in the stomach and dilated first part of the duodenum.

usually the first sign while the degree of abdominal distension is dependent upon the level of the lesion, being virtually absent in the very high atresias. The passage of a small amount of meconium should not discount the diagnosis of an atresia. Abdominal X-rays reveal dilated loops of proximal intestine with air-fluid levels (Fig. 2.4).

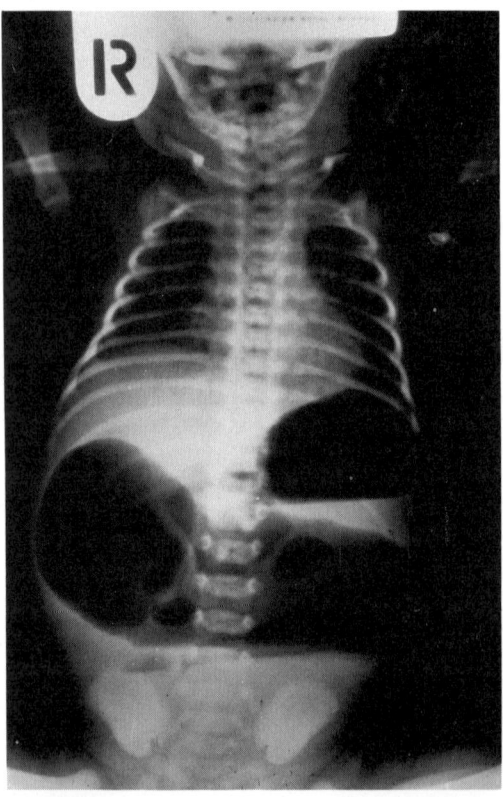

Fig. 2.4 Intestinal atresia. Plain erect abdominal X-ray showing dilated loops of proximal intestine with air/fluid levels. There is an absence of bowel gas shadows in the pelvic region.

Treatment consists of limited resection (Nixon, 1966) of the proximal and distal ends of the intestine adjacent to the atresia and end-to-end anastomosis which can be achieved even in the presence of gross discrepancy in the size of the bowel. It is important to exclude additional atresias in the distal intestine.

Hirschsprung's disease. The absence of parasympathetic ganglion cells in the affected segment causes a functional obstruction due to defective peristalsis. The distal rectum is always affected and the abnormality extends proximally to a varying extent. In 90% of cases the abnormality is confined to the rectosigmoid region while in 5% of cases the entire colon is affected.

The most constant presenting feature is delayed passage of meconium (Swenson et al, 1973). This is usually accompanied by abdominal distension and bile-stained vomiting. The obstruction may be temporarily relieved by the passage of a meconium plug. A small percentage of cases present initially with enterocolitis. There is profuse diarrhoea in association with subacute intestinal obstruction and if unattended it rapidly leads to dehydration and hypovolaemic shock.

The barium enema in the neonatal period is notoriously unreliable. It may reveal a narrow spastic and hypertonic aganglionic rectum. Confirmation of the diagnosis requires the demonstration of a complete absence of ganglion cells together with hypertrophic nerve trunks in a biopsy of the distal rectum. The most convenient method of obtaining this biopsy is by means of a suction biopsy instrument (Noblett, 1969).

Treatment consists of a defunctioning colostomy in ganglionic intestine. This requires frozen-section histopathology. The definitive treatment is usually delayed until the infant is 9–12 months of age when the affected segment is either resection (Swenson, 1948; Rehbein, 1958) or bypassed (Duhamel, 1960; Soave, 1966). All these procedures and their results are described in great detail in Holschneider's monograph on Hirschsprung's disease (1982).

Anorectal anomalies. A clear precise differentiation between high (supralevator) and low (translevator) anomalies is vitally important to the acquisition of continence. A simplified diagnostic scheme for this differentiation is presented below (Stephens & Smith, 1971) (Fig. 2.5).

The clinical diagnosis is sufficient in the majority of cases. Where doubt exists, a lateral inverted X-ray of the pelvis may be helpful in establishing the level of the agenesis (Berdon et al, 1968).

Low lesions are treated by an anoplasty while high lesions require an initial defunctioning colostomy followed 6–9 months later by a pull-through procedure in which the rectum is rerouted anterior to the puborectalis sling.

A wide variety of associated anomalies occur with anorectal anomalies. In addition to congenital cardiac defects and duodenal atresia, the VATER association encompasses most of the anomalies (V = vertebral, A = anorectal, T = tracheal, E = esophageal, R = renal, radial).

Malrotation. During the early weeks of fetal life, elongation and development of the intestine takes place in the physiological umbilical hernia. Between the 10–12 week re-entry into the peritoneal cavity takes place with the duodenum and the caeco-ileal loop undergoing a 270° anticlockwise rotation. Fixation of the intestine in the fully-rotated position then takes place. Failure to achieve the full 270° rotation results in a typical malrotation where the entire midgut is suspended from the posterior peritoneum by a narrow vascular pedicle and abnormal bands cross and compress the second part of the duodenum (Ladd's bands).

Uncomplicated malrotation presents with intermittent bile-stained vomiting. Volvulus around the narrow-based mesentery is heralded by the

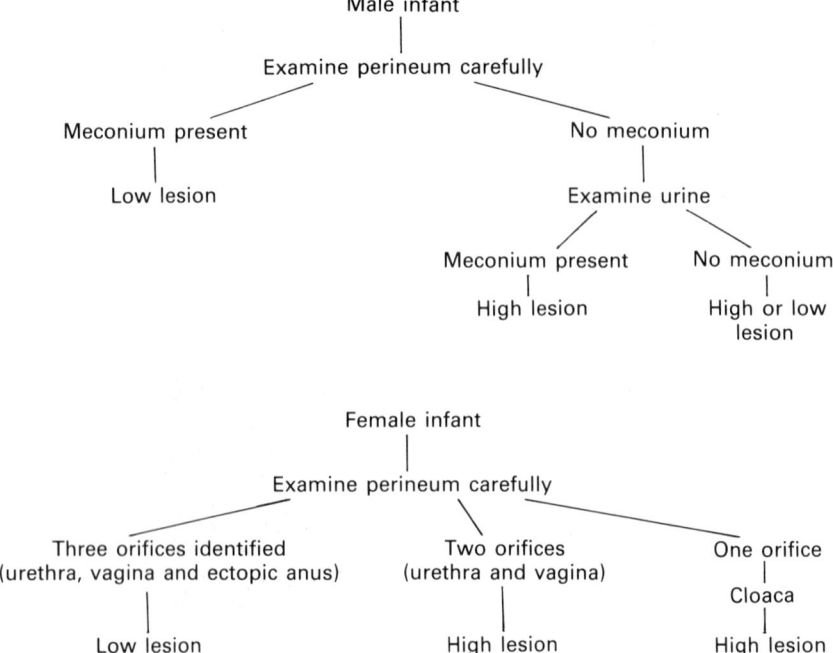

Fig. 2.5 Anorectal anomalies

passage of dark red blood per rectum, continuous bilious vomiting, abdominal tenderness and hypovolaemic shock.

The diagnosis may be suspected on plain abdominal X-ray which reveals a double-bubble appearance and a paucity of gas in the rest of the intestine (Fig. 2.6a). Confirmation of the diagnosis is obtained on either upper or lower gastrointestinal contrast studies which show the abnormal configuration of the duodenum (Simpson et al, 1972) (Fig. 2.6b) and the abnormal position of the caecum and appendix respectively (Berdon et al, 1970).

The treatment of a malrotation should be regarded as a surgical emergency. Derotation of the volvulus, widening of the midgut mesentery and positioning of the duodenum in a downward direction and the caecum in the left hypochondrium is the operative procedure of choice (Ladd's procedure). Any gangrenous intestine should be resected and if possible an end-to-end anastomosis fashioned (Filston & Kirk, 1981; Andrassy & Mahour 1981).

Inguinal hernia. Inguinal herniotomy is the single most common surgical procedure carried out in the neonatal period. The hernia is a result of failure of obliteration of the processus vaginalis and is invariably of the indirect variety. It may present merely as a freely-reducible, intermittent swelling in the groin or it may be irreducible on initial appearance. As there is a high incidence of strangulation with likely damage to the ipsilateral

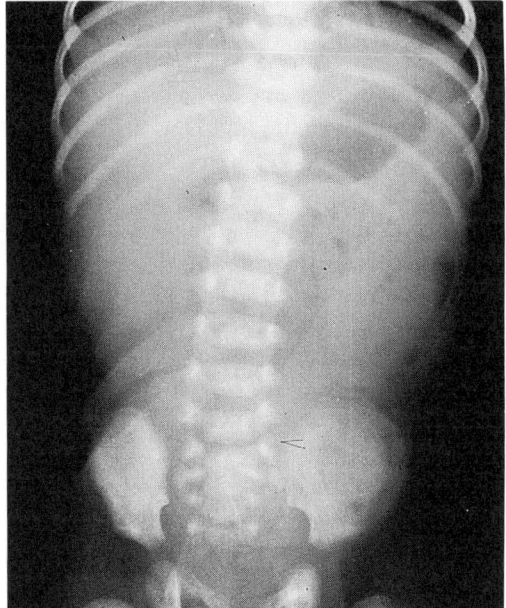

a

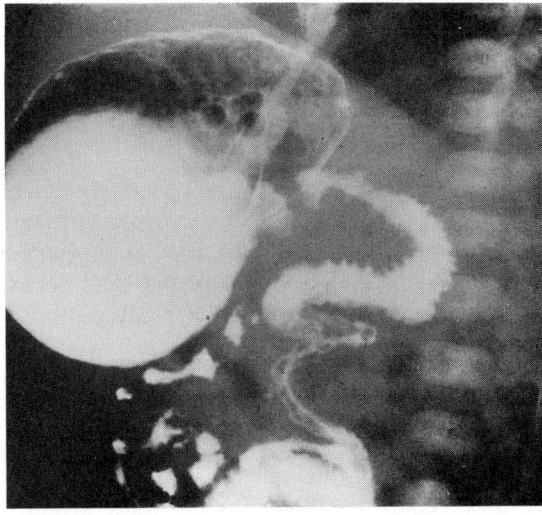

b

Fig. 2.6 Malrotation. (a) Plain abdominal X-ray showing a paucity of bowel gas shadows. This is indicative of a mid-gut volvulus. (b) Barium meal examination showing a 'twisted-ribbon' appearance of the duodenum in the lateral position indicating the presence of a mig-gut volvulus.

testis as well as the intestine, surgical treatment should be regarded as a relative emergency.

The operation, which should be carried out as a day-case, consists of a simple herniotomy, i.e. ligation and division of the hernial sac at the internal inguinal ring. Repair of the muscular anatomy is not necessary.

Necrotising enterocolitis. This relatively recently recognised entity, which is virtually confined to the neonatal period, is due to gas-forming organisms entering the wall of the intestine through mucosa breeches. Perinatal stress, prematurity, septicaemia, exchange transfusion and hyperviscosity are all thought to play an initiating role, but mesenteric vascular ischaemia is considered to be the final common pathway in the pathogenesis of the condition. The pathological lesions vary from pneumatosis intestinalis and mucosal erosions to full-thickness necrosis and gangrene affecting long segments of bowel. The most commonly affected areas are the ileocaecal, splenic and sigmoid colon (Thomas 1982).

The infant presents with abdominal distension, bile-stained vomiting and passes blood and mucus in the stool. The diagnosis is confirmed radiologically by the demonstration of gas within the wall of the intestine (pneumatosis intestinalis) (Fig. 2.7). Pneumoperitoneum signifies an intestinal perforation.

In the early stages of the disease process, conservative treatment is usually successful. This consists of nasogastric decompression, broad-spectrum antibiotics (penicillin, gentamicin, metronidazole) and withholding oral feeds for 14 days during which time parenteral nutrition is administered. The indications of surgical intervention (Kosloske et al, 1980) include evidence of perforation, peritonitis, failure to improve on conservative treatment and late stricture formation. Surgery consists of resection of obviously necrotic intestine and fashioning of proximal and distal enterostomies.

Exomphalos and gastroschisis. These lesions are due to failure of complete regression of the physiological umbilical hernia. Exomphalos major occurs when the defect in the anterior abdominal wall is greater than 5 cm in diameter. There is a high incidence of associated anomalies such as congenital cardiac deformities, chromosomal anomalies and Beckwith — Wiederman syndrome (gigantism, macroglossia, hypoglycaemia). In exomphalos minor, the defect is less than 5 cm in diameter, while in gastroschisis, evisceration of intestine occurs to the right of an apparently normal-appearing umbilical cord. Associated anomalies are rare in these two conditions. Malrotation of the midgut should be regarded as an integral part of all these anomalies. The exomphalos sac consists of outer amniotic membrane and inner peritoneum. Separating these layers are Wharton's jelly.

Exomphalos minor and most gastroschises can be closed directly. The abdominal wall may need to be stretched to accommodate the extruded edematous and thickened intestine of the gastroschisis. Exomphalos major is treated either by painting the sac with an antiseptic solution while

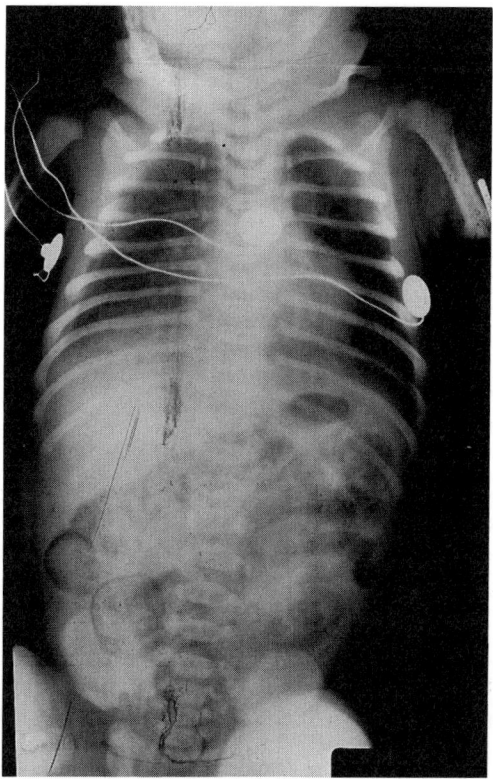

Fig. 2.7 Necrotizing enterocolitis. Plain abdominal X-ray showing pneumatosis intestinalis particularly involving two loops of intestine in the right lower quadrant of the abdomen.

awaiting epithelialisation of the sac (Grob, 1963), or by covering the lesion with prosthetic sheeting (Shuster, 1967).

Spina bifida. Failure of complete closure of the neural tube results in a variety of lesions of varying severity:

(a) Spina bifida occulta occurs when there is failure of closure of the vertebral arches. It may be marked by the presence of an overlying tuft of hair, haemangioma, lipoma, dermoid or sinus.

(b) Meningocoele where the sac contains cerebrospinal fluid without neural tissue.

(c) Myelomeningocoele contains exposed neural tissue. The lower limbs, anal and urinary sphincters are affected to varying degrees.

Except in the very severe case, when surgical closure of the defect would be technically difficult, operative closure should be carried out within 24–48 hours of life in order to prevent neurological deterioration and meningitis. Certain criteria have been proposed to exclude infants with myelomeningocoele from surgical closure (Lorber, 1971). The selection should only be made by doctors experienced in this condition with the realisation that 'selection out' does not necessarily mean that the infant will succumb.

Sacrococcygeal teratoma. These lesions present with a visible swelling varying in extent from a minor polypoid lesion to a tumour the size of the infant's head. The tumour is thought to originate in the notochord and contains tissues arising from all three germ cell layers. It may extend retrorectally into the pelvis and occasionally presents as a dumbbell tumour with a palpable intraabdominal and visible sacrococcygeal mass. Although 99% of these tumours are benign at birth, malignant degeneration rapidly takes place, so that 25% are malignant by 3 months of age and 50% by six months.

Treatment consists of total resection of the tumour en bloc with the coccyx. The procedure may involve considerable blood loss and if total excision is not achieved, recurrences, which may be malignant, may occur.

Urinary tract anomalies. Very few anomalies of the genitourinary tract require urgent surgical attention in the neonatal period. Posterior urethral valves may present either with the total inability to pass urine or dribbling of small amounts of urine continuously or intermittently or the infant may present in renal failure. The bladder may be palpably distended or contracted and rock-hard due to the thickened muscular wall. Unilateral hydronephrosis due to pelvic-ureteric junction obstruction can be safely observed, but bilateral gross hydronephrosis requires urgent drainage, preferably by means of 'pig-tail' nephrostomy catheters. The current approach towards exstrophy of the bladder is to advocate early closure and reconstruction.

Ambiguous genitalia demands early assessment in order to assign the correct gender to the infant.

Urinary tract infection, which may present with septicaemia ane intestinal ileus, requires urgent antibiotic chemotherapy followed by full assessment of the urinary tract to elucidate the cause of the problem and the nature of any underlying abnormality.

REFERENCES

Andrassy R F, Mahour G H 1981 Malrotation of the midgut in infants and children. A 25 year review. Archives of Surgery 116: 158–160

Barnard C N, Louw J H 1956 The genesis of intestinal atresia. Minnesota Medicine 37: 745–753

Berdon W E, Baker D H 1968 The radiological evaluation of imperforate anus. Radiology 90: 466–471

Berdon W E, Baker D H 1970 Midgut malrotation and volvulus. Which films are most helpful? Radiology 96: 375–383

Bishop H C, Koop C E 1957 Management of meconium ileus: Resection, Roux-en-y anastomosis and ileostomy irrigation with pancreatic enzymes. Annals of Surgery 145: 410–414

Brereton R J, Kumar D, Spitz L 1985 Diaphragmatic hernia in Neonates. Zeitschrift fur Kinderchirurgie 40: 75–79

Duhamel B 1960 A new operation for the treatment of Hirschsprung's disease. Archives of Disease in Childhood 35: 38–39

Filston H C, Kirk D R 1981 Malrotation — the ubiquitous anomaly. Journal of Pediatric Surgery 16: 614–620

Girvan D P, Stephens C A 1974 Congenital intrinsic duodenal obstruction. A 20-year review of its surgical management and consequences. Journal of Pediatric Surgery 9: 833–839

Grob M 1963 Conservative treatment of exomphalos. Archives of Disease in Childhood 38: 148–150

Holder T M, Cloud D T, Lewis J E, Pilling G P 1964 Esophageal atresia and tracheoesophageal fistula. A survey of its members by the surgical section of the American Academy of Pediatrics. Pediatrics 34: 542–549

Holschneider A M 1982 Hirschsprung's Disease. Hippokrates Verlag, Stuttgart

Kosloske A M, Papile L A, Burnstein J 1980 Indications for operation in acute necrotizing enterocolitis of the neonate. Surgery 87: 502–508

Lorber J 1971 Results of treatment of myelomeningocoele. An analysis of 524 unselected cases with special reference to possible selection for treatment. Developmental Medicine and Child Neurology 13: 279–303

Nixon H H 1960 An experimental study of propulsion of isolated small intestine and its applications to surgery in the newborn. Annals of the Royal College of Surgeons of England 27: 105–124

Noblett H R 1961 Treatment of uncomplicated meconium ileus by gastrografin enema. A preliminary report. Journal of Pediatric Surgery 4: 190–197

Noblett H R 1969 A rectal suction biopsy tube for use in the diagnosis of Hirschsprung's disease. Journal of Pediatric Surgery 4: 406–409

Park R W, Grand R J 1981 Gastrointestinal manifestations of cystic fibrosis. A review. Gastroenterology 81: 1193–1161

Rehbein F 1958 Intraabdominelle Resektion oder Rektosigmoidektomie bei der Hirschsprungschen Kirarkheit Chirurgie 29: 366–369

Rickham P P, Stauffer U G, Cheng S K 1977 Oesophageal atresia: triumph and tragedy. Australian and New Zealand Journal of Surgery 47: 138–143

Shuster S R 1967 A new method for the staged repair of large omphaloceles. Surgery, Gynecology and Obstetrics 125: 837–850

Simpson A J, Leonides J C 1972 Roentgen diagnosis of midgut malroation: value of upper gastrointestinal radiographic study. Journal of Pediatric Surgery 7: 243–252

Soave F 1966 Hirschsprung's disease: Technique and results of Soave Operation. British Journal of Surgery 53: 1023–1027

Spitz L, Wallis M, Graves H F 1984 Transport of the surgical neonate. Archives of Disease in Childhood 59: 284–288

Stephens F D, Smith E D 1971 Anorectal Malformations in Children. Year Book Medical Publishers Inc, Chicago

Swenson O, Bill A H 1948 Resection of rectum and rectrosigmoid with preservation of sphincter for benign spastic lesions producing megacolon. Surgery 24: 212–220

Swenson O Sherman J O, Firsher J H 1973 Diagnosis of congenital megacolon: an analysis of 501 patients. Journal of Pediatric Surgery 8: 587–594

Thomas D F M 1982 Pathogenesis of neonatal necrotizing enterocolitis. Journal of Royal Society of Medicine 75: 838

Parenteral nutrition — its role in surgical practice

Parenteral nutrition is now available in some form or another in all hospitals in the United Kingdom. Parenteral nutrition can be conveniently considered under two headings — peripheral vein intravenous feeding and total parenteral nutrition. The latter provides fluids of high osmolarity and requires central vein cannulation.

PERIPHERAL VEIN FEEDING — BACKGROUND

Most surgeons and physicians do not realise that peripheral vein feeding is being administered to many of their patients. This is in the form of 5% dextrose which apart from supplying water has potentially powerful and useful metabolic effects.

During the 1940s Dr James Gamble, Professor of Paediatrics at Harvard Medical School carried out a classic series of Life Raft experiments. These studies took place at the Massachusetts General Hospital and also on a raft moored in a small cove off Cape Cod. The purpose of these experiments was to determine the optimum amounts of food and water rations that could be packed into the small space that was available on life rafts. Part of the work related to the amount of glucose per day that was necessary to produce the maximum reduction in urinary nitrogen loss. This amount was found to be approximately 100 g/day for glucose. If we now consider the amount of 5% glucose that is administered to many adult surgical patients this is in the region of 1–2 litres/day or 50–100 G. Thus it can be seen that surgeons are either extremely well educated in the field of nutrition or are fortunate that 5% glucose is a readily available isosmotic solution which does not provide sodium overload to stressed patients!

Attention must now be paid to the body's normal response to starvation. It is clear that most surgical patients are starved perioperatively but equally most seem to make an uneventful postoperative recovery. After hepatic glycogen stores have been utilized in 24–48 hours, the metabolic response to starvation results in a reduction in urinary nitrogen excretion. This reduction in protein breakdown is partly due to increased lipolysis and utilisation of fatty acids. The ketone bodies, acetoacetate and 3-

hydroxybutyrate are also released into the blood and after a few days of starvation are metabolized by the brain with a decreasing need for glucose. Thus there is a reduction in gluconeogenesis from protein. There is also an important reduction in metabolic rate. Thus, the body itself is well able to preserve its protein in short term starvation of a few weeks duration. It has, however, been pointed out by Blackburn et al in 1973 that glucose reduces ketone body production and therefore enthusiasm for its prescription alone for more than a few days needs to be tempered.

The above observations apply to fit healthy adults. Young babies have high glucose and energy requirements for their size and are at risk from hypoglycaemia if starved for more than a few hours. Glucose production and utilisation is much higher in the child than with the adult (Bier et al, 1977). This need for glucose is well known to neonatal surgeons and anaesthetists who avoid long periods of perioperative starvation in their patients. Much nutritional debate will, however, surround the survival of neonates in Mexico in September 1985 who were trapped in hospitals following an earthquake. Some survived for periods up to a week without food or water. This demonstrates the remarkable metabolic adaptations that are brought about in starvation.

Surgical patients, however, undergo a series of contrasting metabolic situations. Patients are often elderly, starved, malnourished and confined to bed. These situations all lower metabolic rate and thus fuel requirements are relatively reduced. Protein turnover and urinary nitrogen excretion similarly decrease. The same patients undergo surgery and may suffer infection. These conditions in contrast cause increases in metabolic rate, fuel requirements, protein turnover and urinary nitrogen excretion. Increased urinary nitrogen loss after injury was first described by Cuthbertson in 1932 and reviewed by him in 1979. The greatest injury that can be received is a large (> 60% surface area) third degree thermal burn. In the past this was associated with very high metabolic rates but given modern burns care, even in this highest of all hypermetabolic states, metabolic expenditure is virtually never more than 2 × basal metabolism rate for age, sex and surface area (Royle & Burke, 1982). Because of the presence of the factors that lower metabolic rate, calorie requirements for most surgical patients are usually only 10% above those of basal metabolism, in the region of 18 000–22 000 cal/day for the average adult.

PERIPHERAL VEIN FEEDING — POSSIBILITIES

Many surgeons feel that if a patient needs parenteral nutritional support this should be total or not at all. This is because of the lack of evidence for the clinical benefits of amino acids, lipid and glucose administered via peripheral veins. The problem with peripheral vein feeding is one of logistics — the isotonic solutions that are required cannot supply enough calories and nitrogen for the patient to reach energy and protein balance without severely overloading the patient with fluid. This problem does not arise with the hyperosmolar solutions that can be given via central veins in a smaller volume of fluid. Similarly, it is a clinical fact that many ill patients have a lack of suitable peripheral veins for repeated cannulation.

Blackburn in the United States in the 1970s was the first of the advocates of the peripheral vein administration of isotonic amino acids. In essence his work shows that nitrogen balance is improved if amino acids are given alone compared with 5% glucose given alone. Nutritionally this is perhaps not surprising. Further help to the cause of peripheral vein feeding was the advent of safe isotonic lipid emulsions that were both of high energy content and also supplied essential fatty acids (Wretlind, 1977). Thus 5% dextrose, 20% lipid and amino acid solutions (5 g N/l) can all be given via peripheral veins. There are also some commercial solutions that contain alcohol which can be a useful energy source supplying 7 cal/g compared with 9 cal/g for lipid and 4 cal/g for carbohydrate and protein. The advantages and disadvantages of alcohol are clear. Some composite solutions contain fructose or sorbitol in addition to alcohol and these are associated with the development of lactic acidosis, particularly in patients with liver disease (Woods & Alberti, 1972). Lactic acidosis is admittedly rare but has a high mortality. These solutions are not recommended for general use.

In contast to adult patients, peripheral vein feeding has found a definite place in neonatal surgery units — though central vein cannulation and hyperosmolar solutions are eventually needed for babies who need feeding for long periods of time.

In the adult the value of peripheral vein feeding is not proven. It is indeed hard to find clinical evidence for improvements in patient morbidity (Hensle, 1978). Peripheral vein feeding can be justified on metabolic grounds in some obese patients and for short periods of time. It, however, has to be stated that nutritionally it is not possible to correct malnutrition in terms of days but only in terms of months of feeding. This is well known from the treatment of malnourished patients in underdeveloped countries. Similarly, it is clear that healthy adults can exist for a month without food. Benedict in 1915 was one of the first to describe the importance of lipid as the major fuel source in the long term starvation. His studies were carried out on a Maltese volunteer (Mr L) who fasted for a month.

TOTAL PARENTERAL NUTRITION

This is the provision of fluid, electrolytes, vitamins, trace elements, calories and protein in sufficient amounts to meet the body's requirements. Total parenteral nutrition (TPN) in man was first shown to be a practical possibility in 1969 by Dudrick. Since then there has been an explosion of interest amongst surgeons. Similar to all treatments, however, it is now clear that there are only certain groups of patients who are likely to benefit from TPN. In some of these patients, TPN will be life-saving.

TPN — what to give

While we may not know precisely the metabolic requirements for individual vitamins, trace elements and amino acids, much has been learned in the last few years.

Similar to Dr Gamble's experiments off Cape Cod in the 1940s, recently Dr J. F. Burke, Professor of Surgery at Harvard Medical School, employing sophisticated techniques using stable non-radioactive isotopes, has demonstrated that there are optimum amounts of glucose that can be given to patients. Too much of a good thing, even glucose, can be bad for the body and glucose when given in excess is simply converted to lipid and carbon dioxide. Thus, optimum rates for the administration of glucose in the adult are 5–7 mg/kg/min. At these rates maximum oxidation of glucose is achieved and maximum reduction of endogenous glucose production ensues together with reduction in protein breakdown (Burke et al, 1979). It is less clear how much lipid and protein to give patients. There is increasing evidence that lipid becomes an important body fuel following trauma or infection (Stoner et al, 1983). Similarly, hyperketonaemia is associated with a reduction in protein breakdown (Smith et al, 1975).

The normal Western diet contains approximately 30% lipid. Many surgeons now give half the non-protein calorie requirements to patients as lipid. A glucose–lipid regimen is well tolerated metabolically (Jeejeebhoy et al, 1976). Lipid emulsions have the great advantage of being Isotonic, contain essential fatty acids and provide many calories in a small fluid volume. In addition to solutions that only contain long chain triglyceride, there will soon be available solutions that contain medium chain triglycerides. The latter appear to be more rapidly metabolized than solutions which contain only long chain triglycerides (Bach & Babayan, 1982).

Most adult patients requiring TPN need about 14 g of nitrogen per day to maintain nitrogen balance. These requirements are increased in the presence of infection or massive trauma but not usually to more than about 21 g/day for any length of time. Some centres favour the use of high glucose, insulin regimens for these patients (Woolfson et al, 1979) but any advantages of a glucose amino acid regimen over a glucose lipid, amino acid regimen in hypermetabolic patients are not proven.

Branched chain amino acids (leucine, isoleucine and valine) are oxidized in muscle in contrast to other amino acids which are metabolized in the liver. Initial experimental studies (Buse & Reid 1975) suggested a possible role for leucine in the regulation of protein breakdown. Clinical studies have, however, so far not shown any clear role for intravenous solutions containing only branched chain amino acids (BCAA) in the management of patients with trauma or liver disease where their administration might be most apt (Madsen, 1983). A practical problem is that BCAA are relatively insoluble and therefore can only supply part of a patients amino acid requirements in order to maintain nitrogen balance if fluid overload is to be avoided.

Hypoalbuminaemia is often noted in patients requiring TPN. The half life of albumin is about 21 days and low plasma albumin concentration is likely to reflect sepsis rather than malnutrition in the surgical patient (Royle & Kettlewell, 1980). Thus, it is prudent for the surgeon to remember that intravenous albumin rather than TPN is by far the most rapid way to correct the hypoalbuminaemia but that surgical drainage of pus is even better at maintaining normal plasma biochemistry.

Low plasma concentrations of vitamin C occur in many patients referred for TPN. The daily provision of water soluble vitamins, all of which have body stores that last only a few weeks appears worthwhile. The daily requirements, even in health are, however, not known for certain. The provision of folic acid which is not present in most multi-vitamin preparation, should also not be forgotten.

Fat soluble vitamins have long term body stores of many months duration. Their provision is not needed unless TPN is given for several weeks. Overdose must be avoided. Fat soluble vitamins can be given conveniently in lipid emulsions once a week. The dose of most fat soluble vitamins required by TPN patients is not known. Vit K requirements are, however, about 0.15 mg per week unless the patient is on antibiotic therapy when prothrombin estimation should be done to gauge any increase in requirements (Hands et al, 1985).

Cases of trace element deficiences, e.g. zinc, copper, selenium have been reported in patients receiving long-term TPN. Thus similar to fat soluble vitamins, trace elements should be provided in patients fed for a week or more.

Table 3.1   Standard TPN regimen — an example

Glucose	250 g: 1000 cal
Lipid	500 ml 20% lipid: 1000 cal
Amino acid	14 g Nitrogen
Sodium	100 mmol
Potassium	100 mmol
Chloride	191 mmol
Calcium	13 mmol
Magnesium	19 mmol
Folic acid	
Water soluble Vitamins	

It has been clearly shown that most adult patients in a general hospital referred for TPN have similar energy requirements (Quebbeman et al, 1982) and can be prescribed a standard TPN regimen (Harper et al, 1983) of equicaloric amounts of carbohydrate and lipid, 14 g of nitrogen, sodium, potassium, chloride, calcium, magnesium, trace elements and water soluble vitamins. An example of a suitable regimen for most patients is shown in Table 3.1 and supplies approx. 2200 cal/day. It will be found that insulin is rarely required to prevent hyperglycaemia with such a regimen. Indi-

Table 3.2 Some metabolic complications of TPN

Fluid imbalance	Abnormal liver function tests — alkaline
Electrolyte imbalance	phosphatase, transaminase, bilirubin
Hyperglycaemia	Increase in blood urea concentration
Hypoglycaemia	Hyperchloraemia
Hyperlipaemia	Hypocalcaemia
Deficiences — vitamin, fatty acid or trace	Hypophosphataemia
elements	

vidual prescriptions are needed for patients with renal, hepatic and respiratory failure. A standard regimen can, however, still be given to most patients receiving renal dialysis. The TPN is given immediately post dialysis. Abnormalities in liver function tests, e.g. a progressive rise in alkaline phosphatase, are common with T.P.N. The cause is not certain and any clinical significance not obvious (Grant et al, 1977). A regimen such as in Table 3.1 together with adequate monitoring, however, should help to avoid most of the metabolic complications in Table 3.2.

TPN — how to give it

TPN has to be administered via a central vein — usually the superior vena cava. The requires cannulation via an infra or supraclavicular route. The former is favoured by most surgeons, the latter by many anaesthetists — this may reflect their overall view of patients! Cannulation is usually performed by a percutaneous technique though surgical exposure of the subclavian or jugular veins avoids the risk of pneumothorax. Cannulation via the infraclavicular route allows for easier subcutaneous tunnelling of the catheter and is recommended. Tunnelling helps in fixation and dressing of the catheter and may reduce infection. The use of a tunnelled silicone catheter should result in a catheter related sepsis rate of only 1–2% (Mitchell et al, 1982). Thus in skilled hands, pyrexias in surgical patients who receive TPN via tunnelled silicone catheters are very unlikely to be due to an infection in the TPN line.

A whole host of technical complications have been reported for the percutaneous cannulation of the superior vena cave (see Table 3.2). The morbidity in practised hands, however, should be very low and quite acceptable. It is, however, essential to obtain an erect chest X-ray immediately after each catheterisation to rule out pneumothorax and misplacement of the catheter. The tip of the catheter must be in the superior vena cava for safe administration of TPN and not in the heart, jugular or axillary veins. It is the responsibility of the doctor who puts in the catheter to see the radiograph before TPN commences (Table 3.3).

TPN solutions are usually sold to hospitals as separate solutions of carbohydrate, lipid and amino acids. There is, however, a great advantage for the nursing staff if they can be administered pre-mixed via a large plastic

Table 3.3 Some complications of percutaneous TPN catheter insertion

---

Technical
  Pneumothorax
  Misplacement of catheter tip e.g. jugular vein, outside venous system
  Vascular — haematoma, arterial, venous, thoracic duct or cardiac damage
  Neurological damage e.g. brachial plexus, phrenic nerve
  Air embolism
  Catheter embolism

Septic
  Septicaemia

Venous thrombosis
  Local or distant

---

bag. Glucose, lipid and amino acids electrolytes and water soluble vitamins can all be mixed together under sterile conditions. This, however, needs a laminar flow hood to produce sterile filling conditions and available and willing pharmacists. Ideally all large hospitals should have this facility.

If 'big bags' are not available to administer TPN, bottles and bags have to be joined together via a series of connectors. This is frustrating for all and the many connections and disconnections are a potential source of infection and air embolism.

The rate of administration of TPN is most accurately controlled by a volumetric infusion pump though there are a variety of other control devices of varying degrees of sophistication and price.

TPN is usually administered over 24 hours. Cyclical feeding with the TPN given while the patient is asleep at night allows the patient to be mobile in the daytime and may be more akin to meal feeding with possible metabolic advantages — this is not, however, proven.

TPN is undoubtedly best administered and monitored via a parenteral nutrition team consisting of interested clinicians, pharmacists, biochemists and most importantly, a parenteral nutrition nurse. The latter supervises dressings and the management of TPN catheters and can act as a most helpful coordinator for the team. As with any other form of surgical practice, a careful TPN audit will reduce morbidity (Nehme, 1980) and control financial expenditure.

TPN — what to measure

The following is feasible in clinical practice:

Haematology   — Twice weekly Hb, WBC, platelets.
              — Weekly — prothrombin time & film.

Biochemistry — plasma: twice weekly — urea, electrolytes, liver function tests, calcium, glucose.

Urine
— daily urine collections for urea and electrolytes.
— daily ward testing for glucose & ketones. If the urine contains glucose patients will need 4–8 hourly blood finger prick samples to test for glucose.

Bacteriology
— Weekly blood cultures.
— Weekly skin culture from catheter entry site into skin.
— blood culture through TPN catheter before removal.
— catheter tips sent for culture on removal.

Fluid balance
— Daily! Fluid overload is a common complication.

Blood Gases
— as necessary, particularly if acidosis or CO_2 retention in suspected.

Nitrogen balance
— an estimate of nitrogen balance can be made if it is assumed that urea contributes 83% of the urinary nitrogen excretion. The measurement of total nitrogen excretion by the Kjeldahl method takes several days and is for research purposes only. Five day nitrogen balances are more meaningful than daily nitrogen balances. The inaccuracy of nitrogen balance estimations lies in the volume of urine excreted per day that is recorded. Many publications indicate positive nitrogen balances of great magnitude. It must be remembered that such positive nitrogen balances are only likely to occur under exceptional circumstances. Thus: urine urea (mmol/l) $\times$ 24 h urine volume (l) $\times$ 0.028 $\times$ 6/5 = urine nitrogen (g/24 h).

Anthropometry
— Body weight, arm muscle circumference, triceps skin fold thickness and grip strength can all be measured on a weekly basis. Rapid changes in body weight, however, reflect changes in water rather than protein. Most anthropometric measurements are useful for research rather than clinical purposes. A poor anthropometric and dynamometric score is, however, related to postoperative complications (Klidjian et al, 1980).

TPN — when to give it

TPN is only indicated when food cannot be absorbed via the gastrointestinal tract either orally or via nasogastric tube or jejunostomy. Despite the fact that many surgical patients are malnourished (Hill et al, 1977a), the absolute indications for TPN cannot be easily given. The following, however, may be used as guidelines.

Trauma

TPN is indicated in the management of patients with severe full thickness thermal burns as soon as a stable cardiorespiratory state has been achieved by the infusion of plasma, colloid and blood. TPN may be needed for several weeks until sufficient calories and protein can be given via the gastrointestinal tract to meet nutritional requirements. Metabolic expenditure in such patients may remain elevated to 50% above basal metabolic rate for weeks.

Gastrointestinal surgery

TPN plays a major role in the management of enterocutaneous fistulae. Provided that there is no distal obstruction, foreign body, major sepsis, tract epithelialization, adjacent cancer or Crohn's disease many enterocutaneous fistulae will close spontaneously with conservative management, i.e. nil by mouth + TPN. This is true occasionally even for some high output fistulae — though they will take longer to close, e.g. 4–6 weeks. TPN thus allows nature to heal a fistula and surgery can often be avoided. The mortality from enterocutaneous fistulae has fallen markedly since the increased use of TPN in their management (MacFadyen et al, 1973; Monod-Broca, 1977; Irving, 1977).

Many patients with inflammatory bowel disease (IBD) are malnourished (Hill et al, 1977b) but the role of TPN in the management of these patients is not yet clear. TPN has been advocated as primary treatment (Mullen et al, 1978), used with steroids as part of a 5-day regimen for an acute attack of inflammatory bowel disease (Truelove et al, 1978), used perioperatively for nutritional support in elective surgery for IBD and finally used as home TPN for patients with the short gut syndrome after massive resection of IBD. TPN is usually of greater use in the management of Crohn's disease rather than ulcerative colitis. There are, unfortunately, no satisfactory controlled trials to report upon.

TPN is frequently used in some centres for the preoperative and/or postoperative nutritional support of patients with upper gastrointestinal tract obstruction or malignancy. The rationale is to correct preoperative nutritional deficiences and provide postoperative metabolic support. These aims are worthy but hard evidence of clinical benefits for patients is difficult to come by (BMJ, 1979). These has been one study from Germany (Muller et al, 1982) indicating a reduction in postoperative morbidity in gastric cancer patients who were fed intravenously preoperatively. Further substantiation has, however, not appeared. It is not in dispute that TPN improves nitrogen balance and may correct immunological impairment (Law et al,

1973), it is however not clear that TPN reduces time in hospital, and improves morbidity and mortality in large groups of patients undergoing major gastrointestinal surgery, whether malnourished or not. In fact TPN would increase time in hospital if given in sufficient amounts preoperatively — as it would take several weeks to improve many patients malnourished state. This is not clinically possible. Preoperative correction of fluid and electrolyte balance, water soluble vitamins, albumin and haemoglobin are, however, all feasible, sometimes forgotten and likely to be of more benefit to the patient than three or four days of TPN.

If a stormy or prolonged postoperative course is, however, anticipated, the insertion of a TPN feeding line in the operating theatre is prudent and may give the surgeon the same help with sleep as an abdominal drain. It might, however, be said that excellent technical surgery might reduce the need for both TPN and abdominal drains.

TPN has a definite role to play in the management of severe acute pancreatitis. It is, however, difficult to predict which of these patients will remain 'nil by mouth' for more than a week. As with many other ill gastrointestinal patients, the absence of peripheral veins to cannulate and the inability of the patient to take food by the intestine should make the surgeon think in terms of TPN both for vasculr access as well as nutritional support. A lipid, glucose, amino acid regimen is quite suitable but with careful monitoring of blood glucose concentrations and a check to make sure that lipaemia is not persistent.

Finally, TPN may be needed for those patients with the short bowel syndrome whether from necrotising enterocolitis in the neonate or inflammatory bowel disease or mesenteric infarction in the adult. There are now several centres throughout the United Kingdom which manage home TPN patients. It is now well proven that these patients can be supported rather like home renal dialysis patients (Irving et al, 1985). TPN is infused overnight at home and the catheter is heparin locked in the daytime allowing patients to carry out normal activities. A week's supply of TPN solutions can be stored in a fridge at the patients home and the catheter, dressings and controlling pump are all managed by the patient following a period of inpatient instruction supervised by a TPN nurse. Initial problems have included exactly who pays for the home TPN patients — hospital, district, region etc.

CONCLUSIONS

TPN has an extremely useful and lifesaving role to play in surgical practice. Every general hospital in the country would benefit from a TPN team, however small and however unofficial. This would reduce morbidity from intravenous feeding and almost certainly provide financial savings due to rational standard prescribing policies for those selected patients who really do benefit from its use — namely those with enterocutaneous fistulae and those who, for whatever reason, cannot absorb food by the gastrointestinal tract for periods of a week or more. The patient with massive burns and the neonatal surgical patient are likely to be in specialist centres and together with the patients with renal and hepatic failure need individual TPN regimens. A simple understanding of the metabolic changes that occur in surgical patients should make TPN prescribing straight forward to all and not a mystery.

TPN is unlikely to prevent gastrointestinal anastomoses from falling apart — only good technical surgery will reduce that sort of postoperative problem. TPN may, however, be a true 'life-line' when disease or surgery bring about serious gastrointestinal complications.

REFERENCES

Bach A C, Babayan V K 1982 Medium chain triglycerides: an update. American Journal of Clinical Nutrition 36: 950–962

Benedict F G 1915 A study of prolonged fasting. Carnegie Institution of Washington Publication, no. 203, Washington D.C., U.S.A.

Bier D M, Leake R D, Haymond M W, Arnold K J, Gruenke L D, Sperling M A, Kipnis D M 1977 Measurement of 'true' glucose production rates in infancy and childhood with 6-6-dideuterated glucose. Diabetes 26: 1016–1023

Blackburn G L, Flatt J P, Clowes G H A, O'Donnell T E 1973 Peripheral intravenous feeding with isotonic amino acid solutions. The American Journal of Surgery 125: 447–454

British Medical Journal (Editorial) 1979 Parenteral nutrition before surgery? British Medical Journal 2: 1529–1530

Burke J F, Wolfe R R, Mullany C J, Mathews D E, Bier D M 1979 Glucose requirements following burn injury: parameters of optimal glucose infusion and possible hepatic and respiratory abnormalities following excessive glucose intake. Annals of Surgery 190: 274–285

Buse M G, Reid S S 1975 Leucine: A possible regulator of protein turnover in muscle. Journal of Clinical Investigation 56: 1250–1261

Cuthbertson D P 1932 Observations on the disturbance of metabolism produced by injury to the limbs. Quarterly Journal of Medicine NSI: 233–246

Cuthbertson D P 1979 Alterations in metabolism following injury. Injury 11: 175–189, 286–303

Dudrick S J, Wilmore D W, Vars H M, Rhoads J E 1969 Can intravenous feeding as the sole means of nutrition support growth in the child and restore weight loss in an adult? Annals of Surgery 169: 974–984

Gamble J L 1947 Physiological information gained from studies on the life raft ration. Harvey Lectures 42: 247–273

Grant J P, Cox C E, Kleinman L M, Maher M M, Pittman M A, Tangrea J A et al 1977 Serum hepatic enzyme and bilirubin elevations during parenteral nutrition. Surgery, Gynecology and Obstetrics 145: 573–580

Hands L J, Royle G T, Kettlewell M 1985 Vitamin K requirements in patients receiving total parenteral nutrition. British Journal of Surgery 72: 665–667

Harper P H, Royle G T, Mitchell A, Greenall M S, Grant A, Winsley B et al 1983 A three year audit of the work of a parenteral nutrition service: the value of a standard regimen. British Medical Journal 286: 1323–1327

Hensle T W 1978 Protein sparing in cystectomy patients. Journal of Urology 119: 355–358

Hill G L, Blackett R L, Pickford I, Burkinshaw L, Young G A, Warren J V, Schorah C J, Morgan D B 1977(a) Malnutrition in surgical patients, an unrecognised problem. Lancet I: 689–692

Hill G L, Blackett R L, Pickford I R, Bradley J A 1977b A survey of protein nutrition in patients with inflammatory bowel disease — a rational basis for nutritional therapy. British Journal of Surgery 64: 894–896

Irving M 1977 Local and surgical management of enterocutaneous fistulas. British Journal of Surgery 64: 690–694

Irving M, White R, Tresadern J 1985 Three year's experience with an intestinal failure unit. Annals of the Royal College of Surgeons 67: 2–5

Jeejeebhoy K N, Anderson G H, Nakhooda A F, Greenberg G R, Sanderson I, Marliss E G 1976 Metabolic studies in total parenteral nutrition with lipid in man: comparison with glucose. Journal of Clinical Investigation 57: 125–136

Klidjian A M, Foster K J, Kammerling R M, Cooper A, Karran S J 1980 Relation of anthropometric and dynamometric variables to serious postoperative complications. British Medical Journal 281: 899–901

Law D K, Dudrick S J, Abdou N I 1973 Immunocompetence of patients with protein calorie malnutrition. The effects of nutritional repletion. Annals of Internal Medicine 79: 545–550

MacFadyen B V Jr, Dudrick S J, Ruberg R L 1973 Management of gastrointestinal fistular with parenteral hyperalimentation. Surgery 74: 100–105

Madsen D C 1983 Branched-chain amino acids: metabolic roles and clinical applications. In: Johnston I D A (ed) Advances in Clinical Nutrition. MTP Press Ltd, Lancaster, p 3–23

Mitchell A, Atkins S, Royle G T, Kettlewell M G W 1982 Reduced catheter sepsis and prolonged catheter life using a tunnelled silicone-rubber catheter for total parenteral nutrition. British Journal of Surgery 69: 420–422

Monod-Broca P 1977 Treatment of intestinal fistulas. British Journal of Surgery 64: 685–689

Muller J M, Brenner U, Dienst C, Pichlmaier H 1982 Preoperative parenteral feeding in patients with gastrointestinal carcinoma. Lancet i: 68–71

Mullen J L, Hargrove W L, Dudrick S J, Fitts W T J R, Rosato E F 1978 Ten years experience with intravenous hyperalimentation and inflammatory bowel disease. Annals of Surgery 187: 523–529

Nehme A E 1980 Nutritional support of the hospitalised patient. The team concept. Journal of the American Medical Association 243: 1906–1908

Quebbeman E J, Ausman R K, Schneider T C 1982 A re-evaluation of energy expenditure during parenteral nutrition. Annals of Surgery 195: 282–286

Royle G T, Burke J F 1982 Substrate requirements in burn patients In: Grant A, Todd E (eds) Handbook of Enteral and Parenteral Nutrition. Blackwell Scientific, Oxford, p 139–143

Royle G T, Kettlewell M G W 1980 Liver function tests in surgical infection and malnutrition. Annals of Surgery 192: 192–194

Smith R, Fuller D J, Wedge J H, Williamson D H, Alberti K G M M 1975 Initial effect of injury on ketone bodies and other blood metabolites. Lancet i: 1–3

Stoner H B, Little R A, Frayn K N, Elebate E A, Tresadern J, Gross E 1983 The effect of sepsis on the oxidation of carbohydrate and fat. British Journal of Surgery 70: 32–35

Truelove S C, Willoughby C P, Lee E G, Kettlewell M G W 1978 Further experience in the treatment of severe attacks of ulcerative colitis. Lancet ii: 1086–1088

Woods H F, Alberti K G M M 1972 Dangers of intravenous fructose. Lancet ii: 1354–1357

Woolfson A M J, Heatley R V, Allison S P 1979 Insulin to inhibit protein catabolism after injury. New England Journal of Medicine 300: 14–17

Wretlind A 1977 Lipid emulsions and technique of peripheral administration in parenteral nutrition. In: Greep, Soeters, Wesdorp, Phaf and Fisher (eds) Current concepts in parenteral nutrition. Martinus Nijhoff, The Hague, p 273–297

FURTHER READING

Grant A, Todd E (eds) 1982 Enteral and Parenteral Nutrition — A clinical handbook. Blackwell Scientific, Oxford

Silk D B A (ed) 1983 Nutritional Support in Hospital Practice. Blackwell Scientific, Oxford

Johnston I D A (ed) 1983 Advances in Clinical Nutrition. MTP Press Ltd, Lancaster

Gastro-oesophageal reflux and management of reflux induced strictures

INTRODUCTION

Episodes of gastro-oesophageal reflux occur daily in the vast majority of normal people. These are most frequent in the upright position, particularly after meals and during exercises which increase intra-abdominal pressure, but are extremely uncommon during sleep. In normal circumstances the refluxed material is cleared from the oesophagus by swallowing. A variety of defence mechanisms exist to prevent reflux, clear the refluxate and avoid the development of reflux oesophagitis. Factors such as lower oesophageal sphincter pressure, oesophageal clearance, potency and volume of refluxed material and oesophageal mucosal resistance are important in determining whether a subject will develop oesophagitis.

Symptomatic gastro-oesophageal reflux is common. In a study of 385 hospital staff Nebel et al (1973) found that reflux symptoms were present in 36%, of whom 7% experienced heartburn daily, 14% weekly and 15% had heartburn at least once a month. Only a minority of symptomatic subjects seeks medical advice and of these most can be controlled with a combination of postural and dietary manoeuvres, supplemented by simple medications where necessary. Only a small proportion of patients will require intensive medical treatment and an even smaller number will require anti reflux surgery.

Reflux oesophagitis has a multifactorial aetiology and variations in the results of investigations and response to treatment are found between different groups of patients. Detailed oesophageal investigation is only necessary in those patients who fail to respond to simple medical treatment. It may be possible to select the most appropriate drug regime for an individual patient on the basis of these investigations (e.g. poor oesophageal clearance — bethanechol; gastric acid hypersecretion — H2 receptor blockers). Failure to respond to intensive medical treatment or the development of complications such as stricture formation, a Barrett's oesophagus or haemorrhage are indications for anti reflux surgery in patients with no other medical contraindications.

PATHOPHYSIOLOGY OF REFLUX OESOPHAGITIS

Winkelstein (1935) was the first to suggest that oesophagitis was the result of reflux of gastrointestinal contents into the oesophagus, although the term 'reflux oesophagitis' was not generally adopted until the 1950s (Allison, 1951). In many patients with reflux symptoms a hiatus hernia was demonstrable radiologically and in the 1940s and 1950s it was believed that this was responsible for their symptoms. Operations were designed to correct the hiatal hernia. However, not all patients with a hiatus hernia have reflux symptoms and, conversely, reflux can occur in the absence of a hiatus hernia (Cohen & Harris, 1971). The factors involved in gastro-oesophageal reflux and the development of reflux oesophagitis are listed in Table 4.1

Table 4.1 Factors involved in the development of reflux oesophagitis

1. Efficiency of the anti-reflux mechanism
2. Volume and composition of refluxed material
3. Oesophageal clearance
4. Decreased oesophageal mucosal resistance
5. Delayed gastric emptying

Anti-reflux mechanism

A positive pressure gradient exists between the abdomen and thorax which increases further with all activities which raise intra-abdominal pressure. Continuous reflux would occur if there was no physiological obstacle at the gastro-oesophageal junction. The lower oesophageal sphincter (LOS), initially described by Fyke et al in 1956, is the principal barrier to gastro-oesophageal reflux. Anatomical factors such as the phreno-oesophageal ligament, right crus of the diaphragm, a segment of intra-abdominal oesophagus and the angle of His are less important than was believed previously. However, there is some evidence that they do augment the LOS, thus contributing to reflux prevention (Dodds et al, 1976).

The LOS is a physiological, rather than anatomical, sphincter which relaxes on swallowing, oesophageal distension and vagal stimulation. Some workers have described the existence of a zone of thickened circular muscle in the lower oesophagus at the point which corresponds to the LOS (Liebermann-Meffert et al, 1979). Tonic contraction of the LOS circular muscle is responsible fot the lower oesophageal sphincter pressure (LOSP) which can be measured manometrically. These circular smooth muscle cells of the LOS have a lower resting membrane potential (-40 mV) than the cells in the body of the oesophagus or stomach (-50 to -60 mV) and this partial membrane depolarisation is responsible for the tonic contraction. Calcium antagonists, such as verapamil, reduce the inward leakage of calcium ions across the cell membrane thus reducing this partial depolarisation and causing a fall in LOSP (Goyal & Rattan, 1980). Although basically myogenic in origin the LOSP is affected by neural and hormonal stimuli and by drugs. It is innervated by inhibitory and excitatory autonomic nerves whose function is to initiate and maintain sphincter relaxation in response to swallowing. Inhibitory nerves predominate. Transmission is via cholinergic vagal fibres but sympathetic inhibitory nerves have also been demonstrated. Atropine administration causes a fall in LOSP, indicating the existence of a significant cholinergic input to the LOS. In pharmacological doses the hormones gastrin, motilin, pancreatic polypeptide and bombesin all increase LOSP. Secretin, cholecystokinin, VIP, GIP and glucagon all cause a fall. In physiological doses these gastrointestinal hormones probably only have a minor role in determination of LOSP. It is possible that they may regulate changes in post prandial LOSP.

In health the LOSP is not constant and marked fluctuations, due to changes in muscle tone and inhibitory and excitatory neural stimuli, can occur, even within short periods of time. The LOS must prevent gastro-oesophageal reflux for the majority of the time but must relax after swallowing to permit passage of a luminal bolus from oesophagus to stomach. The early supposition that gastro-oesophageal reflux is the result of LOS hypotension does not apply to all patients. Many patients with reflux oesophagitis have a normal LOSP (Demeester et al, 1976). In these patients reflux occurs in relation to inappropriate, transient LOS relaxations which are not associated with swallowing (Dent et al, 1980). Gastro-oesophageal reflux is uncommon following swallow-initiated LOS relaxation. Transient sphincter relaxation can occur almost immediately after LOS recovery following a normal swallow-induced relaxation and also in association with tertiary contractions in the body of the oesophaus or after multiple rapid swallows. They are uncommon during sleep. Only 60% of transient LOS relaxations are followed by reflux but these account for over 90% of acid reflux episodes in normal subjects. The reflux occurs during the short period when LOSP is effectively zero and the intraoesophageal and intragastric pressures are equilibrated. The stimulus which initiates non-swallow associated, and therefore inappropriate, LOS relaxations is presently unknown.

These inappropriate transient LOS relaxations explain why some patients with reflux oesophagitis have a normal resting LOSP, why there is overlap is basal LOSP values between patients with reflux oesophagitis and asymptomatic controls, and how reflux occurs in normal subjects with a normal LOSP. In general, patients with severe reflux oesophagitis and those who require surgery tend to have a lower resting LOSP than patients with milder oesophagitis. They have more frequent reflux episodes than control subjects (Demeester et al, 1976). Some patients have a low frequency of gastro-oesophageal reflux and in them other factors must be responsible for the development of reflux oesophagitis.

Oesophageal clearance

Refluxed material is cleared from the oesophagus by a combination of gravity, when the patient is upright, by secondary peristalsis in the body of the oesophagus and, most importantly, by swallowing. During waking swallowing occurs approximately once a minute and is almost completely abolished during sleep. It clears the oesophagus by initiation of peristalsis and brings the slightly alkaline saliva into contact with the refluxate. Disorders of oesophageal motility delay oesophageal clearance and increase the contact time of the refluxed material with the oesophageal mucosa. Nocturnal reflux may result in a prolonged delay in oesophageal clearance because of temporary cessation of swallowing. Oesophageal peristalsis has a high fractional emptying capacity and saliva helps restore oesophageal pH to normal when only a small amount of luminal acid remains (Kjellen & Tibbling, 1978). Salivary flow decreases with age and this may be a factor in the development of reflux oesophagitis in the elderly.

Volume and potency of the refluxed material

The principal substances refluxed into the oesophagus are acid and pepsin, both of which have been shown to produce oesophagitis experimentally (Goldberg et al, 1969). Duodenogastric reflux, which results in the addition of bile salts and pancreatic enzymes to the gastric juice, produces a very potent mixture for oesophagitis production (Gillison et al, 1972). Gastric volume is determined by a number of factors including volume of ingested material, rate of gastric secretion and gastric emptying and the frequency and volume of duodeno-gastric reflux. Forty per cent of patients with reflux oesophagitis may have delayed gastric emptying (McCallum & Berkowitz, 1978). Duodenal ulcer patients have a higher prevalence of reflux oeso-phagitis (Flook & Stoddard, 1985) which may be partly due to increased gastric acid production. Ingested food and fluid have a marked effect on gastric volume and pH. Certain foods increase acid production (milk, coffee, beer), others have an intrinsically low pH (Coca-Cola, pH 2.3).

Mucosal resistance

Oesophageal stratified squamous epithelium does have a capacity to resist injury from refluxed material but is less resistant to damage than other types of gastrointestinal epithelium. Severe oesophagitis with oesophageal desquamation results in replacement of the squamous epithelium with columnar epithelium, a condition known as a Barrett's oesophagus. Less severe oesophageal damage results in increased thickness of the basal cell layer of the epithelium and increased cell turnover.

Summary

Many factors are involved in the development of reflux oesophagitis. Different factors are operative in different individuals, hence the marked variations that can occur in the results of oesophageal investigations and treatment. Effective drug therapy should be based on the results of oesophageal investigations for those patients who fail to respond to simple measures. No single drug regime will effectively cure reflux oesophagitis in all patients.

METHODS OF INVESTIGATION

Intensive oesophageal investigation is inappropriate for the majority of reflux patients whose symptoms are mild and easily controlled by simple measures. These investigations should be reserved for patients with severe symptoms or complications of reflux and should be used to determine a rational plan of treatment.

Barium studies

Barium swallow is the simplest and most readily available technique for oesophageal assessment but is relatively insensitive. Only 50% of patients with reflux oesophagitis have detectable reflux during a standard cineradiographic examination. This may be related to absence of LOS relaxation during the radiological assessment or because of differences in the physical properties of barium and normal gastric contents. Although generally poor in the assessment of gastro-oesophageal reflux and oesophagitis a barium swallow will adequately demonstrate anatomical abnormalities such as a hiatus hernia to oesophageal stricture (Fig. 4.1).

Upper gastrointestinal endoscopy

This is the mainstay of oesophageal assessment and all patients with significant reflux symptoms should undergo endoscopy. It permits direct visualisation of the oesophageal mucosa; quantitative assessment of the length of a hiatus hernia, oesophagitis and columnar metaplasia; biopsy of, and endoscopic guide-wire placement through, a reflux-induced stricture and, finally, allows endoscopic assessment of the stomach, pylorus and proximal duodenum.

Oesophageal manometry

The technological advances of the last decade which have resulted in the production of intraluminal transducers and low compliance infusion systems for use in manometric testing have improved the precision, quantitation and

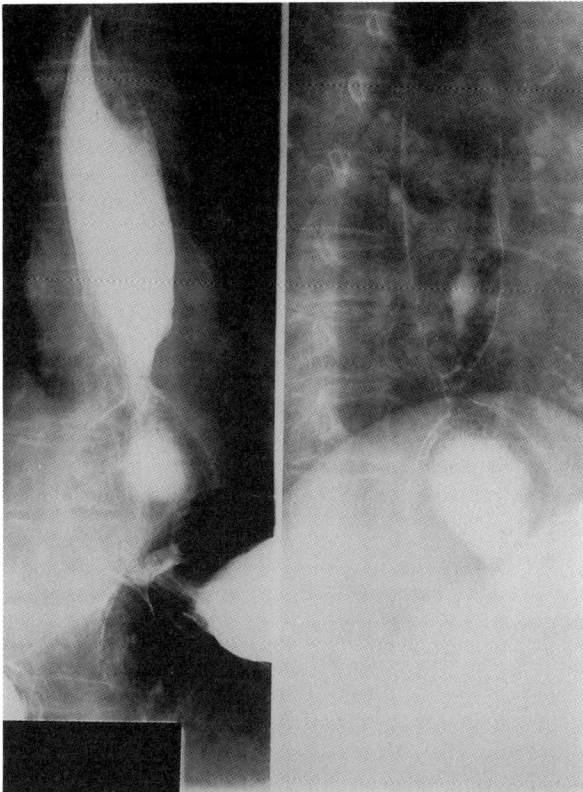

Fig. 4.1 Barium swallow showing a sliding hiatus hernia and a radiologically benign stricture at the gastro-oesophageal junction

reproducibility of oesophageal pressure studies. Although oesophageal manometry is useful in the investigation of patients with chest pain, dysphagia and those in whom achalasia is suspected it is of little value in the evaluation of patients with reflux symptoms (Castell, 1982). Manometry contributes to the understanding of the pathophysiological processes responsible for reflux in a given patient but the technique lacks diagnostic capabilities with respect to reflux symptoms (Pope et al, 1981). It is of value in the research laboratory in the pre and postoperative assessment of patients undergoing prospective evaluation of different anti-reflux procedures.

Intra-oesophageal pH monitoring

Oesophageal pH monitoring for the detection and quantitation of the frequency and duration of acid reflux episodes has increased in popularity in the last 10 years. Post-prandial, 12 and 16 hours recordings have been advocated but 24 hour pH monitoring is the most reliable. Recordings with large diameter pH electrodes connected to a pH meter and pen recorder at the patients bedside have been superceded by ambulatory pH monitoring. Monitoring of pH in hospital significantly underestimates the true extent of reflux which occurs when patients are performing their usual daily activities (Branicki et al, 1982). Ambulatory monitoring has followed the developments and improvements in pH electrodes and recorders. A radiotelemetric capsule, fine glass or antimony electrode can be positioned 5 cm above the manometrically determined LOS and connected to a portable recording unit which is worn on a waist belt that weighs less than 1 kg. During ambulatory pH monitoring patients are free to sleep, eat and perform their usual duties, including manual work. Recordings can be analysed visually and the frequency of reflux episodes and the total time during which intra oesophageal pH is less than 3, 4 or 5 calculated (Fig. 4.2). Computerised data analysis is available for most systems. Using this type of recording it has been shown that patients with reflux symptoms experience longer and more frequent reflux episodes when upright or supine than asymptomatic controls. Patients with mild oesophagitis have increased acid exposure predominantly in the upright position whereas those with severe reflux, ulcerative oesophagitis or strictures have increased acid exposure in both the erect and supine positions and also decreased oesophageal clearance. This technique has certain limitations for only acid, and not biliary or alkaline, reflux episodes are detected and secondly the electrode will not record the volume of refluxed material. Despite these limitations 24 hour pH monitoring is the best method available for quantitation of reflux episodes.

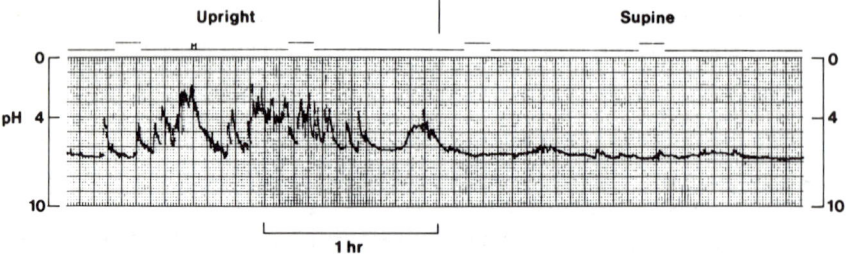

Fig. 4.2 Part of a 24 hour ambulatory pH recording. The patient has frequent reflux episodes in the upright position but there are no episodes of supine reflux.

Ambulatory oesophageal pH monitoring is not necessary in all patients, even those with severe endoscopic oesophagitis in whom the diagnosis is not in doubt. It is particularly useful in the assessment of patients with mild or atypical reflux symptoms or in patients with severe symptoms but no significant endoscopic abnormality. It is also valuable in determining the appropriate drug therapy for patients whose symptoms did not respond to simple medication, in the evaluation of drug efficacy on reflux control and finally pre and post operatively when different anti-reflux operations are being compared (Demeester et al, 1980).

Radionucleotide scanning

The rate of oesophageal clearance in the supine position, which effectively assesses oesophageal motility, can be measured by radionucleotide scanning. The patient is given a liquid bolus of [99m] technetium sulphur colloid and the time taken to clear 90% of the initial dose is measured with a gamma camera. Clearance is delayed in patients with motility disorders, particularly achalasia, and in some, but by no means all, patients with reflux oeso-phagitis. Transit studies may yield useful information is patients with motility disorders but have no place in routine assessment of reflux patients. Alternatively the sulphur colloid can be instilled into the stomach and the gamma camera used to measure gastro-oeosophageal reflux. Because of a number of variables, including gastric emptying, the technique only provides semi-quantitative information on the volume of refluxate. Although the method had limitations it is non-invasive, which can be useful in reflux assessment in children who would not tolerate intubation. It will detect reflux episodes and also pulmonary aspiration.

Investigation and treatment plan

Acknowledging that the pathogenesis of reflux oesophagitis is multifactorial the following plan for investigation and treatment of patients with reflux symptoms is suggested. Those with mild or moderate symptoms should be given advice about postural and dietary control plus antacids if necessary. Patients with severe symptoms, or those who fail to respond to simple treat-ment, require upper gastrointestinal endoscopy and biopsy. A barium swallow is indicated prior to endoscopy in patients with dysphagia to prevent endoscopic misdiagnosis of motility disorders, to identify the position and length of any oesophageal stricture and to look for an oeso-phageal carcinoma. If macroscopic oesophagitis is present medical treatment with H2 receptor blockers, Gaviscon or bethanechol, either singly or in combination, should be instituted. Patients with no oesophagitis require 24 hour pH studies to confirm the suspected diagnosis of pathological reflux and then commenced on medical treatment. The indications for anti-reflux surgery are discussed below.

SURGERY FOR GASTRO-OESOPHAGEAL REFLUX

Indications for surgery

It should be re-emphasized that the majority of reflux patients can be successfully managed with medical treatment. Polk & Zeppa (1969) reviewed 7000 patients with a radiologically demonstrable hiatus hernia and found that only 90 (1.3%) eventually underwent surgery. However, surgery should not be postponed indefinitely until a complication of oesophagitis develops. Severe perioesophagitis, due to longstanding reflux, or the presence of an oesophageal stricture may make the anti reflux procedure technically more difficult, thus increasing the risk of peri and postoperative complications and reducing the success rate of operation.

Table 4.2   Indications for anti-reflux surgery

Failed medical treatment
Complications of reflux
Oesophageal stricture
Barrett's oesophagus
Acute/chronic bleeding
Reflux induced oesophageal spasm

The principle indication for surgery is failure of medical treatment (Table 4.2). The degree to which patients will tolerate reflux symptoms varies enormously. Some with severe endoscopic oesophagitis are content to continue with medical treatment whereas others with minimal oesophagitis specifically request surgery. Ideally all patients considered for anti-reflux surgery should have complied with their postural, dietary and social advice, have had an adequate trial of medical treatment, have endoscopic oesophagitis and confirmation of excessive reflux of pH monitoring. Complications of reflux (oesophageal stricture, Barrett's oesophagus, acute or chronic blood loss from the oesophagus) are indicative of severe reflux and patients with these complications should be considered for surgery. Reflux induced oesophageal spasm may present diagnostic problems. The patients are frequently middle-aged males whose oesophageal pain is mistakenly thought to be myocardial in origin. Often this results in repeated hospital admissions with 'chest pain' and in the imposition of strict physical and social penalties. If the correct diagnosis of oesophageal pain secondary to reflux is made the patient should be treated with the usual anti reflux measures. However, the response to medical treatment is generally poor and careful cardiological assessment of these patients is mandatory to exclude coronary artery disease and myocardial ischaemia. If the cardiac assessment is normal and excessive gastro oesophageal reflux is proven by pH monitoring, then the patients who have failed to respond to medical treatment should be offered surgery.

Choice of operation

Major changes in gastro-oesophageal reflux surgery have occurred in the last 30 years. Reflux symptoms are no longer attributed to an anatomical abnormality, a hiatus hernia, and it is acknowledged that reflux is a physiological problem. As a result 'physiological' operations with increase the pressure at the lower end of the oesophagus have been developed and become popular at the expense of 'anatomical' operations, such as gastropexy, which merely reduce the hiatus hernia and fix the gastro-oesophageal junction below the diaphragm.

The large number of different operations that have been described, often only minor modifications of other techniques, indicates that the results of anti-reflux surgery are not perfect. Both transthoracic and transabdominal procedures have been advocated. The transthoracic approach permits better mobilisation of the oesophagus, which is advantageous is patients with a large hiatus hernia, acquired oesophageal shortening or after previous upper abdominal surgery. However, operation time, postoperative hospital stay and morbidity are greater than after laparotomy. Post-thoracotomy neuralgia is a persistent, troublesome problem in 10 to 15% of patients. These disadvantages are not encoutered after a transabdominal anti reflux procedure which has the added advantage that co-existent intra-abdominal problems (e.g. gall stones, peptic ulcer) can be treated at the same operation. Three basic steps are common to most of the current anti reflux procedures irrespective of approach:

1. Oesophageal mobilisation and re-establishment of a segment of intra-abdominal oesophagus

2. Approximation of the margins of the right crus to narrow the diaphragmatic hiatus.

3. Fixation of the gastric fundus around the lower oesophagus — the fundoplication.

The three most popular are a total fundoplication (Nissen, 1961) or alternatively a partial fundoplication performed through the chest (Belsey, 1980) or the abdomen (Lind et al, 1965). The occurrence of postoperative complications with any of these operations can be reduced by careful surgical technique.

Operative technique

My preference is for a transabdominal anti-reflux operation, reserving the transthoracic approach for patients with a hiatus hernia greater than 8 cm in length or those who have had 2 or more previous attempts at surgical control of reflux. A transabdominal operation through an upper mid-line incision is facilitated by use of a sternal retractor which improves access to the oesophageal hiatus. The lower oesophagus and fundus of the stomach are mobilised by sharp dissection, particularly in the angle of His. It is not necessary to mobilise the left lobe of the liver or to divide any of the short gastric vessels to perform a satisfactory fundoplication. The long-bladed St.Mark's rectal retractor with a lip is ideal for retracting the liver and exposing the diaphragmatic hiatus. Inadvertent damage to the spleen is three times commoner with transabdominal anti reflux operations and significantly increases the morbidity of operation, particularly the occurrence of a subphrenic abcess (Polk, 1976). Damage to the vagus nerves should be avoided and no attempt to begin the repair should be made until at least the lower 6 cm of oesophagus has been mobilised.

The oesophagus is lifted forwards with a tape or rubber catheter. If more than two fingers can be passed through the hiatus the margins of the right are approximated behind the oesophagus (Fig. 4.3a). Two or three interrupted non-absorbable linen or silk sutures are usually necessary. When the approximation is complete it should still be possible to pass the index finger through the hiatus alongside the oesophagus. The crural repair reduces the risk of displacement of the fundoplication into the chest or the development of a postoperative paraoesophageal hernia.

Finally the fundoplication is performed. This may be a total fundoplication or some form of partial fundoplication. My preference is for a partial fundoplication as described by Lind et al (1965). Although definitive proof from a prospective, controlled clinical trial is awaited it appears that the success rate of partial and total fundoplication is similar in terms of reflux control but the former has a lower incidence of post operative dysphagia and 'gas-bloat' symptoms (personal observations). The fundoplication should be 3 cm in length and constructed without tension using non absorbable sutures. The posterior fundus is first anchored to the right lateral side of the oesophagus (Fig. 4.3b). The anterior fundus is then attached to the left lateral side of the oesophagus (Fig. 4.4a) and finally attached to the

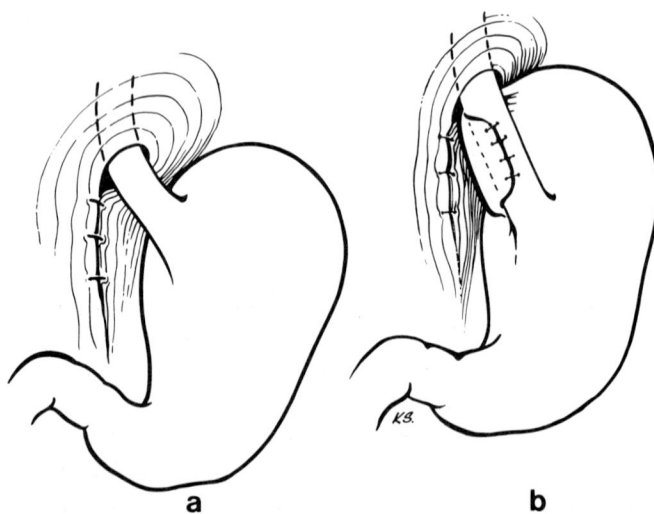

a   b

Fig. 4.3 Stages in a transabdominal partial fundoplication — the Lind operation. After mobilisation of the hiatus hernia and lower oesophagus the margins of the right crus have been opproximated (a). The posterior fundus has been sutured to the right antero lateral wall of the oesophagus (b).

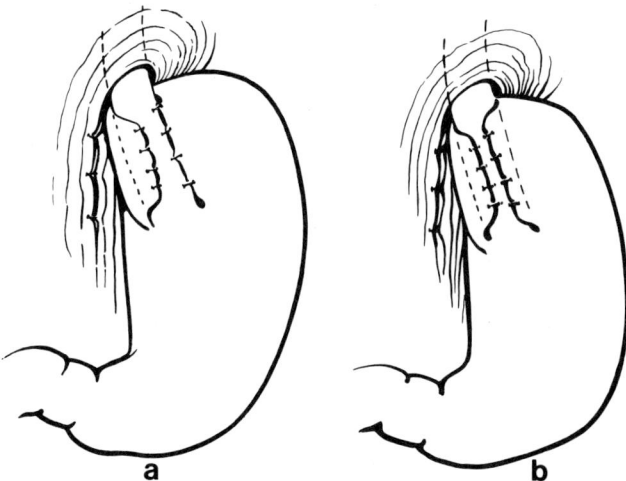

Fig. 4.4 The gastric fundus is sutured to the left lateral wall of the oesophagus (a). The fundus is sutured to the anterior oesophagus completing the fundoplication (b).

anterior wall as a third layer (Fig. 4.4b) leaving a 1 cm strip of oesophagus exposed. The sutures should pass through the gastric and oesophageal seromuscular layers but not the mucosa for fear of bacterial contamination in the area. A Nissen fundoplication should be constructed with an F36 or F40 oesophageal dilator through the gastro oesophageal junction to avoid making the repair too tight. When the dilator is withdrawn it should then be possible to insert an index finger beneath the wrap, between it and the oesophageal wall. A 'Nissen fundoplication' is not a standardized operation and many minor variations of Nissen's original technique have been described (Jamieson & Duranceau, 1984).

Results of anti-reflux surgery

The mechanism by which an anti-reflux procedure controls reflux is not completely understood. The pressure in the high pressure zone is increased and this is probably achieved by a buttressing effect of the fundoplication on the LOS. Satisfactory reflux control is achieved in approximately 90% of patients judged both subjectively and objectively (Bushkin et al, 1977). The success rate of crural repair or gastropexy was only 70 to 75%. Prospective evaluation of the Nissen, Belsey and Hill operations by pH monitoring showed that the Nissen procedure was the most effective in controlling reflux (Demeester et al, 1974). Most operative failures occur within 3 years of operation and late recurrence is uncommon. The majority of patients with a symptomatic recurrence have an intact anatomical repair. Absence of anatomical recurrence of a hiatal hernia is no guarantee that reflux is not occurring. With long term follow up some patients have deteriorating histological changes and clear evidence of reflux despite persistent symptomatic improvement and general satisfaction with the operation (Brand et al, 1979). Incomplete relief of symptoms may be due to an incorrect preoperative diagnosis rather than operative failure e.g. confusion of coronary artery disease with reflux oesophagitis.

Duodenal ulceration is the commonest coincidental finding in patients undergoing anti-reflux surgery, being present in 10 to 20%. Addition of a vagotomy, particularly vagotomy and drainage, reduces the success rate of the anti-reflux operation. Delay in gastric emptying postvagotomy increases the risk of reflux and postoperative duodenogastric reflux may, in turn, be responsible for biliary/alkaline oesophagitis. Highly selective vagotomy is not complicated by biliary reflux but lesser curve gastric ulceration with subsequent perforation, attributed to a relative lesser curve ischaemia, has been described.

The most frequent postoperative complication is dysphagia (Skinner, 1977). This is commonest after total fundoplication, occurring in up to 50% of patients. It is usually mild and transient, beginning within a week of surgery when solid food is introduced into the diet and resolving within 3 weeks as the local oedema around the oesophageal hiatus resolves. Only 5% of patients have dysphagia 6 months postoperatively and by one year this has fallen further to around 2%. Persistent dysphagia has a number of different aetiologies, including a tight crural repair or fundoplication (Stoddard, 1986). Dysphagia due to extrinsic compression at the lower end of the oesophagus which fails to respond to repeated dilatation may require re-exploration of the hiatus with revision of the crural repair or fundoplication.

The 'gas-bloat syndrome' is characterised by post-cibal epigastric discomfort and distension associated with an inability to eructate and/or vomit. It is commonest after total fundoplication and is due to a super-competent wrap which traps swallowed air in the stomach. The symptom is generally mild and has a pronounced tendancy to disappear with longer term follow up. Nevertheless 1 to 2% of patients have disabling symptoms which necessitate dismantling of the fundoplication. The prevalence of this side-effect is diminished by performing a Nissen fundoplication with an oesophageal dilator in position.

Re-operation for recurrent or persistent reflux has been said to carry a much greater mortality and morbidity than primary anti-reflux surgery (Zucker et al, 1982) although this is not my personal experience. The risk of persistent reflux after a second operation is higher than after initial surgery. When further surgery is required and redissection around the hiatus is considered hazardous an alternative surgical approach which has been reported to give good results is antrectomy with Roux-en-Y reanastamosis (Washer et al, 1984). This operation reduces gastric acid secretion and prevents duodenal contents from reaching the oesophagus.

ANGELCHIK PROSTHESIS

Fundoplication can be a difficult operation in an obese patient, has a reported success rate of 80 & 85% which is, to a certain extent, operator dependent and may be complicated by recurrent symptoms, dysphagia and the gas bloat syndrome. Because of these problems Angelchik introduced an anti-reflux device in the 1970s and has reported his results after 10 years experience (Angelchik et al, 1983). The prosthesis is a silicone collar which is positioned around the mobilised intra-abdominal oesophagus and held in position by tieing the two ends of a reinforced Dacron tape which encircles it. A clip or ligature is applied to the ligated tapes to prevent separation. The prosthesis lies loosely around the oesophagus and is not attached either to the oesophagus or the stomach. A radio opaque marker within the tape allows postoperative X-ray localisation of the device.

A number of unique complications are associated with use of this prosthesis. Initial problems of tape disruption and intraperitoneal migration of the prosthesis have been solved by modification of the original design and attaching the securing tapes to the entire circumference of the device. Migration up the oesophagus into the mediastinum results in angulation of the prosthesis and severe dysphagia which can only be cured by its removal. Migration downwards over the stomach produces early satiety and vomiting. These risks of prosthesis migration can be reduced by approximation of the margins of the right crus if the diaphragmatic hiatus is large and by avoiding excessive mobilisation of the gastro-oesophageal junction. The prosthesis is a foreign body and as such should not be used in the presence of sepsis or where there is a possibility of contamination from the gastrointestinal tract. Sepsis may lead to abscess formation and erosion of the prosthesis into the lumen of the stomach or oesophagus. This is an extremely rare, but well documented complication.

Failure to control reflux symptoms and the gas bloat syndrome may also occur, as after fundoplication, and should be treated with long term medical therapy or alternatively, removal of the prosthesis and conventional anti-reflux surgery. However, the main postoperative problem associated with the use of the Angelchik prosthesis is dysphagia. Up to 70% of patients have mild dysphagia immediately after operation. In many this is transient and resolves within a few weeks but upto 30% of patients still have mild dysphagia 1 year postoperatively and a further 10% have moderate or severe dysphagia which requires removal of the prosthesis (Wale et al, 1985). Dysphagia may improve for up to 12 months after operation but there is little likelihood of further improvement thereafter.

The concept of the Angelchik prosthesis is an attractive alternative to fundoplication. It is easy to insert in normal and obese patients, even for the relatively inexperienced anti-reflux surgeon, operation time is short and the operation should produce results which have the lowest operator dependence. However, the most recent studies suggest that athough the results are satisfactory in 80% of patients the complication rate associated with the prosthesis is too high to recomment its regular use. Fundoplication should be regarded as the primary operation for gastro-oesophageal reflux until the results of long term clinical trials of the Anglechik prosthesis are published (Durrans et al, 1985). The device may have a place when previous anti-reflux surgery has failed and when revisional surgery is made difficult by dense fibrous adhesions.

COLUMNAR LINED (BARRETT'S) OESOPHAGUS

A columnar lined (Barrett's) oesophagus is an acquired condition and is not associated with a congenitally short oesophagus as Barrett first believed when he described the condition in 1950. In almost all patients it develops secondary to gastro-oesophageal reflux (Berardi & Devaiah, 1983). However, neither acid or pepsin nor a prolonged history of reflux are necessary for the development of a Barrett's oesophagus. It can occur after damage to the oesophageal mucosa by ingested caustic materials, after total gastrectomy, the oesophageal damage being due to alkaline reflux, and has also been described in children.

Patients with a columnar lined oesophagus have a longer period of acid exposure and greater number of reflux episodes on 24 hour pH monitoring, and a lower LOSP on manometry, than normal subjects and patients with oesophagitis and a squamous lined oesophagus (Iascone et al, 1983). This implies that a Barrett's oesophagus develops in those patients with the most severe gastro-oesophageal reflux. It is not an uncommon condition but its true incidence is often underestimated because the position of the squamo-columnar junction is not carefully identified at endoscopy. Of patients undergoing routine fibreoptic endoscopy of the upper gastrointestinal tract between 20 and 25% have macroscopic oesophagitis and of these patients 10 to 12% have a columnar lined oesophagus (Naef et al, 1975; Rothery et al, 1986). A Barrett's oesophagus is important because of its malignant poten-

tial. Between 8 and 10% of patients develop a primary oesophageal adeno-carcinoma (Fig. 4.5). In some surgically biased series the prevalence of ade-nocarcinoma in Barrett's patients reached 40%.

Clinical features

Typically patients with a columnar lined oesophagus present with symp-toms of reflux or with dysphagia due to a benign stricture or a carcinoma. Alternatively it may be discovered as an incidental finding at endoscopy for peptic ulcer disease. The triad of features which are associated with the condition are:

— a columnar lined oesophagus
— a benign oesophageal stricture
— an oesophageal ulcer.

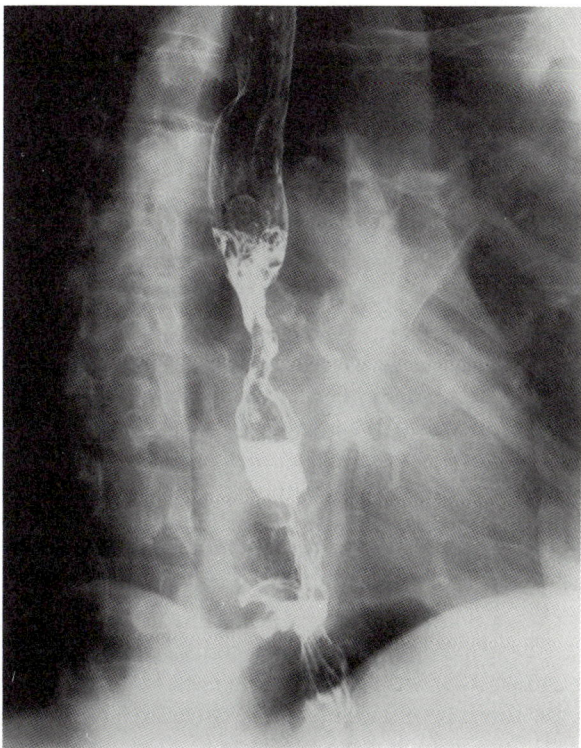

Fig. 4.5 A barium swallow showing a carcinoma in the middle third of the oesophagus in a patient with a sliding hiatus hernia and Barrett's oesophagus

Over 80% of patients have a sliding hiatus hernia, 40 to 50% an oeso-phageal stricture and 30 to 40% an oesophageal ulcer. The stricture in-variably occurs at the squamo-columnar junction which may be located anywhere in the oesophagus from just below the cricopharyngeus to within a few centimetres of the gastro-oesophageal junction. Patients with a stric-ture tend to have more severe reflux and a more extensive columnar lined oesophagus, thus the stricture is often found 25 to 30 cm from the teeth. A benign stricture in the middle third of the oesophagus well above the gastro-oesophageal junction is almost always associated with a Barrett's oesophagus. The strictures are usually short, annular and dilate with rela-tive ease although long, rigid strictures may sometimes occur.

The diagnosis is based on the endoscopic appearance with conclusive proof coming from histological examination of a biopsy specimen from the lower oesophagus. It is not uncommon to find columnar mucosa extending 1 to 2 cm above the gastro-oesophageal junction in normal subjects. For a diagnosis of Barrett's oesophagus the columnar mucosa must extend for a distance of at least 5 cm above the gastro-oesophageal junction. Columns of linear oesophagitis are frequently seen in the squamous epithelium above the squamo-columnar junction.

Histological and histochemical features

Histologically three different types of columnar epithelium may be found within the oesophagus: junctional type epithelium with cardiac mucous glands, an atrophic fundic epithelium which may contain parietal and chief cells and specialised columnar cells resembling either small or large intestinal epithelium. More than one type of epithelium may be present in different parts of the oesophagus in the same patient at the same time. The origin of the atypical mucosa is controversial. Severe damage to the oesophageal mucosa is followed by regeneration of columnar epithelium rather than the normal stratified squamous epithelium. This may originate by epithelial metaplasia, cranial migration of the cardiac junctional mucosa or upward migration from the subepithelial cardiac mucous glands. The normal sequential epithelial change in the upper gastrointestinal tract is stratified squamous, junctional, fundic, pyloric, intestinal epithelium. The sequence is often different in the columnar lined oesophagus which makes the theory of cranial migration of the cardiac junctional epithelium unlikely.

Intestinal type epithelium is a common finding in biopsy specimens. This intestinal metaplasia can be subdivided into different types, by histochemical methods, on the basis of the mucin production by the columnar cells. Type 11B epithelium, which resembles colonic epithelium, is characterised by the presence of sulphomucins in the columnar cells. This variant of intestinal metaplasia is associated with the occurrence of well differentiated carcinoma in patients with gastric cancer. Studies have been performed in patients with a Barrett's oesophagus to determine the prevalence of this type of epithelium and its association with oesophageal adenocarcinoma (Rothery et al, 1986). Although type 11B epithelium is common in those patients with an oesophageal adenocarcinoma it is present in over 70% of all patients and identification of this type of epithelium in biopsy specimens is not sufficiently discriminating to identify those patients who may be at particular risk of developing a carcinoma.

Treatment

The aims of treatment should be to provide symptomatic relief and to return the oesophageal epithelium to normal. Intensive medical treatment with H_2 receptor blockers, Gaviscon and metoclopramide, either singly or in combination, will control the reflux symptoms and heal the oesophageal ulcers in most patients. However, there is no convincing published evidence to prove that any medical regimes, even if given for prolonged periods of 1 to 2 years, will result in regression of the columnar epithelium (Stoddard et al, 1984). Regression has been reported following successful anti-reflux surgery in a small number of patients (Brand et al, 1980). Oesophageal strictures should be treated by biopsy and dilatation followed by either medical or surgical control of reflux. Barrett's oesophagus is not a separate clinical entity but should be considered as an end stage of reflux oeso- phagitis. Because of the magnitude and severity of the reflux continuous, intensive medical treatment will be necessary if symptoms are to be controlled non-operatively. Surgery offers the only prospect of regression of the abnormal epithelium and is thus the treatment of choice in patients with no other contraindication to operation. An anti-reflux procedure and not oesophagectomy should be performed. All patients with a Barrett's oesophagus should have regular endoscopy and oesophageal biopsy, prob- ably at annual intervals, looking for evidence of dysplasia. If dysplasia is present, and confirmed by repeat biopsy, the risk of malignant change is ominous and these patients should be considered for oesphagectomy. Radical surgery is the only chance of cure for a patient with an established oesophageal adenocarcinoma although many of these tumours are unre- sectable at the time of operation. The prognosis of these patients is not dissimilar from other patients with oesophageal carcinoma, unless perhaps the tumour is detected at an early stage during endoscopic serveillance. Of 8 patients personally resected by the Ivor Lewis technique for a Barrett's associated carcinoma in the last 4 years, one patient died from post oper- ative pulmonary problems, two have died from recurrent disease and five are alive, and clincally free of recurrence, between 3 months and $3\frac{1}{2}$ years after surgery.

BENIGN OESOPHAGEAL STRICTURES

Over 90% of benign oesophageal strictures are secondary to gastro- oesophageal reflux. Excluding oesophageal obstruction due to extrinsic compression and misdiagnosed oesophageal carcinoma the other major causes are following oesophagogastrostomy (after oesophagogastrectomy), ingestion of caustic substances and healing of an instrumental perforation. The stricture is the result of healing following reflux induced mucosal damage and protects against further reflux to a certain extent. This is the reason why reflux symptoms may improve when the patient develops a benign stricture. Ulcerative oesophagitis leads to transmural oesophageal inflammation and this in turn results in formation of scar tissue at the site of oesophageal damage. Contraction of the scar tissue results in further narrowing of the oesophageal lumen and acquired shortening of the oeso- phagus. Reflux induced strictures either occur just above the gastro oeso- phageal junction or in the mid oesophagus, the latter group often being associated with a columnar lined oesophagus. They are usually short annular strictures only 1 to 2 cm in length although very long strictures may occur.

Clinical features

Patients present with recent onset dysphagia frequently preceded by a long reflux history. Meat, bread and potatoes are the usual foods which produce symptoms. Total dysphagia, of sudden onset, implies bolus impaction at the level of a stricture. In older patients reflux symptoms are often absent. Patients with scleroderma are particularly prone to stricture formation. Reflux is excessive and the absence of effective oesophageal peristalsis results in prolonged mucosal exposure to acid.

Investigation and treatment

Barium swallow should precede endoscopy to look for the cause of the dysphagia and to help exclude oesophageal carcinoma or a motor disorder. *All* patients with an apparently benign stricture should have endoscopy and biopsy of the narrow area. Oesophagitis is usually evident endoscopically above the stricture. A rigid stricture with no oesophagitis is suggestive of carcinoma and if the initial biopsy is negative the endoscopy should be repeated and further biopsies obtained. Rigid oesophagoscopy and biopsy may be required to obtain a better biopsy specimen for histological examination. There are two components to the treatment of reflux induced oesophageal strictures:

1. Dilatation
2. Medical or surgical control of reflux.

Dilatation

A variety of different types of dilators are available for oesophageal dilatation (Fig. 4.6). These dilators may be passed over a guide-wire (Celestin, Eder-Puestow) or without direct visualisation or guidance (Maloney, Hurst). Dilatation via an oesophagoscope is of limited value for the upper limit of dilatation is only F32–F34, the limiting factor being the internal diameter of the oesophagoscope. Use of a guide-wire carries a risk of wire-induced oesophageal or gastric perforation, the possibility that the wire may become knotted in the stomach and for optimum safety should be performed under X-ray control. Maloneys dilators, which are very popular in North America, can be safely used in the outpatient department for dilatation and carry a negligable risk of oesophageal perforation (Stoddard & Simms, 1984). However, they are unsuitable for very tight strictures which should be dilated initially with Celestin dilators, Eder-Puestow dilators are more traumatic physically and psychologically for the patient and their continued and should be reconsidered when other more acceptable types of dilator are available. If the stricture is soft and dilates easily then maximum dilatation upto F60 can be achieved with one dilatation session. If the stricture is rigid, the possibility of carcinoma should be reconsidered

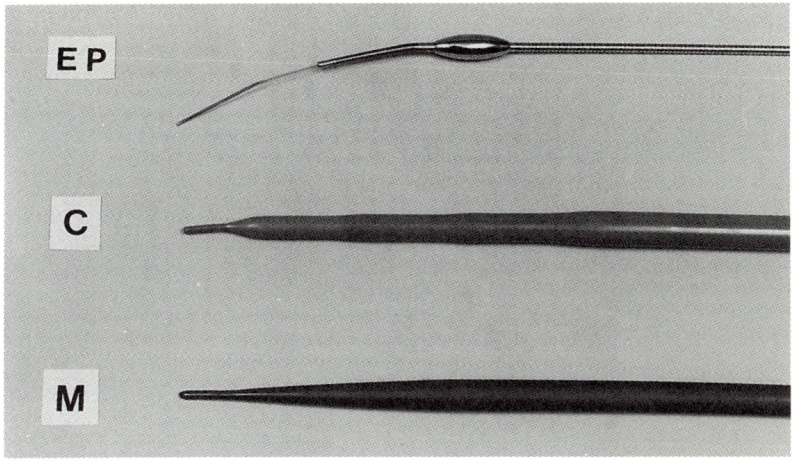

Fig. 4.6 Different dilators for oesophageal dilatation: EP — Eder-Puestow, C — Celestin, M — Maloney

but one should also dilate the stricture gradually over a period of 4 to 6 weeks. Rapid dilatation may result in an oesophageal perforation due to the stricture splitting. Approximately 40% of patients will require only one oesophageal dilatation but the others will require multiple dilatations (Patterson et al, 1983). The interval between dilatations increases with the passage of time.

Reflux control

The first line of treatment is by dietary and postural measures followed by drug treatment. Patients with a benign oesophageal stricture have major reflux and thus will need medical treatment with drugs such as the H2 blockers, metoclopramide or Gaviscon. Antacids alone are insufficient. Elderly patients who are poor candidates for surgery should be maintained on long term medical treatment with periodic oesophageal dilatation when dysphagia recurs. Surgical treatment should be offered to patients with a benign oesophageal stricture and who have no other contraindication, including age, to surgery. Over recent years there has been a trend towards more conservative surgery (Moghissi, 1979). Resection of the stricture is unnecessary in most patients and following adequate dilatation the only surgery that is required is an anti-reflux procedure. Difficulty may be encountered with a severe stricture or the stricture with marked oeso-phageal shortening. Bowel interposition has been advocated by some but the results are not impressive and the morbidity and mortality rates unaccept-ably high. If there is significant oesophageal shortening the oesophagus may be 'lengthened' by performing a transthoracic gastroplasty followed by total fundoplication for reflux control (Henderson, 1983).

The presence of an oesophageal stricture makes the surgical procedure more difficult and increases the risks of surgery. Whenever possible anti reflux surgery should be offered to patients who have severe reflux or who are only poorly controlled by medical treatment before the complication develops.

REFERENCES

Allison P R 1951 Reflux oesophagitis, sliding hiatal hernia and the anatomy of repair. Surgery, Gynecology and Obstetrics 92: 419–431

Angelchik J P, Cohen R, Kravetz R E 1983 A ten year appraisal of the anti-reflux prosthesis. American Journal of Gastroenterology 78: 671–673

Belsey R H R 1980 Gastro-oesophageal reflux. Americal Journal of Surgery 139: 775–781

Berardi R S, Devaiah K A 1983 Barrett's oesophagus. Surgery, Gynecology and Obstetrics 156: 521–538

Brand D, Eastwood I R, Martin D, Carter W B, Pope C E 1979 Oesophageal symptoms, manometry and histology before and after anti-reflux surgery. Gastroentrology 76: 1393–1401

Brand D L, Ylvisaker J T, Gelfand M, Pope C E 1980 Regression of columnar oesophageal (Barretts) epithelium after anti reflux surgery. New England Journal of Medicine 302: 844–848

Branicki F J, Evans D F, Ogilvie A L et al 1982 Ambulatory monitoring of oesophageal pH in reflux oesophagitis using a portable radiotelemetry capsule. Gut 23: 992–998

Bushkin F L, Neustein C L, Parker T H, Woodward E R 1977 Nissen fundoplication for reflux peptic oesophagitis. Annals of Surgery 185: 672–677

Castell D O 1982 Clinical applications of oesophageal manometry. Digestive Diseases and Science 27: 769–770

Cohen S, Harris L D 1971 Does hiatus hernia affect competence of the gastro-oesophageal sphincter? New England Journal of Medicine 284: 1053–1056

Demeester T R, Johnson L F, Kent A H 1974 Evaluation of current operations for the prevention of gastro-oesophageal reflux. Annals of Surgery 180: 511–522

Demeester T R, Johnson L F, Joseph G J 1976 Patterns of gastro oesophageal reflux in health and disease. Annals of Surgery 184: 459–470

Demeester T R, Wang Ching I, Wernly J A et al 1980 Techniques, indications and clinical use of 24-hour oesophageal pH monitoring. Journal of Thoracic and Cardiovascular Surgery 79: 656–670

Dent J, Dodds W J, Friedman R H et al 1980 Mechanism of gastro oesophageal reflux in recumbent asymptomatic human subjects. Journal of Clinical Investigation 65: 256–267

Dodds W J, Hogan W J, Helm J F, Dent J 1981 Pathogenesis of reflux oesophagitis. Gastroenterology 81: 376–394

Dodds W J, Hogan W J, Miller W N 1976 Reflux oesophagitis. American Journal of Digestive Disease 21: 49–67

Durrans D, Armstrong C P, Taylor T V, 1985. The Angelchik anti-reflux prosthesis — some reservations. British Journal of Surgery 72: 525–527.

Flook D, Stoddard C J 1985 Gastro-oesophageal reflux and oesophagitis before and after vagotomy for duodenal ulcer. British Journal of Surgery 72: 804–807

Fyke F E Jr, Code C F, Schlegel J F 1956 The gastro-oesophageal sphincter in healthy human beings. Gastroenterologia 86: 135–150

Gillison E W, De Castro V A M, Nyhus L M, Kusakari K, Bombeck C T 1972 The significance of bile in reflux oesophagitis. Surgery, Gynecology and Obstetrics 134: 419–424

Goldberg H I, Dodds W J, Gee S 1969 Role of acid and pepsin in acute experimental oesophagitis. Gastroenterology 56: 223–230

Goyal R K, Rattan S 1980 Effects of sodium nitroprusside and verapamil on lower oesophageal sphincter. American Journal of Physiology 238: G40–44

Henderson R D 1983 Management of the patient with a benign oesophageal stricture. Surgical Clinics of North America 63: 885–903

Iascone C, Demeester T R, Little A G, Skinner D B 1983 Barretts oesophagus. Archives of Surgery 118: 543–549

Kjellen G, Tibbling L 1978 Influence of body position, dry and water swallows, smoking and alcohol and oesophageal acid clearing. Scandinavian Journal of Gastroenterology 13: 283–288

Lieberman-Meffert D, Allgower M, Schmid P et al 1979 Muscular equivalent of the lower oesophageal sphincter. Gastroenterology 76: 31–38

Lind J F, Burns C M, MacDougall J T 1965 Physiological repair for hiatus hernia — a manometric study. Archives of Surgery 91: 233–237

Jamieson G G, Duranceau A 1984 What is a Nissen fundoplication? Surgery, Gynecology and Obstetrics 159: 591–593

McCallum R W, Berkowitz D M 1978 The frequency of delayed gastric emptying in patients with gastro-oesophageal reflux (GER) and its response to metoclopramide (M) and bethanechol (B). Gastroenterology 74: 1135

Moghissi K 1979 Conservative surgery in reflux stricture of the oesophagus associated with hiatal hernia. British Journal of Surgery 66: 221–225

Naef A P, Savary M, Ozello L 1975 Columnar lined lower oesophagus. An acquired lesion with malignant predisposition. Journal of Thoracic and Cardiovascular Surgery 70: 826–835

Nebel O T, Fornes M F, Castell D O 1973 Symptomatic gastro oesophageal reflux: incidence and precipitating factors. Digestive Diseases 21: 953–956

Nissen R 1961 Gastropexy and fundoplication in surgical treatment of hiatal hernia American Journal of Digestive Diseases 6: 954–961

Ogilvie A L, Ferguson R, Atkinson M 1980 Outlook with conservative treatment of peptic oesophageal stricture. Gut 21: 23–25

Patterson D J, Graham D Y, Smith J L et al 1983 Natural history of benign oesophageal stricture treated by dilatation Gastroenterology 85: 346–350

Polk H C 1976 Fundoplication for reflux oesophagitis. Misadventures with the operation of choice. Annals of Surgery 184: 645–652

Polk H C, Zeppa R 1969 Fundoplication for uncomplicated hiatal hernia. Annals of Thoracic Surgery 7: 202

Pope C E, Meyer G W, Castell D O 1981 Is measurement of lower oesophageal sphincter pressure clinically useful. Digestive Diseases and Science 26: 1025–1030

Rossetti M, Hell K 1977 Fundoplication for the treatment of gastroesophageal reflux in hiatal hernia. World Journal of Surgery 1: 439–443

Rothery G W, Patterson J E, Stoddard C J, Day D W, 1986 Histological and histochemical changes in the columnar-lined (Barrett's) lower oesophagus. Gut (in press).

Skinner D B 1977 Complications of surgery for gastroesophageal reflux. World Journal of Surgery 1: 485–491

Stoddard C J, Patterson J E, Flook D, 1984 Is a columnar lined oesophagus reversible with medical treatment? Gut 25: A1150–1151.

Stoddard C J 1986 Complications of anti-reflux surgery In: Kirk R M, Stoddard C J Complications of surgery of the upper gastrointestinal tract 1st Edition. Bailliere-Tindall, Eastbourne, p: 120–147

Stoddard C J, Simms J M 1984 Dilatation of benign oesophageal strictures in the outpatient department. British Journal of Surgery 71: 752–753

Vansant J H, Baker J W 1976 Complications of vagotomy in the treatment of hiatal hernia Annals of Surgery 183: 629–633

Wale R J, Royston C M S, Bennett J R, Buckton G K 1985 Prospective study of the Angelchik anti-reflux prosthesis. British Journal of Surgery 72: 520–524

Washer G F, Gear M W L, Dowling B L, Gillison E W, Royston C M S, Spencer J 1984 Randomised prospective trial of Roux-en-Y duodenal diversion versus fundoplication for severe reflux oesophagitis. British Journal of Surgery 71: 181–184

Winkelstein A 1935 Peptic oesophagitis. A new clinical entity. Journal of the American Medical Association 104: 906–909

Zucker K. Peskin G W, Saik R P 1982 Recurrent hiatal hernia repair, Archives of Surgery 117: 413–414

Staging and management of gastric cancer

INTRODUCTION

The results of treatment of gastric adenocarcinoma have shown no improvement over the last 50 years. In England and Wales during 1982 there were 10 211 deaths for gastric cancer, a total exceeded only by deaths from carcinoma of the bronchus, large bowel and breast (OPCS, 1983). More than 90% of these deaths occurred within 5 years of the primary treatment.

These poor results have created a fatalistic approach to the management of the patient with gastric cancer which is reflected in the pessimism expressed in much of the Western literature. This contrasts with the reports from Japan where several factors have been responsible for a significant improvement in the results of treatment over the past 20 years. Gastric cancer is the commonest form of malignancy in Japan and in the 1960's much work was devoted to increasing the percentage of cases with early disease (Kajitani & Takagi 1979). In addition, in order to introduce standardisation of the description of the pattern of disease at presentation and the type and results of treatment, the Japanese Research Society for Gastric cancer was organised. This group subsequently published the General Rules for Gastric Cancer Study in Surgery and Pathology in 1962. The concept of stage-related treatment was thus developed.

The results of treatment of gastric cancer in the United Kingdom are unlikely to improve dramatically without a significant increase in the rate of detection of early disease. However, the adoption of the approach advocated by the Japanese does appear to be the most appropriate method of at least standardising the management of the patient with gastric cancer if not improving survival.

STAGING GASTRIC CANCER

Classification of stage

The assessment of the spread of a tumour forms an integral part of the management of any patient with malignancy and is dependant on an understanding of the natural history of the disease. In gastric cancer the primary lesion arises in the stomach wall before initial spread to local nodes and thence to distant nodes. In addition, there is local involvement of adjoining tissues, blood borne dissemination to distant organs and trans-coelomic spread to peritoneal covered organs.

Conventional classifications have been dependant on the histological assessment of the depth of penetration and the involvement of potentially involved tissues. In 1966, the International Union Against Cancer adopted the TNM classification. The extent of the tumour was defined in terms of the primary tumour (T), the regional nodes (N) and distant metastases (M) (Table 5.1). In a report of a collaborative study using the TNM system, Kennedy (1970) demonstrated that the results of treatment were dependant on the penetration of the tumour with 80% surviving for 5 years when the tumour was confined to the mucosa. Once spread had occurred to regional lymph nodes there was a marked decrease in 5 year survival from 60% without nodal metastases to 18% for those with N1 involvement and 8% with N2 involvement.

Table 5.1 TNM classification of gastric cancer (UICC, 1982)

Extent of tumour penetration

T1	Confined to mucosa
T2	Involvement of submucosa but not penetrating the serosa
T3	Penetrating the serosa
T4	Diffusely involving the stomach wall

Extent of lymph node involvement

N0	None
N1	Perigastric nodes in immediate vicinity of primary
N2	Perigastric nodes distant from the primary

Extent of distant metastases

M0	None
M1	Present

The General Rules for Gastric Cancer Study (1973) differed in that the classification was based on macroscopic findings (Table 5.2). The extent of disease was described in greater detail than the TNM classification particu-larly with respect to mucosal penetration, lymph node and distant metas-tases. Lesions confined to the mucosa and submucosa ('early gastric cancer') were subdivided into three types. Type I included protruding lesions, type II were superficial lesions which were further classified as IIa elevated, IIb flat and IIc depressed and type III were excavating lesions. Lymph nodes were classified in tiers according to the distance from the primary lesion (Table 5.2).

The results of treatment reported from Japan confirmed a better prog-nosis for those with early disease with 90.4% surviving for 5 years (Kajitani & Takagi, 1979). In addition a good correlation has been found between the clinical or macroscopic assessment of disease and subsequent histo-

Table 5.2   Japanese Research Society for Gastric Cancer Staging Classification (1973)

Macroscopic assessment of serosal invasion
S0	No invasion
S1	Invasion to serosa is suspected
S2	Definite invasion of serosa
S3	Infiltration into other organ(s)

Macroscopic nodal involvement
N0	No nodal involvement
N1	Involvement of epigastric nodes within 3 cm of primary
N2	Involvement of nodes around the coeliac axis and the left gastric, common hepatic and splenic arteries
N3	Involvement of hepatoduodenal and retropancreatic nodes and nodes in the root of the mesentery
N4	Involvement of nodes at the porta hepatis and para aortic nodes

Macroscopic assessment of peritoneal metastases
P0	No disseminating metastases to any serosal surface except gastric serosa
P1	Disseminating metastasis to local peritoneum (above the transverse colon and including the greater omentum)
P2	Few metastases to distant peritoneum
P3	Numerous metastases to distant peritoneum

Macroscopic involvement of the liver
H0	No metastasis
H1	Metastasis limited to one lobe
H2	Few scattered metastases to both lobes
H3	Numberous scattered metastases to both lobes

Stage 1	S0	N0	P0	H0
Stage II	S1	N1, N2	P0	H0
Stage III	S2	N3	P0	H0
Stage IV	S3	N4	>P0	>H0

Table 5.3   Clinicopathological staging of gastric cancer (Fielding et al, 1984)

Stage	Clinical	Pathology
I	Radical resection (T1 N0 M0)	Muscularis propria − Serosa − Node −
II	Radical resection (T2–4 N0 M0)	Muscularis propria + Serosa +/− Node −
III	Radical resection (TX-4 N1–3 M0)	Muscularis propria +/− Serosa +/− Node +
IV A	Palliative resection (TX-4 NX-3 M0-1)	Residual disease
IV B	No resection (TX-4 NX-4 M0-1)	Positive histology

logical grading (Miwa, 1979). The increased precision of nodal classification demonstrated that nodal metastasis was an independant prognostic factor and survival decreased with increasing nodal tier involvement. The 5 year survival rates for those with N0, N1, N2, N3 and N4 nodes were 80%, 39%, 23%, 11% and 8% respectively. Such information could not be derived from the TNM classification as the N2 group contained N2, 3 and 4 nodes for the Japanese classification. Nevertheless, in a discussion of the different methods of staging, Takagi (1981) described a good correlation between the TNM and the General Rules staging systems.

In an attempt to modify the TNM system by including both clinical or intraoperative findings and pathological features, Fielding and colleagues (1984) have proposed a clinicopathological system (Table 5.3). In stage I, II and III, radical surgery has resected all macroscopic disease. In stage IV there is residual macroscopic disease and this has been subdivided into IVA to include those undergoing a palliative resection and IVB in whom no tumour has been removed. The age-adjusted survival for 13 175 patients classified in this way is shown in Figure 5.1.

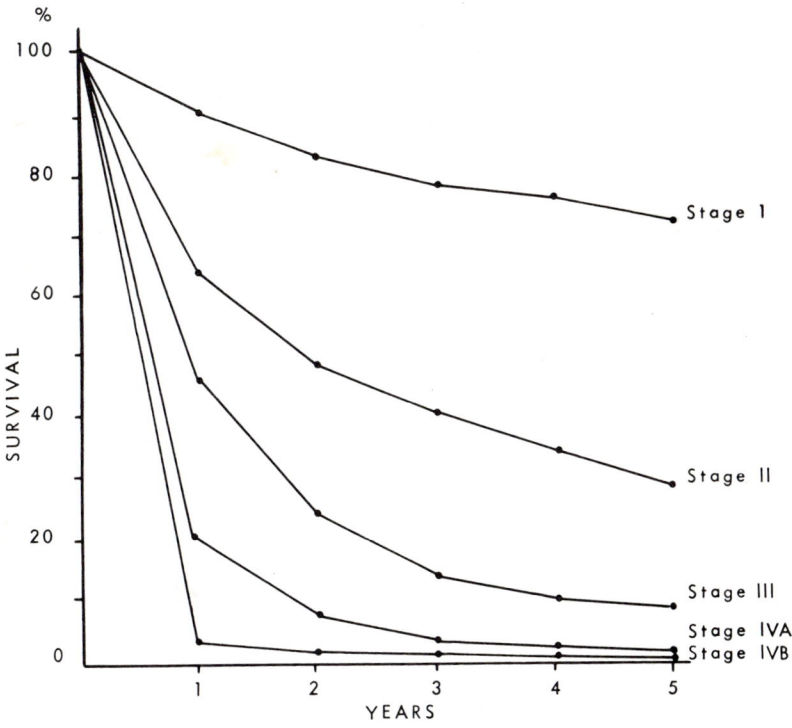

Fig. 5.1 The age adjusted survival of 13 175 cases of stomach cancer by stage

Methods of staging

Clinical assessment

Clinical assessment of the patient with gastric cancer is limited to the discrimination between localised and advanced disease. Large series have defined a number of factors which have prognostic significance. Although dyspepsia as a presenting symptom is associated with both early (Friesen et al, 1962) and advanced lesions (Swynnerton & Truelove, 1952), loss of weight is less frequently seen in patients with early lesions (Fielding et al, 1980). Similarly, patients with a short history tend to have a worse prognosis than those with a long history which suggests a more localised lesion (Brookes et al, 1965; Fielding et al, 1980).

Physical examination identifies sites of gross metastatic disease such as the liver, pelvic peritoneum and supraclavicular lymph nodes. The frequency, however, of such findings in patients at presentation is low as Kennedy (1970) described irregular hepatomegaly in 6.1% and enlarged supraclavicular nodes is 4.1% of 1 241 patients included in a multicentre review.

Laboratory investigations

In gastric cancer a specific haematological or biochemical parameter that indicates the extent of disease has yet to be defined. Serum Carcinoembryonic Antigen (CEA) has been measured preoperatively and despite assay variability, levels greater than 40 mg/ml are strongly suggestive of metastatic disease and an associated poor prognosis. Intermediate (10–40 mg/ml) and normal levels (<10 mg/ml) are of less value and although early disease may be present, equally more widespread disease may also be present (Hine et al, 1978). Studies of the pepsin precursor, pepsinogen I, have shown significantly low levels in patients with the so-called premalignant conditions of intestinal metaplasia (Stemmerman et al, 1978) and chronic atrophic gastritis (Varis et al, 1979). Furthermore, 15/48 patients presenting with advanced disease had a fall in serum pepsinogen I 45 months before diagnosis (Nomura et al, 1980). These studies, however, have been restricted to selected populations and it remains to be seen whether this marker can correlate with the stage of disease.

Imaging techniques

Conventional radiological techniques have been limited to diagnosis and demonstrating gross secondary disease. Much of the Japanese early detection programme was based on the typical appearances of double contrast studies. Irregularity or breaks in the contrast coating the gastric folds close to an ulcer were considered suggestive of mucosal and submucosal infiltration (Shirakabe et al, 1966). However, these appearances do not necessarily reflect Stage I disease, as 4.2% and 14.5% of these lesisons limited to the mucosa and submucosa respectively had lymph node metastases (Sogo et al, 1979).

Recent improvements in isotope and ultrasound scanning and computerised axial tomography (CT) have increased the resolution of metastatic deposits and have also been used to indicate the local extent of primary tumours.

Hepatic metastases. Comparative studies of the three modalities (isotope scans, ultrasound and CT scans) demonstrated accuracy rates of approximately 80% for each method in the detection of secondary liver disease (Smith et al, 1982; Schreve et al, 1984). Each of the techniques is limited by size of the deposit, the critical diameter being 2 cm. Schreve and colleagues (1984) described 10 lesions less than 2 cm in diameter; 5 were correctly identified by CT, 3 by ultrasound and 2 by isotope scanning. This limitation of the techniques by lesion size is particularly significant as Ozarda & Pickren (1962) reported from an autopsy series that 30% of liver metastases were less than 2 cm in diameter. Nevertheless because of the complimentary nature of the techniques, investigation of clinical suspicions of hepatic metastases should initially be investigated by isotope scanning and subsequently by ultrasound or CT (Cosgrove & McCready, 1978; Snow et al, 1979).

Lymph node metastases. Both ultrasound scanning and CT have been evaluated in the detection of enlarged intraperitoneal lymph nodes (Husband & McCready 1979). Ultrasound scanning is limited as lymph nodes often have similar ultrasonic characteristics to loops of bowel and discrimination is thus difficult (Tyrell et al, 1972). CT appears more reliable as nodes of 1–2 cm in diameter have been identified because of density differences from surrounding fat (Lee et al, 1978). Infiltration of a node, however, does not necessarily enlarge the node and equally nodes may become enlarged by inflammation rather than tumour. The inability of CT to detect architectural changes within nodes thus limits the assessment of invaded intra-abdominal nodes.

Locally invasive disease. Neither the accumulation of apparently tumour specific radioisotopes such as Gallium (Edwards et al, 1967) nor the characteristic ultrasonic features of gastric tumours (Walls, 1976) have proved valuable in the assessment of the extent of local disease. Early results with CT, however, have been encouraging. Characteristic changes in the morphology of the bowel wall by tumour infiltration were described in both gastric and colorectal cancer (Kressel et al, 1978). Subsequently, Moss and colleagues (1981) described a staging classification based on CT appearances (Table 5.4) which was found to have a good colleration with the findings at operation. More recently Dehn and colleagues (1984) have demonstrated that infiltration of three or more associated organs by primary gastric cancer implies inoperability. Unfortunately, involvement of two or less did not necessarily confirm operability. Whether more advanced machines with bet-

Table 5.4   Computerised tomographic staging of gastric cancer (Moss et al, 1981)

Stage I	Wall of normal thickness with polypoid lesion protruding into the lumen
Stage II	Local thickening of stomach wall by plaque-like or nodular lesion. No extension beyond stomach wall
Stage III	Local thickening of stomach wall with direct extension into surrounding tissue. Local or regional node enlargement but without distant metastases
Stage IV	Distant metastases irrespective of local extension

ter resolution will allow precise evaluation of small tumour volumes remains to be seen.

Invasive techniques

The contribution of endoscopy and histological examination of biopsied lesions has been similar to that of double contrast radiology with respect to diagnosis. Following the widespread use of upper gastrointestinal endoscopy the incidence of Stage I disease has increased not only in Japan (Takagi, 1981) but also in the Western World (Elster et al, 1975). Nevertheless, accurate assessment of the stage of disease can only be made at laparotomy, although laparoscopy can influence management in selected cases.

Laparoscopy. Studies of laparoscopy in the management of gastric cancer have supported the use of the technique in unfit patients with suspected advanced disease. Laparoscopy has a minimal morbidity and in the reported series a reasonable accuracy. Cuschieri (1980) described the correct assessment of local disease which was resectable in 75% of patients and of advanced disease which was unresectable in 67%. Similarly, Gross and colleagues (1984) were able to resect 16 of 19 tumours considered to be free from metastatic disease. They were unable, however, to remove the stomach in 2 patients with posterior extension into areas inaccessible to the laparoscope.

Laparotomy. Accurate staging of gastric cancer can only be achieved at laparotomy, by assessing the macroscopic appearance and spread of the disease and by biopsy of potentially involved areas for histological examination. The two determinants of radical resectability are the extent of local infiltration and the presence of distant metastases. Local disease can be difficult to define as microscopic tumour can be detected distant from the edge of a macroscopic lesion (Coller et al, 1941; Zinnager & Collins, 1949). Techniques such as frozen section examination (Papachristou et al, 1980) and cytological study (Keighley et al, 1981) of resection margins have therefore been advocated to assess microscopic spread intraoperatively. A recent study has emphasised the adoption of such techniques as patients with positively involved resection margins survived for a shorter time stage for stage than those with uninvolved resection lines (Hockey et al, 1984).

The identification of distant metastases is accomplished by macroscopic inspection and intraoperative frozen section examination or cytological assessment of potentially involved sites. Examination for liver metastases is limited by the size and the site of the lesion. Superficial lesions may be undetectable if situated on an inaccessible surface. Nevertheless, the accuracy of palpation has been estimated as approximately 90% (Ozarda & Pickren 1962). Differentiation of infiltrated and inflammatory lymph nodes is possible by cytology and frozen section examination. In a study of aspiration cytology Morris and colleagues (1982) described a good correlation with conventional paraffin section examination. More recently it has been suggested that the initial step at laparotomy for gastric cancer should be the sampling of infracolic preaortic (N4) nodes for frozen section examination (Keighley et al, 1984). Evidence of involvement of these nodes should preclude a radical resection as such patients have a very poor prognosis.

MANAGEMENT OF GASTRIC CANCER

Surgery offers the only possibility of cure for the patient with gastric cancer. It is pertinent therefore to consider preoperative preparation, the aims and methods of surgical treatment and the place of adjuvant modalities and follow-up after operation.

Preoperative preparation

Patients with stomach cancer are frequently malnourished and even cachexic at presentation. The influence of the cachectic state on the eventual outcome of treatment is difficult to assess. Correction of preoperative anaemia and of severe hypoalbuminaemia are obviously essential. Hyperalimentation however for one or two weeks before surgery by the elemental or the parenteral route has not been proven to be of significant benefit (Johnston, 1981) despite claims of the efficacy of nutritional support in the control of malignancy disease (Copeland et al, 1977; Muller et al, 1982). It would seem therefore more appropriate to assess each patient on his overall nutritional merit rather than recommend the routine use of nutritional support.

Aims and methods of surgical treatment

Laparotomy and the techniques already described to evaluate the spread of disease should be considered prerequisite to the management of all patients with gastric cancer. Surgical treatment is determined by the pattern of spread of disease and the pattern of recurrence.

Spread of disease

The traditional belief, derived from the impression of early gastric surgeons, that the pylorus was not transgressed by intramural spread is still prevalent today. In a multicentre prospective study, Hockey and colleagues (1984) have shown that there has been little improvement in the surgeon's ability to achieve microscopic clearance when compared with results reported 40 years ago (Coller & McIntyre, 1941). Several groups, however, have suggested that macroscopic clearance of at least 6 cm is associated with a low incidence of resection line involvement (Papachristou et al, 1980). This obviously involves extending the resection into the duodenum for antral lesions and into the oesophagus for cardia lesions with an associated thoracotomy.

The lymphatic spread of metastases to the tiers of nodes described in the General Rules (1973) is considered to be consistent with advancing disease. This concept of the natural history of lymphatic spread has formed the basis for the definition of radical surgery. In the General Rules, gastrectomies were classified as types R1, R2 and R3 according to the extent of the associated lymph node resection (i.e. an R1 resection excises N1 nodes etc.). Absolute curative resections were defined as en-bloc resections with clear margins including tiers of nodes beyond those involved. A sub-group of relative curative resections were classified as en-bloc resections with clear margins but including only the tier of nodes involved. Non-curative resections were divided into relative, in which residual disease was suspected, and absolute, in which residual tumour was definite. The 5-year survival rates for these different resections as performed by Japanese surgeons were 77% for absolute curative resections, 40% for relative curative resections, 22% for relative non-curative resections and 6% for absolute non-curative resections (Miwa, 1979). Since most lymphatic metastases are initially limited to the N1 or N2 tiers, the R2 and R3 resections are equivalent to the absolute curative procedures. Adoption of these procedures in the West have only been described in personal series. However, the initial results are certainly better than the standard limited gastrectomy of the R1 type reported in most series. Cuschieri has described a cumulative 3-year survival of 46% for those having a potentially curative R2 resection (Diggory & Cuschieri, 1985). It remains to be seen whether such survival rates can be equalled or even improved by groups of interested surgeons.

Sites of recurrent disease

Details of the sites involved by recurrent disease have been derived from post-mortem series, which reflect the end stage of the malignant process and from reoperation series, which demonstrate the pattern of disease in selected asymptomatic patients. In a post mortem series of 92 patients after 'curative' subtotal gastrectomy, loco-regional recurrence was found as a component in 74 (80.4%) with involvement of perigastric lymph nodes or the gastric bed in 48 (52%) (McNeer et al, 1951). Distant recurrence was seldom found to be the only site and was usually associated with substantial loco-regional disease. A similar picture was described by Gunderson & Sosin (1982) from their 'second look' laparotomy series. Loco-regional recurrence was a component in 72 of 82 patients (87.8%) and the sole site in 44 (53.7%). In addition 30% had recurrence in the gastric remnant either alone or as a component. These findings further support the use of extensive local resection together with en-bloc removal of structures involved by direct spread via the omenta such as the transverse colon or tail of the pancreas.

Advocates of total gastrectomy for all patients emphasise the significance of remnant recurrence. However, in a review of the literature total gastrectomy was associated with a higher perioperative mortality which adversely affected overall survival (Longmire, 1980). Nevertheless large series from surgeons with a special interest in gastric cancer have described postoperative mortalities of 9.3% (Pichlmayer & Meyer, 1981) and of 6.2% (Kajitani & Miwa, 1979).

Surgical technique

Radical resection (R2). The precise location of the N1 and N2 nodes varies according to the site of the primary (Fig. 5.2). Lesions in the distal 2/3 of the stomach should be treated by subtotal gastrectomy with en-bloc excision of the omentum and N1 and N2 nodes together with removal of the right cardiac, common hepatic and coeliac axis nodes. Lesions in the upper 1/3 should be treated by total gastrectomy with en-bloc removal of the omenta and N1 and N2 nodes.

The mobilisation of the stomach and lymphadenectomy are accomplished by firstly detaching the greater omentum from the duodenum and the transverse colon. The anterior leaf of the mesocolon and the pancreatic capsule, or serous floor of the lesser sac, are removed prior to ligating the right gastroepiploic vessels. The gastroduodenal artery is next isolated, ligated and divided. The lesser omentum is detached from the left lobe of the liver and dissected downwards to identify the right gastric vessels. These are ligated and divided, removing the appropriate lymph nodes.

The duodenum can now be divided to allow the distal stomach with attached omenta to be reflected out of the left costal margin of the incision. The retro-pancreatic glands and the glands along the common hepatic artery are dissected en-bloc from left to right through the foramen of Winslow. The coeliac axis nodes are included in this part of the dissection. The left gastric artery is isolated, ligated and divided with removal of the related nodes. The suprapancreatic nodes are cleared from the splenic vessels as are the splenic nodes from the splenic hilus. Finally detachment of the lesser omentum from the cardia and the gastric omentum up to the point

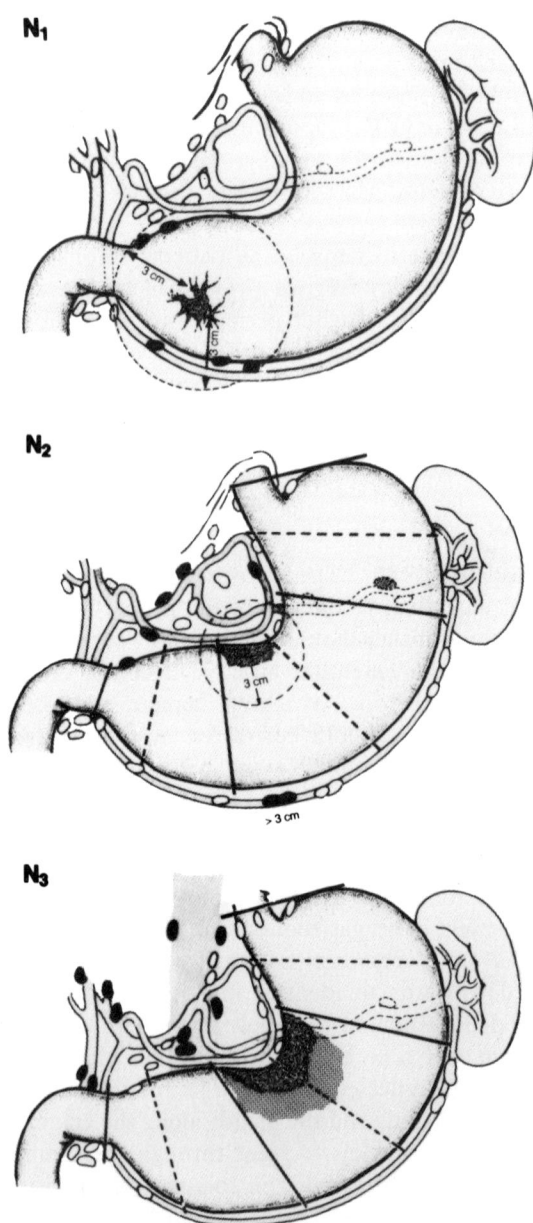

Fig. 5.2 The tiers of lymph nodes in the TNM system (N1 within 3 cm of tumour, N2 perigastric nodes, N3 distant nodes)

of gastric resection completes the mobilisation of the stomach and the lymphadenectomy. Partial or total gastrectomy can now be performed.

Reconstructive techniques. The surgical procedure is not limited to adequate excision of the primary lesion and the sites of present or potential spread. It is imperative that careful consideration be given to the restoration of gastrointestinal continuity as significant morbidity after a curative operation for cancer represents failure of the primary procedure. After a subtotal gastrectomy, either a gastroduodenal (Billroth I) or a gastrojejunal (Billroth II or Polya) anastomosis may be performed. Although the gastroduodenal anastomosis is more physiological, the small remnant of a radical resection is more likely to be associated with problems of bile reflux. These can be minimised by providing effective biliary diversion by a Roux-en-Y technique, which is appropriate for reconstructing both partial and total gastrectomies. Investigations with radiolabelled HIDA scanning demonstrated that biliary reflux after total gastrectomy was related to the length of the diverting jejunal limb. Limbs of 40 cm or more were associated with least reflux (Donovan et al, 1982) and it is suggested that such reconstruction is used after both total and partial gastrectomy.

Palliative treatment

Although radical resection of the R2 type offers the best chance of cure, only 20% of patients will have tumours appropriate for such surgery. In a review of the pattern of disease at presentation 80% of patients had lesions suitable for palliation only (Allum et al, 1985) (Fig. 5.3). Few of these patients survived for longer than 2 years after diagnosis. However, those who underwent a palliative resection fared significantly better than

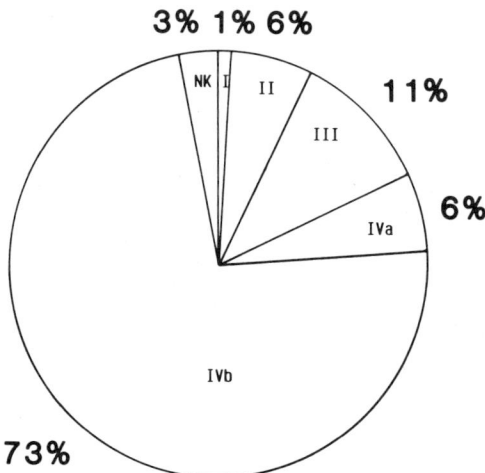

Fig. 5.3 The percentage distribution by stage of 13 175 patients with gastric cancer

those treated by a bypass procedure or by intubation (Fig. 5.4). Furthermore, this improvement was maintained even in the presence of hepatic, peritoneal or multiple site metastases.

Many patients are denied surgery because of concern for the associated high operative mortality. Review of the postoperative mortality demonstrated that those undergoing resection had a lower mortality rate than those treated by the other palliative measures (Fig. 5.5). Thus, all patients should be considered not only for laparotomy but also for resection to palliate disease causing pyloric obstruction, bleeding or pain.

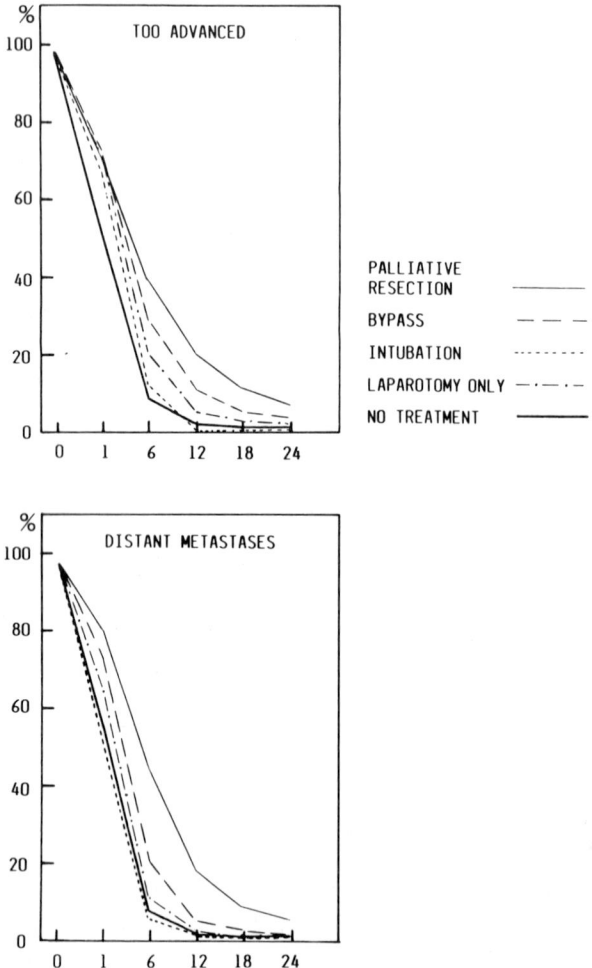

Fig. 5.4 The age adjusted survival over 24 months after palliative treatment in the presence of locally advanced disease and distant metastases

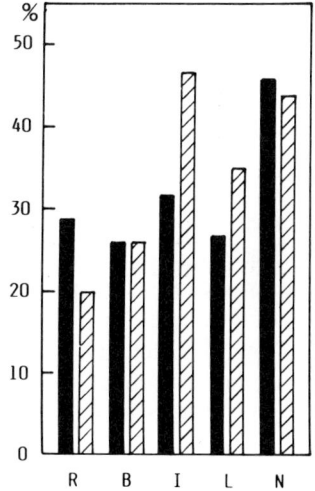

R   RESECTION
B   BYPASS
I   INTUBATION
L   LAPAROTOMY ONLY
N   NO TREATMENT

Fig. 5.5 The 30-day mortality by treatment for locally advanced disease and distant metastatic disease

Adjuvant therapy

The present pattern of disease suggests that surgery alone is often insufficient to eradicate all disease. This failure of surgery indicates a potential role for other treatment modalities. Numerous chemotherapeutic agents have been evaluated alone or in combination (Earl et al, 1984). However, these trials have frequently been uncontrolled and the assessment of response has been equivocal. Response rates of up to 20% have been described for 5-fluorouracil (Carter & Comis, 1977). Mitomycin C (Frank & Osterbury, 1960) and carmustine (BCNU) (Moertel 1973). However, such response rates have not been associated with any improvement in survival. Multicentre trials of combination chemotherapy have been undertaken both in the USA and the United Kingdom with conflicting results. The three most active single agents, 5-FU, adriamycin and mitomycin C have been combined in different regimes. In the American Study with FAM, there were 42% partial response rates in patients with advanced tumours (MacDonald et al, 1980). However, in a prospective controlled study in the UK with mitomycin C and 5-FU no survival advantage was observed over surgery alone (Fielding et al, 1983).

An implication from the 'second look' operation series was that the distribution of locoregional recurrence could be encompassed in a radiation portal (Gunderson & Sosin, 1982). Although response rates have been observed in patients with minimal residual disease after resection (Gunderson & O'Connell, 1984), adjuvant radiotherapy has yet to be demonstrated of value in a controlled study. It is possible that components of radiotherapy and chemotherapy may be superior to either alone.

Follow-up

Regular review of patients after primary surgery for gastric cancer is essential to seek and palliate recurrent disease, to manage postoperative complications other than recurrence, to provide support and reassurance for the patient and to assess the results of the primary treatment. Most are reviewed on a symptomatic basis. However, recent evidence suggests that regular endoscopic review can detect local remnant recurrence at an earlier stage in asymptomatic patients than investigation of symptomatic patients (Allum et al, 1984). Whether further resection is possible depends on associated locoregional disease; only 1 of 7 patients in the series cited was suitable for conversion from partial to total gastrectomy.

Any patient undergoing gastric resection is prone to the established complications of gastrectomy, in particular weight loss, bile vomiting and reflux oesophagitis. Such symptoms require careful reassurance and symptomatic management. Supplemental iron and vitamin B12 are required for life, especially for those having total or radical subtotal gastrectomy.

Finally the high incidence of advanced primary disease is unfortunately accompanied by a very poor short term survival. The majority of these patients will require adequate analgesia which occasionally entails coeliac axis nerve block and palliative radiotherapy to alleviate the discomfort of extragastric extension or enlarging liver metastases.

FUTURE PROSPECTS IN GASTRIC CANCER

Japanese experience of gastric cancer has clearly demonstrated that the disease can be managed effectively. In the UK interested surgeons have begun to consider trials based on the surgical approaches advocated by the Japanese. The results of such trials will be eagerly awaited. However, a major problem likely to be present in these studies will be the limited numbers of cases suitable for radical resection of the R2 type. Increase in the numbers of patients with suitable disease can only be achieved by earlier detection. Although mass screening on the Japanese scale is not justifiable, identification of those at greatest risk such as in certain occupations and environments may improve the rate of diagnosis of early lesions. A study of screening high risk patients has already been started by the British Stomach Cancer Group and its results will indicate the place of modified screening programmes in the UK.

REFERENCES

Allum W H, Hockey M S, Fielding J W L 1984 Gastric remnant recurrence — detection and implications for the management of gastric cancer. Clinical Oncology 10: 333–339
Allum W H, Roginski C, Fielding J W L, Powell D J, Waterhouse J A H, Brookes V S 1985 All gastric cancer should be resected. European Journal of Surgical Oncology 11: 101

Brookes V S, Waterhouse J A H, Powell D J 1965 Carcinoma of the stomach: a 10 year survey of results and of factors affecting prognosis. British Medical Journal I: 1577–1583

Carter S K, Comis R L 1977 Gastric cancer: current status of treatment. Journal of the National Cancer Institute 58: 567–578

Coller F A, Kay E B, MacIntire R S 1941 Regional lymphatic metastases of carcinoma of the stomach. Archives of Surgery 43: 748–761

Copeland E M, Daly J N, Dudrich S J 1977 Nutrition as an adjunct to cancer treatment in the adult. Cancer Research 37: 2451–2456

Cosgrove D O, McCready V C 1978 Diagnosis of liver metastases using ultrasound and isotope scanning techniques. Journal of the Royal Society of Medicine 71: 652–657

Cuschieri A 1980 Laparoscopy in general surgery and gastroenterology. British Journal of Hospital Medicine 24: 252–258

Dehn T C B, Reznek R H, Nockler I B, White F E 1984 The preoperative assessment of advanced gastric cancer by computed tomography. British Journal of Surgery 71: 413–417

Diggory R T, Cuschieri A 1985 R2/3 gastrectomy for gastric carcinoma: an audited experience of a consecutive series. British Journal of Surgery 72: 146–148

Donovan I A, Fielding J W L, Bradby H, Sorgi M, Harding L K 1982 Bile diversion after total gastrectomy. British Journal of Surgery 69: 389–390

Earl H M, Coombes R C, Schein P S 1984 Cytotoxic chemotherapy for cancer of the stomach. In: Wrigley P F M, Timothy A R (eds) Clinics in Oncology 3:2 Cancer of the Stomach. W B Saunders Company, London, p 351–369.

Edwards C L, Hayes R L 1969 Tumour scanning with 67 Gallium citrate. Journal of Nuclear Medicine 10: 103–105

Elster K, Kolaczek F, Shimamoto K, Freitag H 1975 Early gastric cancer — experience in Germany. Endoscopy 7: 5–10

Fielding J W L, Ellis D J, Jones B G, Paterson J, Powell D J, Waterhouse J A H, Brookes V S 1980 Natural history of 'early' gastric cancer: results of a 10 year regional survey. British Medical Journal 218: 965–967

Fielding J W L, Roginski C, Ellis D J, Jones B G, Powell D J, Waterhouse J A H, Brookes V S 1984 Clinicopathological staging of gastric cancer. British Journal of Surgery 71: 677–681

Fielding J W L et al 1983 An interim report of a prospective, randomized, controlled study of adjuvant chemotherapy in operable gastric cancer: British Stomach Cancer Group. World Journal of Surgery 7: 390–399

Frank W, Osterberg A E 1960 Mitomycin C (NSC-26980) — an evaluation of the Japanese reports. Cancer Chemotherapy Reports 9: 114–119

Friesen G, Docherty M B, Remine W H 1962 Superficial carcinoma of the stomach. Surgery 51: 300–312

Gross E, Bancewicz J, Ingram G 1984 Assessment of gastric cancer by laparoscopy. British Medical Journal 288: 1577

Gunderson L L, Sosin H 1982 Adenocarcinoma of the stomach: Areas of failure in a reoperation series (second or symptomatic look) clinicopathological correlation and implications for adjuvant therapy. International Journal of Radiation, Oncology, Biology and Physics 8: 1–11.

Hine K R, Booth S N, Leonard J C, Dykes P W 1978 Carcinoembryonic antigen concentrations in undiagnosed patients. Lancet II: 1337–1340

Hockey M S, Fielding J W L, Kelly K A, Ward L, Brookes V S, Craven J L, Mason M C, Winsey H S 1984 Resection line disease in stomach cancer. British Stomach Cancer Group. British Medical Journal 289: 601–603

Husband J E, McCready V R 1979 Scanning: which technique? British Journal of Hospital Medicine 21: 618–626

Japanese Research Society for Gastritic Cancer 1973 The General Rules for the Gastric Cancer Study in Surgery. Japanese Journal of Surgery 3: 61–71

Johnston I D A 1981 Nutritional support for the cancer patient. In: Fielding J W L, Newman C E, Ford C H J, Jones B G (eds) Advances in the Biosciences Vol. 32: Gastric Cancer. Pergamon, Oxford, p 149–158

Kajitani T, Miwa K (eds) 1979 Treatment results of stomach carcinoma in Japan, 1963–1966 (WHO-CC Monograph 2). Who, Tokyo

Keighley M R B, Moore J, Lee J R, Malins D, Thompson H 1981 Peroperative frozen section and cytology to assess proximal invasion in gastro-oesophageal carcinoma. British Journal of Surgery 68: 73–74

Keighley M R B, Moore J, Roginski C, Powell D J, Thompson H 1984 Incidence and prognosis of N4 node involvement in gastric cancer. British Journal of Surgery 71: 863–867

Kennedy B J 1970 TNM Classification for stomach cancer. Cancer 26: 971–983

Kressel H Y, Callen R W, Montague J P, Korobkin M, Goldberg H I, Moss A A, Arger P H, Margulin A R 1978 Computed tomographic evaluation of disorders affecting the alimentary tract. Radiology 129: 451–455

Longmire W P 1980 Gastric carcinoma: is radical gastrectomy worthwhile. Annals of the Royal College of Surgeons of England 62: 25–30

Lee J K Y, Stanley R J, Sagel S S, Levitt R G 1978 Accuracy of computed tomography in detecting intra-abdominal and pelvic adenopathy in lymphoma. American Journal of Roentgenology 131: 311–315

Macdonald J S et al 1980 5-Fluorouracil, doxorubicin and mitomycin (FAM) combination chemotherapy for advanced gastric cancer. Annals of Internal Medicine 93: 533–536

McNeer G, Vandenberg H, Donn F Y, Bowden L A 1951 A critical evaluation of subtotal gastrectomy for the cure of cancer of the stomach. Annals of Surgery 134: 2–7

Miwa K 1979 Cancer of the stomach in Japan. Gann Monograph on Cancer Research 22: 61–75

Moertel C G 1973 Therapy of advanced gastrointestinal cancer with nitrosoureas. Cancer Chemotherapy Reports (Supplement) 4: 27–34

Morris D L, Moore J, Thompson H, Keighley M R B 1982 Peroperative lymph node imprint cytology for staging gastric carcinoma. British Journal of Surgery 69: 282

Moss A A, Margulis A R, Schnyder P, Thoeri R F 1981 A uniform, computed tomography based staging system for malignant neoplasms of the alimentary tract. American Journal of Roentgenology 136: 1251–1252

Muller J M, Dienst C, Brenner U, Pichlmaier H 1982 Preoperative parenteral feeding in patients with gastrointestinal carcinoma. Lancet I: 68–71

Nomura A M Y, Stemmerman G N, Samloff I M 1980 Serum pepsinogen I as a predictor of stomach cancer. Annals of Internal Medicine 93: 537–540

Office of Population Censuses and Surveys 1983. Mortality Statistics: Cause 1982. London, HMSO

Ozarda A, Pickren J 1962 The topographic distribution of liver metastases. Its relation to surgical and isotope diagnosis. Journal of Nuclear Medicine 3: 149

Papachritou D N, Agnanti N, D'Agostino H, Fortner J G 1980 Histologically positive oesophageal margin in the surgical treatment of gastric cancer. American Journal of Surgery 139: 711–713

Pichlmayr R, Meyer J J 1981 Patterns of recurrence in relation to therapeutic strategy. In: Fielding J W L, Newman C E, Ford C H J, Jones B G (eds) Advances in the Biosciences Vol 32, Gastric Cancer. Pergamon, Oxford, p 171–190

Schreve R H, Terpstra O T, Ausema L, Lameri J S, van Seijen A J, Jeckel J 1984 Detection of liver metastases. A prospective study comparing liver enzymes, scintigraphy, ultrasonography and computed tomography. British Journal of Surgery 71: 947–949

Shirakabe H, Ichikawa H, Kamakura K, Nishizawa M, Higurashi K, Hayakawa H, Murakami T 1966 Atlas of X-ray diagnosis of early gastric cancer. Igaku-Shoiu Ltd, Tokyo

Smith T J, Kemeny M M, Sugarbaker P H, Jones A E, Vermess M, Shawker T H, Edwards B K 1982 A prospective study of hepatic imaging in the detection of metastatic disease. Annals of Surgery 195: 486–491

Snow J H, Goldstein H M, Wallace S 1979 Comparison of scintigraphy, sonography and computed tomography in the evaluation of hepatic neoplasms. American Journal of Roentgenology 132: 915–918

Sogo J, Kobayashi K, Saito J, Fujimak M, Moto T 1979 The role of lymphadenectomy in curative surgery for gastric cancer. World Journal of Surgery 3: 701–708

Stemmerman G N, Ishidata T, Samloff M, Masuda H, Walsh J H, Nonmura A, Yamakawa H, Glober G 1978 Intestinal metaplasia of the stomach in Hawaii and Japan. A study of its relation to serum pepsinogen I, Gastrin and parietal cell antibodies. American Journal of Digestive Diseases 23: 815–820

Swynnerton B F, Truelove S C 1952 Carcinoma of the stomach. British Medical Journal
    I: 287–292
Takagi K 1981 The incidence of gastric cancer since the advent of endoscopy. In: Fielding
    J W L, Newman C E, Ford C H J, Jones B G (eds) Advances in the Biosciences Vol 32,
    Gastric Cancer. Pergamon, Oxford, p 159–170
Tyrell C J, Cosgrove M O, McCready V R, Peckham M J 1977 The role of ultrasound in
    the assessment and treatment of abdominal metastases from testicular tumours. Clinical
    Radiology 28: 475–481
UICC (International Union against Cancer) 1982. TNM Atlas — Illustrated guide to the
    classification of malignant tumours. Springer Verlag, Berlin
Varis K, Samloff I M, Ihamaki T, Siurala M 1979 An appraisal of tests for severe atrophic
    gastritis in relatives of patients with pernicious anaemia. Digestive Diseases and Sciences
    24: 187–191
Walls W J 1976 The evaluation of malignant gastric neoplasms by ultrasonic B-scanning.
    Radiology 118: 159–163
Zinnager M M, Collins W T 1949 Extension of carcinoma of the stomach into duodenum
    and oesophagus. Annals of Surgery 130: 557–566

The management of stones in the common bile duct

INTRODUCTION

When stones are discovered in the bile duct they should be completely removed as soon as conveniently possible. Whilst they remain the patient can develop obstructive jaundice or cholangitis at any time. Cholangitis may still be rapidly fatal whilst severe jaundice substantially increases the risks of removing the stones. On the other hand stones in the bile duct may cause no symptoms for many years and only come to light when the patient develops a complication. Sometimes these symptoms can be trivial or confusing particularly in the elderly. Mild transient jaundice and septicaemic collapse are two examples. Occasionally abnormal liver function tests often done for other reasons leads to the discovery of stones in the bile ducts but the most common time to find them is during a cholecytectomy.

DIAGNOSIS

Peroperative cholangiography

Over 40 000 cholecystectomies are performed each year in England and Wales and stones will be removed from the bile ducts during the operation in approximately 5000 patients. The incidence of gall stones increases with age and so does the proportion of patients with stones in the bile ducts. Under the age of 50 years only one in 20 patients will have a stone in the duct but this increases to one in five patients over the age of 70 years (McSherry & Glenn, 1980). These patients can sometimes be predicted if, for instance, they have had an episode of jaundice in the past or the bile duct is 10 mm or more in diameter at laparotomy (Edholm & Jonsson, 1962). Sometimes the stones can be seen or felt within the bile duct but whatever the findings the younger surgeon when removing a gall bladder should always obtain an operative cholangiogram. Some surgeons prefer to select those patients who need a cholangiogram. They complain about the time taken to obtain the pictures and more significantly that an average of two out of every five ducts explored as a consequence of an abnormal cholangiogram do not contain stones. It is true that with increasing experience the investigation can sometimes be omitted but the quickest and most accurate results will always be obtained with careful attention to detail and constant practice.

It is best to cannulate the cystic duct with a fine plastic tube although a small Foley balloon catheter may be better for a grossly dilated cystic duct. Small stones must first be removed from the cystic duct otherwise they will be pushed into the common bile duct. For the same reason injection of contrast into and then compression of the gall bladder is unwise. When the cystic duct is very small or cannot be found such as after a previous cholecystectomy then a direct injection into the bile duct itself will outline the anatomy as well as any stones. However, the needle hole will leak for several hours and a drain is essential.

It is easiest to control the speed and the volume of injection using an image intensifier but most surgeons are only able to take two separate pictures. The dye should be dilute enough to reveal small stones but dense enough to provide adequate contrast (25% Hypaque is suitable). Air bubbles must be rigorously excluded from the syringe and cannula as they look like stones on the pictures. For the first exposure 3–6 ml (approximately half the diameter of the common bile duct in millimetres) should be injected and a total of 10–30 ml of contrast (approximately twice the diameter of the duct) for the second.

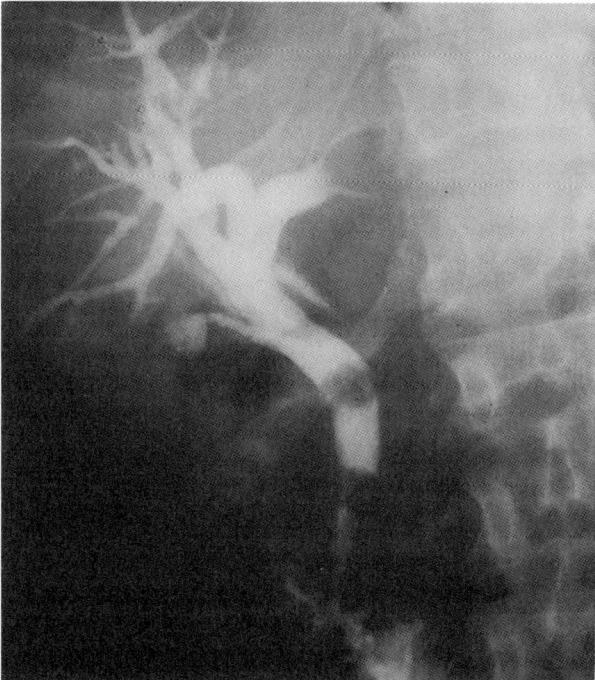

Fig. 6.1 Operative cholangiogram to show stones in the common bile duct

It is not always easy to interpret the pictures (Fig. 6.1). Stones sometimes hide within the intrahepatic ducts which may not fill if there is rapid flow into the duodenum. Overlying gas shadows can mimic stones and excess contrast in the bowel may obliterate the lower end of the duct. Ampullary spasm as well as stones can prevent free flow of contrast into the duodenum and this can be caused by certain anaesthetic drugs, particularly fentanyl. If this is suspected further pictures must be taken after the administration of an antispasmodic.

One development of cholangiography has been to measure pressure in the bile duct and flow through the ampulla (Ribeiro et al 1980). However the technique is intricate and interpretation of the figures complicated so that few surgeons use manometry to diagnose stones in the bile duct even though they could, with cholangiography, reduce the number of negative duct explorations.

Ultrasound examination

Developments in ultrasound technology have made it possible to demonstrate stones in the gall bladder with accuracy and without irradiation (Cooperberg & Burhenne 1980). Provided the ultrasonographer is skillful and experienced most surgeons will undertake a cholecystectomy on a suitable patient following an abnormal ultrasound examination without requiring an oral cholecystogram. Cholecystography has been the standard examination for many years but it does not demonstrate the bile ducts and in the past if information about the ducts was needed before operation then an intravenous cholangiogram was necessary. This investigation has a significant morbidity and was rarely done particularly as operative cholangiography provided better pictures. Nowadays cholecystography and cholangiography have both been replaced by the ultrasound probe which will image both the gall bladder and the bile duct. Most patients with gall bladder stones will have normal ducts and this might provide an objective reason for omitting an operative cholangiogram. For those patients in whom ultrasound demonstrates definite dilatation or stones in the ducts there may be a place for removing these stones endoscopically first.

For the patient who comes into hospital with jaundice or cholangitis ultrasound examination of the bile ducts is the first and most important investigation. The presence of dilated ducts establishes an extrahepatic obstructive cause for the jaundice. Dilatation will not be present in the early stages of an obstruction and if doubt remains the examination should be repeated one week later. Cholangitis is almost always accompanied by dilatation of the bile ducts. Stones in the bile ducts can sometimes be seen (Fig. 6.2) but at present ultrasound will identify the site of obstruction in only two-thirds of patients and the cause in one-third (Baron et al, 1982). This is not a great disadvantage as a contrast study which will identify the site and the cause is always needed next. If the gall bladder is still present

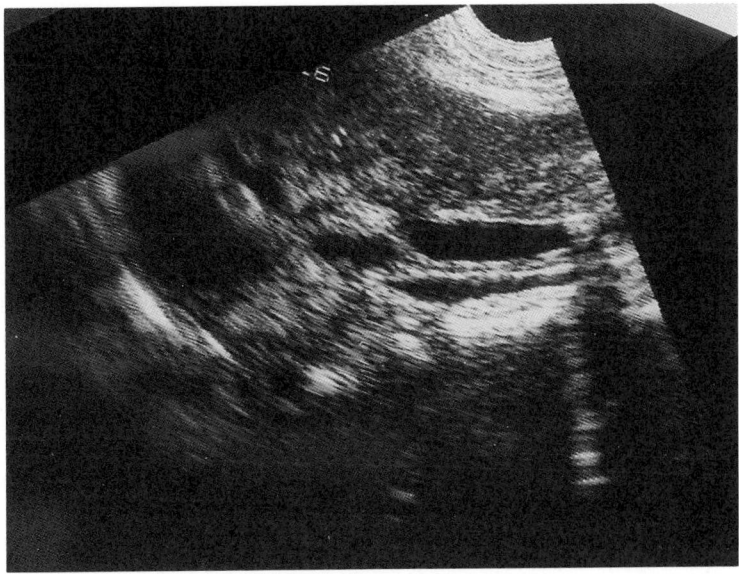

Fig. 6.2 Ultrasound examination showing dilated common bile duct containing a stone with the typical ultrasonic shadow (Courtesy of Dr D Lindsell)

and cholecystectomy is appropriate then an operative cholangiogram can be done. In other circumstances an endoscopic or percutaneous cholangiogram should be obtained.

Endoscopic retrograde cholangio-pancreatography (ERCP)

The introduction of ERCP has made the diagnosis and the treatment of biliary and pancreatic disease very much easier. With experience it is possible to manipulate a long side viewing endoscope into the second part of the duodenum so that the endoscopist looks directly at the ampulla. Anatomical abnormalities such as a previous Polya gastrectomy or pyloric stenosis may make this difficult or impossible but there are no absolute contraindications. On the other hand technical skill is required and the reader is referred to a specialist text for a detailed description of the procedure.

Adequate sedation is necessary and if it is known that the bile duct is obstructed then suitable antibiotics must be given before an attempt is made to cannulate the ampulla. The pancreatic duct and the bile duct run away from the ampulla in different directions but nevertheless patience and perserverance as well as constant slight changes of position are often needed to outline the required duct. Even so it is only possible to cannulate one or both of the ducts in 90% of the patients (Cotton, 1977). Correct dilution of the contrast medium and the elimination of all air from the syringe and cannula are once again essential. The whole biliary tree must be outlined.

Contrast sometimes enters the cystic duct selectively if the gall bladder is still present and the cannula is lodged at the ampulla. The tip of the cannula must then be advanced beyond the opening of the cystic duct to outline the intrahepatic ducts and tilting the patient head down may help. Sometimes the lucent whirlpool that develops when contrast is injected under pressure through a narrow cannula into a broad bile duct can look very like a stone but the artefact will disappear when the contrast has completely mixed with the bile. Good quality radiographs are essential. These require co-ordination and co-operation between the endoscopist and the radiologist. Certainly no operative procedure should be started until lucencies consistent with stones are definitely seen on the pictures (Fig. 6.3).

Percutaneous transhepatic cholangiography (PTC)

The development of the fine flexible Chiba needle has made percutaneous cholangiography a safe and widely available investigation which is most useful in patients with extrahepatic obstructive jaundice. The needle will enter a bile duct in perhaps 99 out of every 100 patients with a dilated

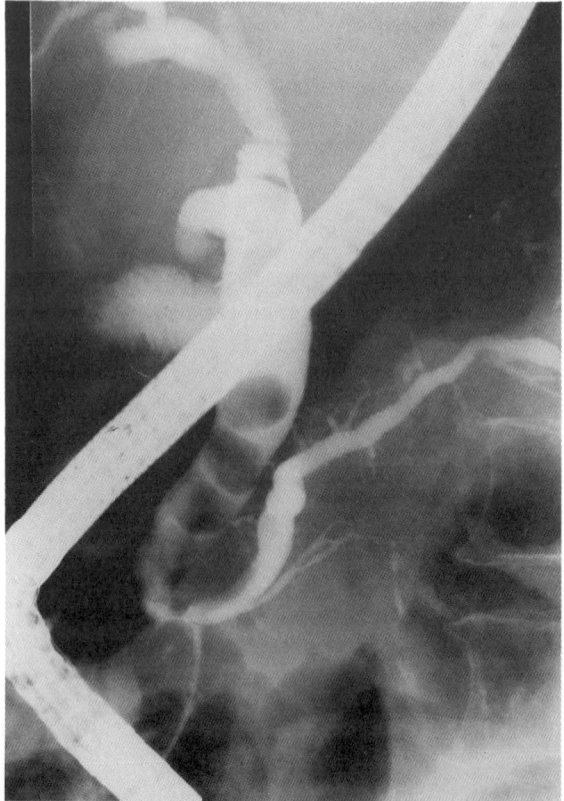

Fig. 6.3 ERCP picture showing multiple stones in the common bile duct

system. Complications such as infection, usually cholangitis, haemorrhage or a bile leak occur in just over 3% of patients (Gold et al, 1979). Mobile stones are easily identified but if contrast will not pass beyond an impacted stone the meniscus can sometimes be mistaken for a stricture. If a totally obstructed system is punctured then some procedure to decompress the ducts must be performed promptly. This is a disadvantage of percutaneous cholangiography as it is not practical to remove stones from the bile duct through the liver and, unless an endoscopic sphincterotomy can be done, surgery will be necessary.

TREATMENT

Until recently stones could only be removed from the bile duct at a laparotomy. Such operations are technically quite difficult and require at least two weeks in hospital. Nowadays the stones can also be removed through the divided ampulla into the duodenal lumen following an ERCP whilst stones left behind after surgery can be extracted along the t-tube track. Nevertheless at present surgery is still the commonest method.

Surgery

Prophylactic antibiotics must be given before the bile duct is explored because bacteria will be present in the bile in 80% of these patients. A second essential preliminary is full mobilisation of the second part of the duodenum and the head of the pancreas off the posterior abdominal wall. There are then two possible approaches to the bile duct. The supraduodenal route is slightly safer but the initial exploration is blind because of the right angled approach to the duct. There is also the risk of a retained stone which is not a problem when the ampullary sphincter is divided. For this reason the transduodenal route may be more appropriate if a choledochoscope is not available but the bowel is opened and manipulation of the pancreatic duct sometimes causes pancreatitis. It is the best operation when the bile ducts are narrow or when there is a small stone impacted in the ampulla. Such a stone is impossible to remove from above and pushing it on into the duodenum is unsatisfactory and unreliable.

Transduodenal sphincteroplasty

If the ampulla can be felt through the duodenal wall a short longitudinal duodenotomy can be accurately placed. If it cannot be felt it is usually possible to locate the papilla with a finger tip once the bowel is open. Access is then simpler if a stay suture is inserted through the bowel wall just beyond the ampulla. Both the pancreatic and the bile ducts must be identified with a probe. One blade of a pair of fine scissors is inserted into the bile duct and the ampullary sphincter is divided. This is best done in stages placing interrupted stitches of fine catgut to approximate the duodenal mucosa to the bile duct epithelium at each stage. These sutures should be tied only when it is certain that they do not surround the pancreatic duct. Straight Desjardins forceps will remove all the large stones. Any small ones can theoretically be left as they will pass spontaneously but if a choledochoscope is available it is preferrable to check that the ducts are clear. The duodenum is then closed transversely and the abdomen shut with a drain down to the operation site.

Retained stones cannot be easily identified after this operation and they should not cause a problem anyway. For the same reasons some surgeons have advocated creating a choledochoduodenostomy (Schein et al 1978). The operation is quick and easy to do and so avoids a prolonged exploration of the duct which is an advantage in an elderly patient. However, stones, debris and food sometimes collect in the segment of the duct between the fistula and the ampulla and sometimes the fistula stenoses. Both can cause recurrent cholangitis.

Although the incidence of acute pancreatitis after transduodenal sphincteroplasty varies between 1% and 10% at least half the patients with this complication will die (Cave-Bigley et al 1984). The operation is probably best avoided therefore in patients who have had previous pancreatitis. A duodenal fistula develops in a few patients but it will usually close spontaneously. Overall an average mortality for transduodenal exploration of the bile duct would be 5% (Vellacott & Powell, 1979).

Supraduodenal exploration of the bile duct

The bile duct is first exposed for a short distance in the free edge of the lesser omentum and a longitudinal incision is made in the duct just sufficient to remove the largest stone seen on the operative cholangiogram. Some bile should be sent for culture. All the easily accessible stones can then be removed from the duct with angled Desjardins forceps although stones in the retroduodenal portion of the duct can often be manipulated into the choledochotomy by fingers placed along the line of the common bile duct behind the head of the pancreas. Nowadays a choledochoscope should be used next but if this instrument is not available then a conventional exploration must be undertaken.

Firstly it is worthwhile counting the number of stones and noting their position on the X-ray. If some still remain then further exploration with forceps, baskets and balloons is necessary. It is also worthwhile to flush the ducts with saline injected through a catheter passed up and down the duct. Traditionally a bougie is also passed blindly through the ampulla into the duodenum. Since this serves no useful purpose and can create a fistula which is sometimes seen at ERCP it should not be done.

Very occasionally the experienced surgeon can now be certain that no stones remain in the bile duct. If choledochoscopy has also demonstrated a widely patent ampulla the risk of a postoperative bile leak from the duct is minimal and he can close the choledochotomy without a t-tube (Vassilakis et al, 1979). In every other circumstance a t-tube is essential. Some surgeons also obtain a further cholangiogram at this stage but air bubbles which look like stones are so often present that the investigation is probably better omitted. However without choledochoscopy we know that stones will still remain in the ducts once in every seven or eight patients. How these stones are to be removed subsequently must be considered before the operation is finished. If the expertise is available to remove stones along the t-tube track then the t-tube must be at least 14 Fg in size. It should be brought out at right angles to the bile duct, run a straight course to the lateral abdominal wall and leave the skin below the costal margin and behind the anterior axillary line. If endoscopic extraction of any retained stones would be possible then these details are less important.

The t-tube should not be removed before the tenth postoperative day and then only after a cholangiogram has shown free flow of contrast into the duodenum and the absence of stones in the duct. It is wise to occlude the tube for 24 hours before it is removed. If the t-tube is removed too soon bile may leak into the peritoneal cavity and this is the only serious complication of the operation apart from a retained stone.

Overall the mortality rate following supraduodenal exploration of the bile duct is about 3%. However this average figure conceals a significant variation with age. In patients under the age of 50 years the mortality is less than 1% but at 65 it is nearly 5% and this increases again to nearly 25% in patients over the age of 80 years (McSherry & Glynn, 1980). Similar mortality rates apply when the ducts are explored but no stones are recovered. This can be expected in one third of explorations so careful and accurate cholangiography is absolutely essential. All these figures are generally worse if the duct is being explored for the second or third time.

Choledochoscopy. Both rigid and flexible instrument are made and either is perfectly adequate for choledochoscopy. Two lengths of the rigid instruments may be needed for a complete examination but together they are still very substantially cheaper than a fibreoptic choledochoscope. Warm saline under adequate pressure is necessary for a good view. Distension of the ducts can be helped by crossing over the stay sutures and thus closing the small choledochotomy around the instrument. The intrahepatic ducts are easiest to see and should be inspected first. The lower half of the duct is difficult to view, partly because the irrigation fluid leaks away through the ampulla but also because, unlike within the liver, the walls of the duct are not held open by the surrounding structures. It is therefore best to pass the instrument blindly down as far as the ampulla and then to view the lumen on withdrawal. Even so it is easy to miss a stone hidden within the folds of an incompletely distended distal duct. Sometimes keeping the choledochoscope still and using the left hand to move the bile duct and the duodenum over the tip of the instrument is best. This is certainly a good way to pass the instrument through the ampulla into the duodenum when this is possible.

When residual stones are discovered they are often difficult to remove. Sometimes the jet of saline from the end of the choledochoscope itself can be directed to wash them out. It will certainly wash out the debris which is usually present and which, if left, could be the start of a recurrent stone. Sometimes removing the choledochoscope and reverting to Desjardins forceps is best but if visual control is needed a basket is the safest tool. Although instrument channels are provided within all the instruments it is often better to pass the basket alongside the choledochoscope as this allows independent manipulation. A balloon catheter may be useful but it is very easy to overdistend the balloon and rupture a bile duct particularly within the liver. Before the endoscope is removed from a supraduodenal chole-dochotomy it is essential to check that stones have not been simply washed past the instrument into the other section of the duct. Very rarely stones can be seen but cannot be safely removed. They should be left. Other methods of removal can be tried later if necessary.

The ability to see within the bile duct is a definite advantage. After the ducts have been cleared by conventional means more stones will be found by choledochoscopy in perhaps 15% of patients (Keighley & Kappas, 1980). Without choledochoscopy about 10% of bile duct explorations leave one or more stones behind (Glenn, 1974) and the difference between these two figures reflects the greater accuracy of choledochoscopy as compared with post-operative t-tube cholangiography. Some surgeons have not left any stones behind at all after using the choledochoscope and some have found it valueless but in most people's hands the incidence of retained stones should fall to about 2% of all bile duct explorations (Finnis & Rowntree, 1977, Feliciano et al 1980).

Retained stones. Everyone leaves a stone behind sometimes. In the past this meant a second and more difficult operation which might damage the bile duct. Nowadays retained stones are generally easy to remove and further surgery is rarely required. Indeed it is not always necessary to do anything. Small stones may pass spontaneously with time and this might be shortened by irrigating the t-tube with saline. Larger stones need to be reduced in size. Heparin, sodium cholate or mono-octonoin infused down the t-tube will dissolve some stones but their effect seems entirely unpredictable.

In fact physical removal of the stones either percutaneously through the choledochotomy or endoscopically through the ampulla is best. Endoscopic extraction can be undertaken as soon as the stones are discovered unless the duodenum has been opened when it is wise to wait for 4 weeks. Percutaneous removal requires a well formed track so that the t-tube must stay for 6 weeks. Then after confirming that some stones are still present the tube is removed and either a steerable catheter or the flexible chole-dochoscope is passed along the fistula and into the bile duct. Radiological control is required with the catheter but the endoscope can be steered by direct vision. A stone is trapped in a dormier basket passed within the instrument and the whole assembly is withdrawn. Repeated passes are necessary to remove multiple stones. Perforation of the fistulous track is the only serious complication. This is more likely if the t-tube is too small or has been incorrectly placed. Nevertheless, Burhenne, who devised the steerable catheter, was able to remove all the retained stones percutaneously in 91% of his patients (Burhenne, 1976).

Endoscopic sphincterotomy

This is the most important therapeutic development of ERCP and a significant advance in the treatment of bile duct stones. After obtaining a cholangiogram the fine plastic cannula used to intubate the ampulla is replaced by a spincterotomy knife. In fact the knife consists of a wire passed down inside a long plastic catheter and attached to the tip. For the last 3cm the wire lies outside the plastic tubing. The ampulla is cannulated in the usual way and the knife must be seen to lie well within the bile duct on the X-ray screen. The tubing is then withdrawn so that half the wire lies outside the ampulla. When the wire is shortened in relation to the outer plastic tubing this bowstrings the exposed portion across the luminal wall of the ampulla (Fig. 6.4). Cutting diathermy divides the sphincter and makes a wide opening into the bile duct.

This is a surgical operation on the ampulla, albeit a small one, and

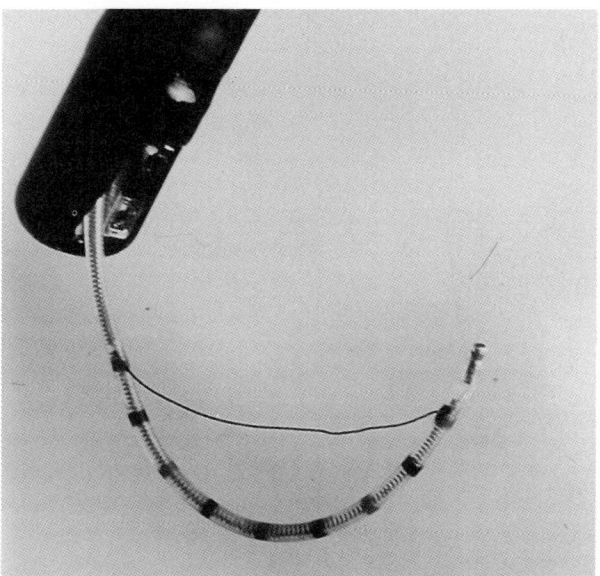

Fig. 6.4 Bowed sphincterotomy knife

haemorrhage, cholangitis and pancreatitis are all recognised complications. They affect about 10% of patients and usually settle with conservative management. Restenosis is rare. Patients in whom the bleeding is not going to stop can often be recognised and prompt laparotomy is required. The operation is identical to a transduodenal sphincteroplasty and the bleeding is controlled with fine catgut stitches taking care once again to avoid the pancreatic duct. It is amongst these patients and those who develop severe acute pancreatitis that the 1% mortality of endoscopic sphincterotomy arises (Cotton & Vallon, 1981). In contrast to conventional surgery this figure is the same for all age groups.

Once the sphincter has been divided all the stones should be removed from the ducts with a balloon or a basket (Fig. 6.5). However most stones will pass spontaneously if given time to do so and it is then only necessary to repeat the ERCP 4 weeks later and confirm that the ducts are clear. With either method an experienced endoscopist can expect to remove all the stones in 80% of the patients. A sphinterotomy cannot be done in half the failures and stones are still present in the other 10% (Cotton & Vallon, 1981, Viceconte et al, 1981).

Large stones and tightly packed facetted stones cause the most difficulty. Absolute size is less important than the diameter of the stone in relation to the size and shape of the proximal common bile duct. If these are incom-

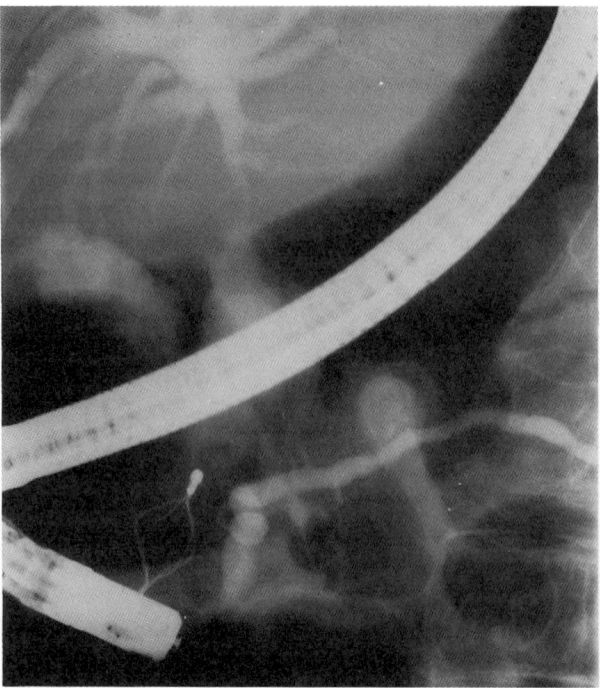

Fig. 6.5 Stone trapped in a basket being removed from the bile duct (same patient as Fig. 6.3)

patible and extraction is attempted it is easy for the basket to become stuck. For this reason attempts have been made to disintegrate large stones with ultrasound, laser light or by mechanical disruption but for the moment these methods are either experimental or unreliable. Dissolution is only slightly more satisfactory. Chemical agents such as mono-octonoin can be infused continuously down a naso-biliary drain left behind at ERCP. After 2 weeks about one-third of the stones are either smaller or softer and can be removed. This takes time, the success rate is poor and patients dislike the tube in their nose.

It is best to identify these difficult stones on the preliminary cholangiogram, not to divide the ampulla and to offer the patients an operation. Some will decline and others are unfit for an operation. Many of these patients are elderly and for this small group excellent palliation can be provided by inserting a permanent biliary stent. This can be easily done endoscopically and drains the duct as well as preventing impaction of the stone.

Indications for endoscopic removal of bile duct stones

Endoscopic removal of bile duct stones is virtually painless, is usually followed by an immediate recovery and involves only a few days in hospital. It is the best treatment for any patient who has had a cholecystectomy in the past and then develops recurrent stones. Whatever the patient's age and whether the indication is jaundice, cholangitis, pancreatitis or simply recurrent pain the risks of endoscopic treatment are always less than the risks of surgery. The same applies to any patient over the age of 65 years who develops complications from stones in the bile duct and still has their gall bladder. Surgery will sometimes be needed when endoscopy fails but very few of the patients in this second group, perhaps 10%, will need a subsequent cholecystectomy (Cotton & Vallon, 1982).

All the remaining patients are under the age of 65 and still have a gall bladder. This will be the source of the symptoms in most patients under the age of 50 years and these patients need a cholecystectomy. Any stones in the duct should be dealt with at the time even if they are discovered beforehand. An endoscopic sphincterotomy would be inadequate and anyway the risks of endoscopy and surgery in this age group are the same.

Between the ages of 50 and 65 years other factors need to be considered. If the symptoms are chronic and the cholecystectomy is likely to be easy this is the treatment of choice. For the patients who present with jaundice, cholangitis or pancreatitis, an urgent endoscopic sphincterotomy followed by a delayed cholecystectomy might be best. Whether this approach should be adopted in patients under the age of 50 is controversial. We do not yet know the long-term complications of destroying the ampulla although surgeons have been doing sphincteroplasties safely for many years. An endoscopic sphincterotomy for a young person with severe gall stone pancreatitis or whose life was threatened by cholangitis might well be best. We must hope that more experience and further trials will give the answer.

REFERENCES

Baron R L, Stanley R J, Lee J K T, Koehler R E, Melson G L, Balfe D M, Weyman P J
1982 A prospective comparison of the evaluation of biliary obstruction using computed
tomography and ultrasonography. Radiology 145: 91–98

Burhenne H J 1976 Complications of non-operative extraction of retained common duct
stones. American Journal of Surgery 131: 260–262

Cave-Bigley D J, Aukland P, Kane J F, Hardy E G 1984 Transduodenal exploration of
the common bile duct in a district general hospital. Annals of the Royal College of
Surgeons of England 66: 187–189

Cooperberg P L, Burhenne H J 1980 Real time ultrasonography. Diagnostic technique of
choice in calculous gall bladder disease. New England Journal of Medicine
302: 1277–1279

Cotton P B 1977 Progress Report ERCP. Gut 18: 316–341

Cotton P B, Vallon A G 1981 British experience with duodenoscopic sphincterotomy for
removal of bile duct stones. British Journal of Surgery 68: 373–375

Edholm P, Jonsson G 1962 Bile duct stones related to age and duct width. Acta Chirurgica
Scandinavica 124: 75–79

Feliciano D V, Mattox K L, Jordan G L 1980 The value of choledochoscopy in exploration
of the common bile duct. Annals of Surgery 191: 649–654

Finnis D, Rowntree T 1977 Choledochoscopy in exploration of the common bile duct.
British Journal of Surgery 64: 661–664

Glenn F 1974 Retained calculi within the biliary ductal system. Annals of Surgery
179: 528–539

Gold R P, Casarella W J, Stern G, Seaman W B 1979 Transhepatic cholangiography: The
radiological method of choice in suspected obstructive jaundice. Radiology 133: 39–44

Keighley M R B, Kappas A 1980 Evaluation of operative choledochoscopy. Surgery,
Gynecology and Obstetrics 150: 357–359

McSherry C K, Glenn F 1980 The incidence and causes of death following surgery for non-
malignant biliary tract disease. Annals of Surgery 191: 271–275

Ribeiro B F, Williams J T, Lees W R, Roberts M, Lequesne L P 1980 An evaluation of
cholangiomanometry with synchronous cholangiography. British Journal of Surgery
67: 863–868

Schein C J, Shapiro N, Gliedman M L 1978 Choledochoduodenostomy as an adjunct to
choledocholithotomy. Surgery, Gynecology and Obstetrics 146: 25–32

Vassilakis J S, Chattopadhyay D K, Irvin T T, Duthie H L 1979 Primary closure of the
common bile duct after elective choledochotomy. Journal of the Royal College of
Surgeons of Edinburgh 24: 156–158

Vellacott K D, Powell P H 1979 Exploration of the common bile duct: a comparative
study. British Journal of Surgery 66: 389–391

Viceconte G, Viceconte G W, Pietropaolo V, Montori A 1981 Endoscopic sphincterotomy:
Indications and results. British Journal of Surgery 68: 376–380

FURTHER READING

Berci G, Hamlin J A 1981 Operative biliary radiology. Williams and Wilkins, Baltimore

Blumgart L H (ed) 1982 The biliary tract. Churchill Livingstone, Edinburgh

Cotton P B, Williams C B 1982 Practical gastrointestinal endoscopy. Blackwell Scientific
Publications, Oxford

Kune G A, Sali A 1980 The practice of biliary surgery. Blackwell Scientific Publications,
Oxford

Matolo N M (ed) 1981 Biliary tract disease. In: Surgical Clinics of North America.
Saunders, Philadelphia.

The role of surgery in pancreatitis

INTRODUCTION

Most patients with either acute or chronic pancreatitis do not warrant surgical treatment. However, almost all patients with acute pancreatitis present with abdominal pain of sudden onset and associated vomiting. They therefore are most likely to be admitted under the care of a surgical department for their emergency treatment. This naturally also applies to patients who suffer from recurrent attacks of acute pancreatitis, while those with chronic pancreatitis are most frequently referred for a surgical opinion in respect to pain which is the predominant symptom of this disease. A minority of patients with chronic pancreatitis warrant direct surgical intervention, usually to provide an alternative drainage to the pancreatic duct system, or to resect the most severely affected areas of the pancreas. It is wrong to believe that this is the only role of surgery in the management of chronic pancreatitis which will be considered later in the chapter.

ACUTE PANCREATITIS

The place of surgical intervention in the management of acute pancreatitis is dependent on a number of factors and it may be considered under the following headings:

— Laparotomy for diagnostic reasons.
— Surgery for removal of necrotic tissue in or around the pancreas.
— Intervention to remove gallstones.
— Surgery for late complications e.g. pseudocyst and abscess.

Laparotomy for diagnostic uncertainty

This type of surgery falls into two separate categories. On the one hand there is the situation where the diagnosis of acute pancreatitis has not been considered, and on the other there is the situation where, despite careful enzyme measurements in blood and urine, genuine diagnostic doubt still lingers in the surgeon's mind. It is the author's impression that the former is numerically more important than the latter, even at the present time when urine 'dip strip' tests are now available, analogous to those that have been used for many years to detect the presence of glucose in urine.

Where a young and inexperienced surgeon finds him or herself within the peritoneal cavity with pointers to acute pancreatitis being evident, then it is wise to call in the help of a more exprienced person to fully assess the situation. In addition to assessing the degree of severity of pancreatitis it will probably be advisable in a significant proportion of patients to remove gall stones from the biliary tree in a comprehensive fashion. Free fluid with a high content of amylase, lipase and albumin (as well as a large number of other substances) may be present. The fluid can range in colour from clear to very dark resembling prune juice, and the darker the colour of the fluid the more severe the attack of pancreatitis. In acute pancreatitis the fluid is likely to be uninfected and should be odourless, but a Gram film should be checked and bacteriological culture carried out (Bradley et al, 1981). In addition an assessment of the content of the common enzymes and albumins is valuable. The gastrocolic omentum should be opened to allow an estimate of the degree of involvement of the body and tail of the gland, and a gentle Kocher's manoeuvre carried out to check whether the findings on the anterior surface of the head of pancreas are similar to those posteriorly.

The terms 'haemorrhagic' and 'necrotising pancreatitis' are somewhat emotive, and in addition are often used inaccurately. At least two groups in the world have found that the term 'necrotising pancreatitis' has been wrongly applied in approximately 50% of patients assessed at laparotomy because the necrosis is confined to the tissue around the pancreas and does not extend to the pancreas itself. A careful description of findings is valuable although the dynamics of acute pancreatitis are such that it should not be assumed that the description which held at the time of laparotomy will necessarily pertain later in the illness. A clear definition of the term 'haemorrhagic pancreatitis' is lacking. Does this relate only to the gland, or to the peritoneal fluid as well? Does it relate to a few limited areas of blood on one segment of the pancreas or to a much more extensive process? For these reasons, as well as a careful description of the operative findings, it is well to relate disease severity to the presence of objective signs such as those depicted in Table 7.1 (Osborne et al, 1981).

Where the pancreas is grossly inflamed and shows areas of superficial haemorrhage or necrosis the minimum that should be done is to place soft sump drains into the lesser sac, and over the the anterior surface of the gland. These drains facilitate peritoneal lavage should this be indicated, e.g. in the presence of renal failure. Removal of necrotic tissue by gentle finger dissection as described later in the chapter may be indicated.

Does early laparotomy represent an additional hazard to the patient? It is probable that in milder forms of pancreatitis, and with current intensive care support more readily available, that direct surgical intervention early

Table 7.1   Glasgow system of prognostic factors (Imrie et al, 1978; Osborne et al, 1981)

1. Leucocytosis — WBC > 15 000/mm^3
2. Blood glucose > 10 mmol/l (in absence of diabetes)
3. Blood urea > 16 mmol/l (even after i.v. fluids)
4. Arterial paO$_2$ < 60 mmHg (8 kPa)
5. Total calcium < 2.0 mmol/l
6. Serum albumin < 32 g/l
7. LDH > 600 international units/l
8. AST > 200 units/l

Presence of any 3 or more within 48 hours indicates severe disease

in the disease is less hazardous than previously. An older paper in which the mortality for both early laparotomy and conservative management was compared (in unselected patients with all forms of acute pancreatitis) no difference in mortality in the two groups was found (Trapnell & Anderson, 1964). However, it must be noted that each group had a mortality of between 23 and 24% and that experience is not paralleled in other centres such as New York and Glasgow. Ranson found that in patients with objective evidence of severe acute pancreatitis there was a mortality rate of 16% for conservative management and 67% for those undergoing early laparotomy (Ranson et al, 1976). Prospective studies by our team in Glasgow have shown a similar increased incidence of complications and death in the patients undergoing early surgery. The most valuable study has been one in which the New York University group found no increased hazard in mild acute pancreatitis for limited operation (aspiration of fluid and placement of drains), but all forms of surgical intervention at the early stage of severe acute pancreatitis added to the likelihood of death (Ranson, 1984)

Where enzyme measurements have been carried out and genuine diagnostic doubt still exists in the surgeon's mind then a check through the list included in Table 7.2 should prove helpful. This embraces most of the conditions where hyperamylasemia might occur in the context of an appropriate clinical presentation, although it is important to appreciate that it is exceptional for *perforated duodenal ulcer* within 5 hours of onset to have an associated gross rise in serum amylase. Furthermore, the clinical and radiological diagnosis of *small bowel obstruction* and *dissecting aortic aneurysm* should not pose any real problem

An unusual differential diagnosis listed on Table 7.2 is that of ectopic pregnancy and the hyperamylasemia in this situation is associated with amylase production from the fallopian tube. A careful history and examination of the patient should not lead to genuine diagnostic doubt; although routine biochemical screening has led some clinicians away from the appropriate diagnosis when they were unaware of the association of raised amylase with ectopic pregnancy. Obviously the appropriate therapy for ectopic pregnancy is surgical intervention.

Table 7.2 Differential diagnosis of acute pancreatitis from other emergencies with hyperamylasaemia

Easier	More difficult
Early perforated DU (< 5 h)	Later perforated DU (> 5 h)
Small bowel obstruction	Mesenteric ischaemia
Ectopic pregnancy	
Dissecting aortic aneurysm	
Renal failure	
(Macroamylasaemia)	

Acute renal failure

Acute renal failure is associated with a rise in serum amylase but standard screening of creatining and urine amylase will usually clarify the situation very quickly. In *macroamylasaemia* the patient always has a raised serum amylase and tends to have very low levels in urine. Therefore a urinary amylase estimation may be virtually diagnostic of this condition in which a very large amylase molecule approaching 200,000 daltons instead of the normal molecule around 45,000 daltons is present. The large molecule does not filter through the renal glomerulus resulting in persistent high levels of serum amylase and minute levels of urine.

Differential diagnosis

The more difficult differential diagnosis occurs usually in patients who have a perforated duodenal ulcer of more than 5 hours duration, or in mesenteric arterial occlusion or venous thrombosis. It has been documented that perforated duodenal ulcers between 5 and 24 hours after onset tend to have much higher serm amylase levels than those before this time (Imrie et al, 1974). In the patients suffering from atrial fibrillation, or a recent heart attack then arterial embolic occlusion of the superior mesenteric artery is likely and an early diagnostic laparotomy would be entirely justified. However, it is important to remember that in the single published study carried out in patients with mesenteric ischaemia only 2 of 34 patients whose serum amylase was examined had elevations greater than twice the top of the normal range (Ottinger, 1978). Our own study of the problem of serum amylase levels in mesenteric ischaemia found a higher incidence than Ottinger (Wilson & Imrie, 1986). Five of 63 patients had an amylase level recorded above 1200 units/litre, while 10 others had a level greater than 600 units/litre representing 24% of our total. It would therefore appear that hyperamylasaemia is a relatively unusual accompaniment of this problem. *Peritoneal aspiration* can be very helpful in both these situations (Bradley et al, 1981) as micro-organisms will probably indicate more rapidly the presence of infection and the need for early laparotomy. In the emergency situation the first step for the surgeon is to smell the aspirate; followed by a rapid Gram film; then bacterial culture. Foul odour or bacteria on the film point to the need for urgent operation as it is unusual for this to occur in severe acute pancreatitis, and usually derives from compromised or ruptured gut.

What should a surgeon do when inside the peritoneal cavity in a patient with gallstone induced pancreatitis? — (a) remove the gall bladder (Table 7.3), and (b) carry out an operative cholangiogram and, if indicated by the radiology, explore the common bile duct.

Table 7.3 Suggested sequence of steps at early laparotomy where acute pancreatitis is the diagnosis

1. Free fluid to both biochemist — amylase, albumin
      and bacteriologist — culture (± Gram film)

2. If gallstones present or 'much suspected' (females; LFT pattern)
   — cholecystectomy
   — do operative cholangiogram
   — explore CBD *if* clear indication
   If possible use supraduodenal approach only;
   If necessary employ transduodenal approach

3. Examine whole of pancreas with care
   — remove infected necrotic tissue

4. Placement of drainage/lavage catheters
   (lesser sac, head pancreas, body and tail panceras)

5. Feeding jejunostomy

Antibiotic cover with Cefuroxime or a similar second generation Cephalosporin is adequate. It is worth remembering that only a small amount of dye should be put into the common duct to prevent obscuring a single stone at the lower end. If this should be identified then gentle removal using a Fogarty balloon catheter is recommended rather than passing metal probes or instruments through the lower end of the common bile duct. It is unusual to require to carry out a transduodenal sphincteroplasty but Figure 7.1 illustrates a patient in whom a gallstone had migrated into the proximal pancreatic duct and was removed by this approach. The operation was carried out within 6 hours of admission to hospital, the clinical diagnosis being suspected empyema of gall bladder.

Any free fluid present at the laparotomy should be sent for both bacteriological and biochemical analysis. As already noted it is most unusual for infection to be present where the primary problem is acute pancreatitis.

Diffuse fat necrosis may well be evident and should be ignored but any area of necrotic tissue around the pancreas (or within its substance) should be removed with care. It may be necessary to carry out a 'bacon slicing procedure' from the distal aspect of the pancreas towards the head to ident-

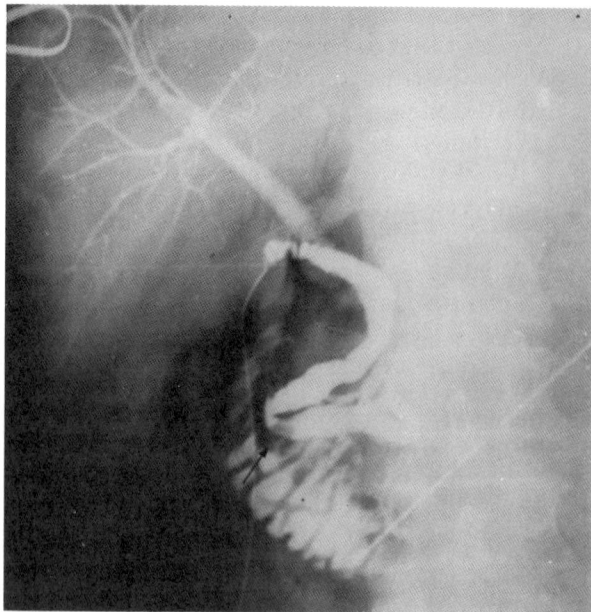

Fig. 7.1 Gallstone (arrowed) demonstrated in the pancreatic duct at operative cholangiogram with 24 hours of onset of symptoms wrongly diagnosed as acute cholecystitis. Acute pancreatitis the main pathology.

ify the extent of necrosis in the more severe instances of acutepancreatitis. Preoperative CT scanning will now delineate this phenomenon and provide guidance to the surgeon when necrosis of the gland is present.

Finally a decision must be taken as to the wisdom or otherwise of inserting a fine bore jejunostomy feeding tube and this is usually a good procedure, as it will minimise or eliminate the need for a central intravenous feeding line, the jejunostomy being more physiological and with less risk of infection. The major points to be considered when inside the abdomen are highlighted in Table 7.3.

Failed or failing conservative treatment

This is an area in which there is increasing interest at the present time. In a patient receiving optimum vigorous supportive therapy including mechanical ventilation and intravenous nutrition failure to improve may be associated with marked pyrexia where cholangitis or infection of pancreatic or peripancreatic necrotic tissue is the source. Cholangitis may be suspected clinically where rigors are present with associated severe pyrexia (temperature in excess of 39°C). In this situation endoscopic sphincterotomy or surgical intervention may well be necessary and is discussed in the next section. Where there is no pointer to the presence of gallstones it may well by that failure to improve is related to an extension of peri-pancreatic necrotic process. CT scanning can be most helpful in this situation and the newer scanners which necessitate a shorter time for the patient to hold his/her breath are obviously preferable. However, many hospitals in the United Kingdom do not have access to a CT scanner and this is true for many other parts of the world. In this situation blood cultures alone might indicate the nature of the problem and a straight direct antero-posterior abdominal X-ray may indicate the presence of gas bubbles in and around the pancreas. Should a CT scan or careful ultrasound scan be available then needle aspiration of the tissue in and around the pancreas will give information as to the presence or otherwise of bacteria. The group of patients who have infected necrotic material have a much poorer prognosis and it is essential that surgical excision with external drainage be carried out. The excision of necrotic tissue is best done by blunt finger dissection or gentle teasing out with forceps. Great care is required when close to large veins. In addition to CT scanning both endoscopic pancreatography and angiography may provide valuable information as to the nature of the problem and thereby guide the surgeon as to the best site for his incision and location of the trouble. It is the author's preference to use a transverse upper abdominal incision for most comprehensive exposure of the pancreas.

Experience with the approach, of combined clinical and CT scan assessment, for the management of complicated acute pancreatitis has come from Boston in the group directed by Banks and from Ulm in West Germany by the group directed by Beger (Bittner et al, 1984) Both claim the invaluable asset of frequent CT scans with modern machinery and a probable lowering of mortality with directed surgical intervention at varying times after the patients' admission to hospital. Each clinical group has found CT of great assistance in pinpointing sites for needle aspiration to base a judgement for or against surgical intervention dependent on the presence of sepsis.

Although recommendations for surgical excision of part or the whole of the pancreas have been made from time to time, and some anecdotal case reports have shown spectacular success associated with this radical approach in younger patients, only surgeons from Finland have reported on any reasonable numbers treated in this way. In an initial report on 30 young patients with a mean age of 37.4 years, Kivilaakso and co-workers performed 24 distal pancreatic resections and six more radical procedures with an overall mortality of 37% (Kivilaakso et al, 1981). Nearly all the patients had alcohol associated disease and were operated on at approximately 48 hours from admission to hospital. They were all judged to be failing with maximum conservative management.

In a further study of 45 patients with the most severe acute pancreatitis, representing less than 6% of all patients admitted to their own hospital, the same workers randomised the patients to maximum conservative supportive therapy including peritoneal lavage, or this treatment with pancreatic resec-

Table 7.4 Relationship between outcome and gross pathological changes in the pancreas (modified from Kivilaakso et al, 1984)

Patient group	Total necrosis	Diffuse necrosis	Local necrosis	Deaths
Resection (18)	7	7	4	4
Lavage (17)	5	10	2	8
Deaths	6	3	3	

tion added. Once again these were young patients with a mean age of 37 years, 30 of whom were male. Although the 18 patients randomised to resectional treatment had a lower mortality it was not statistically significantly different from the group treated without surgery (Table 7.4). In addition, they made an attempt to correlate the degree and extent of necrosis of the pancreas with outcome, but both the patients with total necrosis and local necrosis had a 50% mortality (Kivilaakso et al, 1984). The practice in Finland is not typical of many areas of the world but it does indicate that in the worst patients, provided they are young, the addition of surgical resectional procedures did not increase the mortality compared to their control group. The great difficulty for workers in other countries is to translate this type of experience and the critical question as to the necessity for removing uninfected necrotic material remains unanswered. There can be no debate that infected peripancreatic and pancreatic necrosis requires to be removed, if the patient is to have any prospect of survival. Multiple operations are sometimes required in an individual patient, but failure to operate invariably results in death while adequate surgery will result in approximately two-thirds of patients surviving. In the most severe cases it has been suggested that the abdominal wall should not be closed surgically, and that antiseptic soaked packs be placed within the peritoneal cavity and changed on a regular basis. Such patients are invariably within Intensive Care Units and on ventilator treatment, thus facilitating this form of approach. One of the regular problems with this type of patient is the lack of suitable drainage tubes to allow the necrotic material which may further accumulate after an initial operation, to pass to the exterior.

THE TIMING OF INTERVENTION IN PATIENTS WITH BILIARY ASSOCIATED ACUTE PANCREATITIS

During the last 5 years a number of approaches in timing of interventional procedures have been advocated. These can be subdivided into three categories:

(a) *Immediate intervention* (within 48 hours of hospital admission). This timing has been championed by Acosta and Stone from a surgical standpoint (Acosta et al, 1978; Stone et al, 1981), while a number of groups have suggested that immediate endoscopic sphincterotomy would also be an effective approach (Safrany & Cotton, 1981; Rosseland & Solhaug, 1984)

(b) *Early intervention* (between 2 and 7 days). This approach allows moretime for verification of the presence of gallstones and is favoured by Ranson, Kelly, Tondelli and our own group in Glasgow (Kelly, 1980; Ranson, 1979; Osborne et al, 1981; Tondelli et al, 1982).

(c) *Delayed intervention*. This is the traditional approach which advocates the patients being allowed a complete recovery from the episode of pancreatitis with subsequent planned admission for elective biliary surgery.

In the discussion and controversy which surrounds this subject some authors have not made it clear whether their policy applies 'across the board' to patients with mild and moderate pancreatitis through to the most severe forms of the disease where intensive care, including assisted ventilator therapy is often required within hours of hospital admission. Furthermore, especially in the area of surgical therapy, it is not always clear whether those who advocate the earlier surgical approaches apply them to the oldest group of patients. With these points in mind it is reasonable to cover the problems associated with each of these lines of management.

Immediate intervention

In terms of immediate intervention one of the bigger problems is being sure that the aetiology is attributable to gallstones. The Atlanta group (Stone et al, 1981) relied heavily on an absence of a history of alcohol intake. While Acosta's group took this into account they put great weight on the findings of liver function tests (Acosta et al, 1978). The surgical approach of Stone and his colleagues was a little unusual in that the only opening in the proximal area of the biliary tree was via the cystic duct through which the cholangiogram catheter and subsequently a Fogarty balloon catheter was passed. They created a surgical sphincteroplasty extending 2.0 to 2.5 cm along the lower bile duct and then divided the septum with the pancreatic duct. Reliance was then placed on retrieval of stones within the biliary tree from below using balloon catheters. Although mortality and morbidity were not significantly improved by immediate surgery compared to the group of patients who had delayed therapy, the total stay in hospital was significantly reduced with obvious advantages both to the patient and the community in terms of hospital economy (Stone et al, 1981). Acosta and his colleagues did not have a control group in their study but relied on historical 'controls' and claimed an advantage for immediate surgical intervention (Acosta et al, 1978).

Controlled studies of endoscopic sphincterotomy in acute pancreatitis are under way in various parts of the world and a preliminary report from Leicester in Great Britain (Leese et al, 1985) suggests that this may prove to be a viable option which will obviously be associated with less upset than a major surgical operation to the patients. Nevertheless, it must be remembered that this is a considerable intervention with potential deleterious effects to the patient as well as beneficial. One advantage is that the endoscopist can check whether or not gallstones are present by a diagnostic cannulation prior to any attempt at diathermy sphincterotomy. He, or she, therefore has a major advantage over the surgical approach in this respect. In addition, the respiratory upset of severe hypoxaemia which is a hallmark of acute pancreatitis would be considerably less from the intravenous sedation required to carry out ERCP compared to a general anaesthetic and a full surgical procedure. On balance therefore, it seems that clinicians who favour an early interventional approach will be more likely to utilise the choice of endoscopic sphincterotomy, contingent both on availability of local expertise and the knowledge that a cholecystectomy would be necessary in many patients at a subsequent time.

Early intervention

Those who favour early operation (2 to 7 days) have a considerable advantage in terms of time regarding investigation and delineation of the presence of gallstones. In addition, a selective policy is possible with regard to the patients with the most severe forms of acute pancreatitis being subject to operation or endoscopic sphincterotomy at an agreed time with intensive care clinicians. In our retrospective study it was clear that these patients represented particular problems and in some intances surgery was even delayed until a much later time on account of various system failures (Osborne et al, 1981). At the present stage of information it is difficult to be dogmatic about the optimum timing of intervention for these severely ill patients. While those who advocate immediate intervention and point to some patients who do exceptionally well, they do tend to forget that it is *transient* migration of gallstones which precipitate an attack of pancreatitis. True impaction of stones at the ampulla is a relatively uncommon entity while a case for checking whether or not impaction is present by diagnostic ERCP has already been inferred. With regard to the report from Switzerland (Tondelli et al, 1982) it was clear that immediate surgery was associated with a much higher mortality and for the same reasons both Kelly and Ranson in the United States favour delay of a few days before operation (Ranson, 1979; Kelly, 1980).

All of these clinicians are in little doubt that the advantages to the patient with mild or moderate pancreatitis in having eradication of stones from their biliary tree during the same admission are considerable. The doubts continue regarding an 'across the board' policy for those with the most severe forms of the disease.

All of the groups who have reported on biliary surgery or endoscopic sphincterotomy within 48 hours of hospitalisation have found a much higher incidence of stones within the common bile duct than in patients who have their procedures delayed for a few days or for many weeks. The incidence of CBD stones is in the region of 70% to 95% with the immediate approach and with the delayed approach being 15% and 20%.

Delayed intervention

The older school of thought which favours an appreciable time interval between the episode of pancreatitis and elective biliary surgery cannot be completely discounted as all the studies point to the risk in terms of mortality and morbidity being no higher, with the proviso that a recurrent attack of acute pancreatitis does not supervene in the interval period. The prediction of the onset of these further attacks is obviously an impossibility in terms of providing any guarantee for the patient and this fact, combined with the increased efficiency of the earlier surgical approaches, has resulted in a greater interest in stone eradication at the first admission to hospital.

SURGERY FOR LATE COMPLICATIONS

Pseudocyst

The role of surgery in the management of this condition is currently the most established therapy although for certain patients alternative approaches such as percutaneous aspiration of the pseudocyst are valid. The range of surgical options is considerable and is partly determined by the maturity of the pseudocyst and whether it is specifically a complication of acute or chronic pancreatitis. A major problem in assessing much of the literature on pancreatic pseudocyst is that clarification as to its relationship to acute or chronic pancreatitis is often imprecise. Furthermore, details as to the aetiology of the acute pancreatitis are frequently omitted. This is of considerable importance as it has recently been shown that biliary associated acute pancreatitis has a much higher morbidity and mortality than the more common association of pseudocyst with alcohol abuse and pancreatitis (Imrie & Shearer, 1985). The other major cause of pancreatitis which leads on to pseudocyst formation is pancreatic trauma.

When a pseudocyst develops within 14 to 20 days of an episode of acute pancreatitis there is almost a 50% prospect of spontaneous resolution without intervention. Where the patient's condition is stable it is fully justifiable to monitor the clinical condition and carry out regular ultrasound scans to determine whether the pseudocyst is prgressing or regressing in size. A pseudocyst of at least 5 cm diameter which is unchanging or increasing in diameter should be drained, especially if it has been present for as long as 6 weeks after the onset of the acute pancreatitis. Prospective studies carried out by the author have shown that there is a six times greater incidence of pseudocyst following an attack of acute pancreatitis of alcohol aetiology compared to a gallstone associated attack. The mortality and morbidity is many times greater in the infrequent cases associated with gallstones and this cannot be entirely attributable to the older age of the patient. Haemorrhage and sepsis are particularly daunting complications of such surgery and it is quite reasonable in the older patient with a gallstone associated pseudocyst to consider percutaneous drainage. However, this approach does not tackle the basic problem of the presence of gallstones and the risk of a further attack of acute pancreatitis, and in addition, the pseudocyst may recur, and frequently does, after percutaneous aspiration.

The best surgical approach in my opinion is to aim to drain the pseudocyst by an internal method, usually cystogastrostomy, and at the same procedure remove the gall bladder, carry out an operative cholangiogram and clear the common bile duct. Prophylactic antibiotic therapy given at the time of pre-medication for anaesthesia need not include metronidazole but must include a broad spectrum antibiotic to kill common biliary pathogens. A second or third generation cephalosporin or gentamicin combined with ampicillin is sensible in this situation.

Cystogastrostomy

A longitudinal incision is made in the anterior wall of the stomach and, having secured any bleeding from the edges of that incision the pseudocyst, which is usually adherent to the posterior wall and bulging anterorly, is aspirated. The purpose of aspiration is to determine the type of fluid within the pseudocyst so that in the presence of a blood filled cyst control of the situation is not lost and it should be possible to secure the feeding vessels prior to fully opening the structure. In the normal situation an incision through the posteror wall of the stomach and then through the anterior wall of the pseudocyst is advised to be not less than 5 cm, and preferably nearer 10 cm in length. The aspirates and specimens are taken for bacteriology and also for biochemistry to check both the amylase and albumin content. It is common to find peri-pancreatic slough in the depth of the pseudocyst. If this can be removed by gentle, very gentle, finger dissection then this should be done. However, if it does not mobilise with ease it is better left in situ. The edges of the anterior wall of the pseudocyst and the posterior wall of stomach are then sutured together with interrupted dexon or vicryl and the anterior gastrotomy subsequently closed. Although some prefer to leave a tube through the anterior abdominal wall and the anterior gastric wall into the pseudocyst cavity across the posterior wall anastomosis, e.g. a Foley catheter, this is unnecessary.

Other techniques

In the minority of patients who have pseudocysts not adherent to the posterior wall of the stomach the location of the pseudocyst will determine what is the best treatment. Small lesions in the head of the pancreas may be treated by simple aspiration at laparotomy, while larger ones can be treated by anastomosis to the adjacent duodenal wall, cystduodenostomy.

Larger pseudocysts away from this location can be treated by drainage into a loop of jejunum, or into a Roux loop. All of these methods of internal drainage are associated with better results than external drainage procedures which are complicated by fistula and abscess formation. It should be noted in the patients who do not have a mature and tough pseudocyst wall that external drainage may be the only possible procedure and that the poorer results with this type of drainage may be simply a reflection of the more severely ill patients who tend to have this problem.

Percutaneous aspiration

The exact role of percutaneous aspiration of pancreatic pseudocyst is a little unclear. The two options are either to drain the pseudocyst with a Chiba needle or with a catheter threaded over the needle at the time of the procedure which can be guided by either ultrasonic or CT scanning. The advocates of this approach point to the relatively minor upset to the patient, while acknowledging the frequent need for multiple aspiration to be carried out. It has been contended that the catheter drainage is the more successful approach but the numbers of patients currently published using either percutaneous technique is still limited. Multiple aspirations increase the risk of infecting a sterile pseudocyst and there can be no question that the slough, which is so frequently present in the base of the pseudocyst, will certainly not be removed by this approach and, being dead tissue, is at increased risk of infection. Therefore, from a therapeutic standpoint percutaneous aspiration or catheter drainage is sensible as a temporary measure in a particularly ill patient considered unfit for surgery but cannot be reckoned the best treatment in the present state of knowledge which leaves internal surgical drainage as the desired approach. This is associated with a very low risk and good prospects of cure at the first treatment both in patients whose aetiology is alcohol abuse and traumatic pancreatitis. The results in those with gallstone associated acute pancreatitis complicated by pseudocyst are less good.

Immediately following surgical drainage of a pancreatic pseudocyst elevated serum and/or urine amylase levels will return to normal rapidly and the patient's well being usually improves quite rapidly too. In particular the quite severe catabolic state which accompanies some pseudocysts and necessitates total parenteral nutrition improves very soon after adequate treatment. In the more severely ill patients who may never have recovered a satisfactory clinical condition since the onset of their acute pancreatitis (often those who require an external drainage procedure) a feeding jejunostomy can be of great help in the postoperative management.

Pancreatic abscess

Under the generic heading of pancreatic abscess come two distinct categories of problem with a very different outcome.

Well circumscribed abscess

This may derive from infection occurring in a pseudocyst, or be infected from a very early stage. This type of problem is usually effectively dealt with by external drainage. Occasionally recollection of the abscess may occur and a further drainage procedure be required, but the complication rate of this type of pancreatic or peri-pancreatic abscess is much lower than the second form.

Diffuse sepsis

A diffuse peri-pancreatic, or even pancreatic, sepsis with infection spreading along tissue planes in the retroperitoneal spaces. Often the pancreatic tissue itself is partially or completely necrotic and requires removal together with drainage of all the infected tissue. Complete debridement of compromised tissue, as well as exploration of all possible extensions of the original source of sepsis in or close to the pancreas is mandatory. Neglect of surgical drainage results in 100% mortality and localised drainage procedures invariably result in more operations being necessary, should the patient survive the first one.

An anterior surgical approach is usually essential through either a wide transverse upper abdominal incision or a long paramedian vertical incision. Isotope gallium or labelled leucocyte nuclear medicine scans may be valuable, but ultimately success or failure is often dependent on the care with which a very complete and tedious laparotomy is performed. Full display of all sections of the anterior aspect of the pancreas must be carried out and mobilisation of the posterior aspect of the head of the gland, the lesser sac, and the tissue around the spleen must be carefully performed. The paracolic gutters should be needle aspirated and probed for extensions of pus. Particular difficulty can be encountered in laying open extensions of pus superiorly from the pancreatic bed towards the diaphragm in the retroperitoneal planes. Although relatively unusual, this type of problem frequently complicates the more severe episodes of acute pancreatitis where intensive initial conservative management has resulted in the patient's survival. No surgeon should feel any sense of shame in requiring to perform two or more procedures to drain such infected tissue and persistence of fever, leucocytosis or any other objective signs of recurrent abscess necessitate further laparotomy.

There is a world of difference between a well circumscribed abscess and this type of problem, where even in the most exeprienced centres with specialist care, mortality rates range from 30% to 70%. Intravenous antibiotic therapy tends to be quite ineffective while lavage of the drainage areas through soft plastic catheters and sump drains using antiseptic solution is to be commended. This may be required for many weeks.

Pancreatic fistulae

These often occur following drainage of a pancreatic abscess and may be shown to communicate with the main pancreatic duct, small bowel or large bowel, and less frequently the stomach. The initial management of such problems is usually by total parenteral nutrition using a long central intravenous line. About half the cases will result in spontaneous closure associated with TPN while the remainder require some sort of surgical procedure. Sinograms can be helpful (Fig. 7.2) and surgical disconnection of fistulae or proximal re-routing of the bowel indicated. Fistulae do not represent either numerically, or in terms of severity, nearly the problem of pancreatic sepsis and most patients survive.

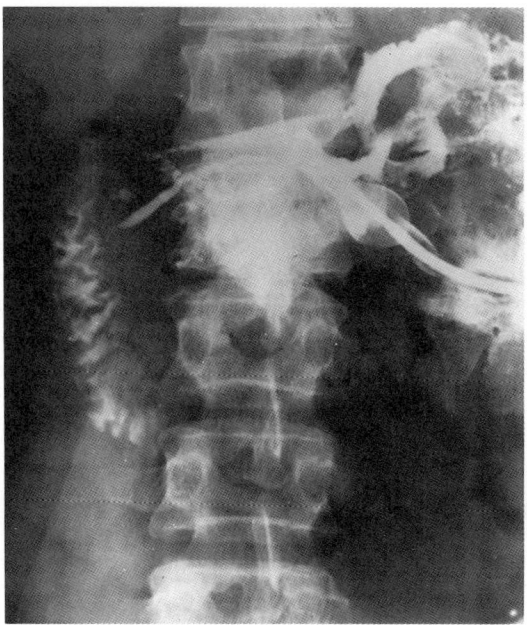

Fig. 7.2 Sinogram via Foley catheter outlining the pancreatic duct, duodenum, distal transverse and proximal descending colon

Pancreatic ascites

This is a relatively unusual complication of either acute or chronic pancreatitis and will usually result from the rupture of a pancreatic pseudocyst which communicates with the main pancreatic duct, or an internal fistula from the main pancreatic duct first to the lesser sac and thereafter the collection of pancreatic juice in the peritoneal cavity occurs. Some have tried to introduce large amounts of Trypsin into the duodenum in an effort to close down the pancreatic function and Somatostatin might be particularly helpful in this context, although I have never used it. An endoscopic pancreatogram can outline the site of disruption at the main pancreatic duct and either controlled drainage of the ducts at the point into a Roux loop or distal resection of the gland from that point may be performed. Sometimes the exact site of the leak may be difficult to pinpoint at operation and simple external drainage, together with a feeding jejunostomy or continued TPN can result in closure of the pancreatic duct leak.

Pancreatic trauma

In blunt abdominal trauma from sporting injuries in games such as football and rugby (as well as steering wheel injuries), complete or partial transection of the body of pancreas against the vertebral column may occur. In this situation a check of blood and urine levels of amylase or lipase may well give an early indication of the nature of the problem. Immediate surgical intervention is indicated as an early operation wil allow fairly easy completion of a partial transection and removal of the distal transected gland. Small traumatic lesions at the tail of the pancreas may occur in association with a ruptured spleen, but the most feared type of blunt abdominal injury is where the head of the gland is involved. This usually occurs together with duodenal injuries and the infection rate is high. Furthermore, it is particularly difficult to carry out a pancreaticoduodenectomy when the bile duct and pancreatic duct are of normal size. Technically the dissection may also be complicated by damage to major blood vessels such as the superior mesenteric vein and splenic vein and several different views have been expressed as to the best line for the surgeon to take in managing this particular problem. None of these is ideal and for the moderately experienced or inexperienced surgeon it is best to simply leave a soft sump drain, or better two, to remove fluid from this area and to arrange transport to a centre of specialist experience in pancreatic surgery.

RECURRENT ACUTE PANCREATITIS

Although it is most usual to find this associated with alcohol abuse or persistence of gallstones, occasionally it has been described as associated with a condition known as pancreas divisum. In this condition the two main pancreatic ducts in development, i.e. that serving the ventral pancreas (duct of Wirsung); and that serving the dorsal pancreas (duct of Satorini) remain separate. In a proportion of patients with this abnormality pancreatitis affects one part of the gland only, usually that drained by the dorsal pancreas through the duct of Santorini. Sphincteroplasty of the duct of Santorini in this situation has been associated with improvement in the problem of recurrent pain and episodes of pancreatitis in some patients, while others have not been helped to all by this procedure (Russell et al, 1984). The results of resectional operations have been unpredictable and quite frequently disappointing (Bradley et al, 1984). The recommendation

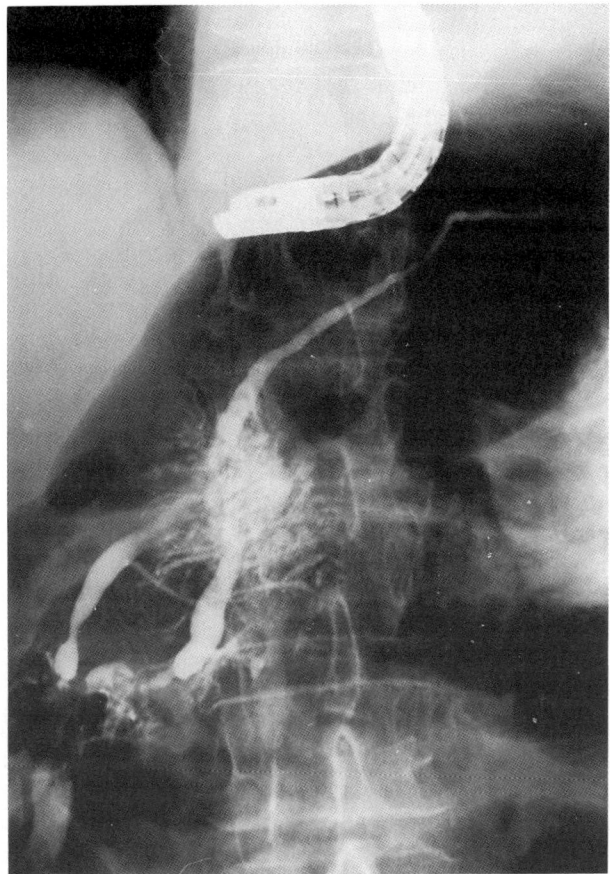

Fig. 7.3 ERCP in patient with pancreas divisum, unusual in that changes of chronic pancreatitis were confined to the ventral pancreas. In this 77 year old patient no operation has been performed.

with regard to surgery in this condition is to proceed very cautiously and to make the patient fully aware of the unpredictable outcome of present therapy. An example of pancreas divisum (or non-fusion of the pancreatic ducts) is shown in Figure 7.3.

SURGERY FOR CHRONIC PANCREATITIS

While there is little debate as to the advisability of surgical treatment for cysts and pseudocysts associated with the presence of chronic pancreatitis where the patient is suffering pain, there is some variation in approach to the management of pain in the majority of patients with this condition.

Where the aetiology of chronic pancreatitis can be established it is most frequently due to long term alcohol abuse, but there remains a significant proportion of patients in whom no aetiology is ever determined. Pain, being a subjective phenomenon, can be difficult to assess, and it is wise to bring these patients into hospital for a period of assessment to determine analgesic requirements as well as to carry out investigations of pancreatic structure and function. A psychiatric assessment and full personality assessment is advisable and the radiological abnormalities which are demonstrated at ERCP must be considered with the patient's clinical history and overall assessment. Approximately 15% of patients with chronic pancreatitis have no pain and the remainder will be troubled by pain of varying severity.

The evidence from the natural history of the disease (Ammann et al, 1984) is that pain usually becomes a lesser problem after a number of years but this is a small consolation to the patient or to those looking after him throughout the years until the pain regresses. The cause of pain may be due to strictures or stones in the main pancreatic duct system causing back pressure in the drainage area of the pancreas. Gross fibrosis associated with chronic pancreatitis may cause nerve damage within the gland and these are considered to be the two major causes of pain. Characteristically the pain comes on about 30 to 40 minutes following a meal and is relieved by the patient leaning forward in a sitting position. However, many patients with this condition suffer episodes of pain which are unrelated to food and vary both in the intensity and duration of the problem. The target of the surgeon involved in the management of such patients is to relieve the pain while conserving the maximum amount of pancreatic tissue. The two major surgical approaches have been to drain the pancreatic duct system behind the obstruction by anastomosing the pancreatic duct to the jejunum either directly or via a Roux loop. The alternative approach has been to resect the most severely diseased pancreatic tissue and usually this approach is used to deal with the small cysts and pseudocysts that can be associated with chronic pancreatitis.

When surgery is considered the only satisfactory method left to treat the pain of chronic pancreatitis it is best to consider all the aspects of the individual patient's problem together and to endeavour to have a course of action based on pancreatogram appearance and the clinical problem, especially the location of the patient's pain. A final decision as to the best therapy in terms of drainage procedure or surgical resection may only be possible at the time of laparotomy. Cancer of the pancreas may be exceedingly difficulty to differentiate from chronic pancreattis, even at operation, although certain useful blood markers which differentiate the two conditions have been described in recent publications. Serum testosterone levels are usually low in carcinoma and normal in chronic pancreatitis in men, who represent the majority of patients (Shearer et al, 1984). Likewise the radio-immunoassay of the commercially available antigen CA 19–9 may also prove a valuable test. Even the pathologist may have difficulty differentiating the two conditions, especially on a frozen section. The problems of a differentiation of the two diseases is highlighted by the presence of a number of patients with carcinoma in most published series of chronic pancreatitis and vice versa.

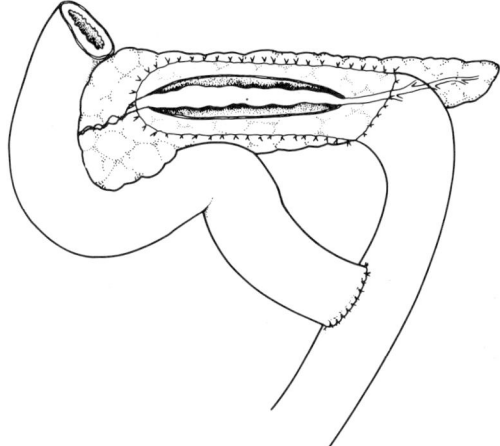

Fig. 7.4 Side to side pancreatico-jejunostomy of the type described by Partington and Rochelle

Improvements to main pancreatic duct drainage

Under this heading there have been many different procedures described.

Side-to-side pancreatico-jejunostomy

In this operation a Roux loop is created and the end of the Roux loop is closed over and a side to side anastomosis made with the hardened pancreatic tissue over an opened duct using interrupted non-absorbable sutures. In this operation the spleen is usually not disturbed and both blood loss and morbidity are low. The success of the operation in relieving pain has now been described by a number of groups and is usually satisfactory when patient selection has been carefully restricted to those with a long area of dilated duct behind a single stricture or a number of dilatations, all of which are laid open. This operation is an improvement on the earlier operation described by Peustow and Gillesby in which the tail and body of the pancreas are invaginated into the end of the Roux loop which was then sutured around the mid section of the pancreas. Although this operation is rarely, if ever, practised today the name of Puestow is often wrongly attributed to all types of drainage procedure.

An alternative type of drainage operation more recently introduced by Lord Smith and popularised by Knight (Fig. 7.5) utilises anastomosis of the end of the Roux loop on to the side of the pancreatic duct at the point of maximum dilatation, sometimes employing a T-tube placed in the pancreatic duct to splint the anastomosis temporarily. The earlier operations which employed anastomosis of the end of the Roux loop onto the cut surface of the distal pancreas are only infrequently used as this method of drainage is less satisfactory and there is also a tendency at a later stage for the Roux loop to become detached from the pancreas.

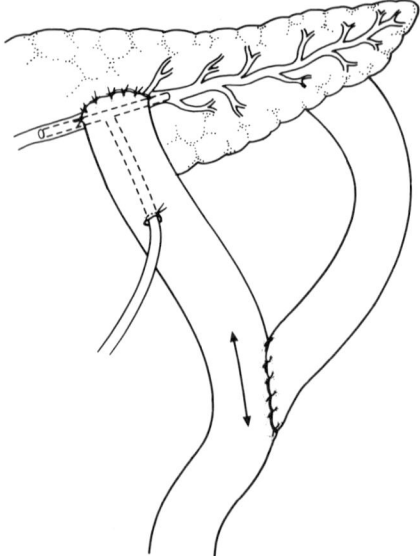

Fig. 7.5 Alternative pancreatico-jejunostomy (Smith and Knight) in which only a small area of the pancreatic duct is anastomosed to the end of the Roux loop

Surgical sphincteroplasty

Surgical sphincteroplasty of the ampulla of vater to lay open the duct of Wirsung was initially practised as a rather empiric procedure for the management of pancratic pain with indifferent and bad results in terms of pain relief. More recently with the important and valuable information derived from preoperative ERCP it has been proposed that a subgroup of patients with chronic pancratitis who have a single stricture at or close to the ampulla may be suitably treated by sphincteroplasty and wide laying open of the ampulla with, or without, extraction of pancreatic duct stones (Hansell et al, 1986). The pancreatic duct stones are largely composed of calcium carbonate with a small amount of phosphate and can be removed by a Dormia basket and even Fogarty catheter, although this tends to be ruptured by the spicules of the calcium carbonate stones. Small artery forceps and even Vokmann's spoon have been employed to remove the stones and results in this small group of patients are promising.

Endoscopic sphincterotomy

Endoscopic sphincterotomy of the pancreatic duct is difficult to achieve because of the angles at which the endoscope tends to lie within the duodenum, whereas satisfactory sphincterotomy of the bile duct is much easier to perform. Furthermore, the removal of stones by an endoscopic approach is beset by the manner in which the stones tend to embed in the walls of the main pancreatic duct.

The introduction of a latex type gel either endoscopically or at operation to block the whole of the main pancreatic duct as a treatment of pain of chronic pancreatitis was popular in Germany a number of years ago, but is now considered unsatisfactory, except for one group of surgeons who carry out the procedure in conjunction with a Whipple operation.

Resectional surgery

Distal pancreatectomy

The most frequently performed operation with the lowest morbidity and mortality is distal resection of chronically inflamed pancreas when the disease is restricted to this area. Both pancreatic cysts and pseudocysts associated with chronic pancreatitis are frequently in the area of the gland anterior or to the left of the vertebral column and this operation can be fairly simply carried out in conjunction with splenectomy. With gross pancreatic inflammation it is virtually impossible to remove the distal pancreas and preserve the spleen because of the adherence of the inflamed tissue of the pancreas to the splenic vessels. While some create a Roux loop and anastomose this to the cut surface of the pancreas it has already been mentioned that such loops tend to part company with the pancreatic tissue after a period of time. It is the author's practice to simply sew over the pancreatic duct with fine vascular suture or a metal clip, and then to close over the cut surface of the gland with interrupted heavy silk sutures (Fig. 7.6). Using this approach pancreatic fistulae have rarely been encountered. When unfortunate enough to be dealing with such a fistula a period of intravenous parenteral nutrition usually is sufficient to encourage the fistula to close.

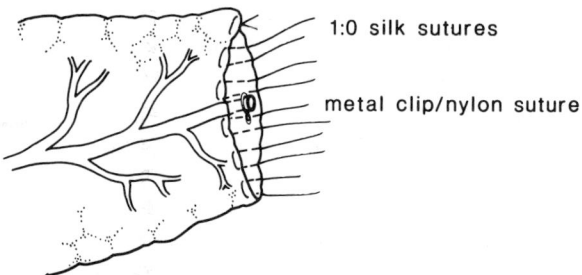

1:0 silk sutures

metal clip/nylon suture

Fig. 7.6 A simple and effective method of closure of the cut surface of the pancreas

Sub-total pancreatectomy

More extensive resections moving across the line of superior mesenteric vein towards the curve of the duodenum carry a higher operative morbidity and postoperative problems associated with diabetes are naturally more frequent. The most extensive operation of this kind, short of a total pancreatectomy, includes the removal of all but a small percentage of the gland lying in the curve of the duodenum. This so-called 95% pancreatectomy or sub-total pancreatectomy can be somewhat hazardous in terms of preservation of the vascularity of the duodenal loop. Some authors have included a fair number of these cases in their personal series (Frey et al, 1976) with good results but the number of patients warranting this approach in my practice has been very restricted. The question must also be asked what is the gain for the patient with chronic pancreatitis as opposed to the simpler operation of total pancreatectomy. The answer is that the diabetes which ensues may be easier to control and the continuity of the alimentary canal is maintained. This latter point obviously means that blind loop problems do not occur and absorption tends to be better.

Whipple's operation

Resection of the head of the gland in the form of a Whipple operation has been most frequently practised in France as a surgical management of chronic pancreatitis. In the patients who have most prolific disease affecting the head of the gland it can be a very satisfactory operaton and it has been argued by Longmire that in such patients whose chronic inflammaory process is predominantly in the head of the gland delay in carrying out surgery results in eventual destruction of the body and tail of the gland. Most surgeons carrying out a pancreatico-duodenectomy for chronic pancreatitis today would attempt to maintain the integrity of the whole stomach and the pylorus, either anastomosing the cut surface of the proximal duodenum to the end of the Roux loop or to its side. Although the number of patients dealt with in this way has so far been small most surgeons carrying out the procedure are impressed with the better long-term results, while conceding that there may be problems in gastric emptying in the initial 6–8 weeks after surgery. The anastomosis between the pancreas and the end or side of the Roux loop in the Whipple operation is the anastomosis which is most prone to complications in terms of leakage and haemorrhage. A technique of buttress suturing with heavy silk sutures which is a modification of a procedure originally described by Warren has been successfully employed with very few complications in our own institution (Fig. 7.7). Others have felt the anastomosis so risky that they have blocked the pancreatic duct and abandoned the exocrine part of the gland, preferring to avoid the risk of this anastomosis

Total pancreatectomy

Total pancreatectomy for chronic pancreatitis has occasionally been practised as a primary procedure but is more frequently carried out as an end stage to a number of lesser operations and the long-term results in terms

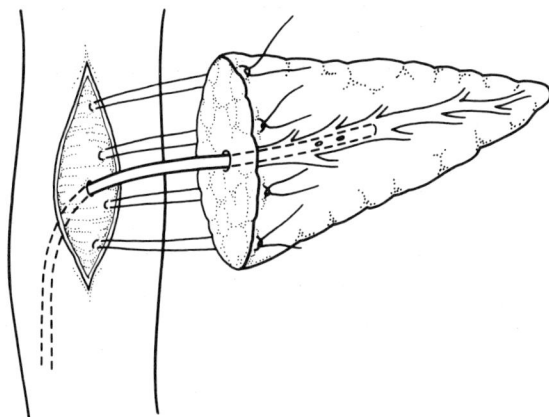

Fig. 7.7 Modified Warren end to side pancreatico-jejunostomy. The incision in the jejunum only includes the serosa and part of the muscle layer. The heavy sutures between pancreas and jejunum of 1/0 silk. Fine vicryl suture between the pancreatic duct and the jejunal mucosa should be placed and final anterior layer of 2/0 silk between the anterior cut surface of the pancreas and the lateral border of the jejunal incision. Pancreatic duct to jejunal mucosa secured with two fine vicryl sutures.

of morbidity and mortality are not encouraing (Braasch et al, 1978). Nevertheless, it may be the best operation for a small proportion of patients and, with developments in pancreatic transplanation may have a greater role in the future. All groups of surgeons carrying out this operation have experienced occasional problems, with severe hypoglycaemia being the most feared. This may be due to the loss of glucagon and other islet hormones such as Somatostatin and the abrupt drops in sugar have been associated with death in some of the patients at varying times from a few weeks to many years after operation. Pancreatic supplementation to make up for the exocrine gland loss at best results in a patient being anything from 12% to 25% below their optimum weight. It is therefore appropriate that the surgeon bears in mind the price to the patient of this radical approach when balancing the equation of pain relief with loss of function.

Coeliac ganglion block or excision

The practice of percutaneous coeliac block using alcohol based solutions by percutaneous or operative means has not been blessed with long-term success in terms of pain relief. At best a period from 2 to 3 years pain relief can be expected and the complications of the procedure which include impotence and lower limb paralysis are such that at least one group has felt that the procedure can not be recommended for use in the management of chronic pancreatitis, especially in young patients; whereas it is certainly a valuable procedure for pain relief in those with carcinoma of pancreas (Leung et al, 1983). Operative excision of the coeliac ganglion is a tricky procedure as the nerve tissue may be adherent to a chronically inflamed pancreas in a patient who has had a number of procedures carried out previously. It can be difficult to dissect away from the adjacent artery and modern carefully monitored studies of the efficacy or otherwise of this approach are yet lacking.

Other surgical procedures

Duodenal bypass

Occasional patients with severe chronic pancreatitis affecting the head of the gland may present with a picture similar to pyloric stenosis due to encroachment upon the neighbouring duodenum, A barium study will show a very narrowed duodenum and gastroenterostomy is the best method of relieving this problem.

Biliary bypass

External compression of the lower CBD by chronically inflamed tissue in the head of the pancreas may present as obstructive jaundice with or without cholangitis. The radiological appearance of the bile duct is characteristic and often described as a 'rat-tail deformity'. In a proportion of patinets this form of jaundice subsides spontaneously and no intervention is required. However, persistence of jaundice or recurrent cholangitis should be dealt with in a positive manner and the most effective one is to perform a choledocho-jejunostomy to Roux loop of jejunum. It is unusual for the bilirubin level to rise above 150 micrograms/ litre from chronic pancreatitis and the usual pattern is to find the bilirubin level in the region of 30–120 micrograms/ litre. It is in this group of patients that particular difficulty may be encountered in striving to differentiate chronic pancreatitis from carcinoma. The blood markers which have been described earlier in the chapter should be utilised and also needle aspiration of the head of pancreas to obtain cytology.

Pancreatic biopsy

The safest method to obtain a biopsy of pancreas is to carry out a fine needle aspiration and to examine the tissue cytologically. The next most popular method is using the Tru-cut biopsy needle, passing it through the lateral wall of duodenum and then the medial wall into either the superior or inferior aspect of the head of the gland. This is considered reasonably safe as fistula formation, which is the major problem associated with biopsy, tends to resolve in a drainage into the duodenum. The desired piece of pancreatic tissue may not be able to be reached by such a method and occasionally a direct needle biopsy of another part of the gland is performed. Should a pancreatic fistula develop then treatment as described earlier should be instituted in the form of parenteral nutrition.

An alternative method of obtaining a satisfactory pancreatic biopsy is to take a scalpel and plane a piece of tissue from the relevant part of the gland.

REFERENCES

Acosta J M, Rossi R, Galli O M R, Pellegrini C A, Skinner D B 1978 Early surgery for acute gallstone pancreatitin: evaluation of a systemic approach. Surgery 83: 367–70

Amman R W, Akovbiantz A, Largiader F, Schueler G 1984 Course and outcome of chronic pancreatitis. Longitudinal study of a mixed medical-surgical series of 245 patients. Gastroenterology 86: 820–828

Bittner R, Beger H G, Block S, Buchler M 1984 The role of infection in pancreatic necrosis. Digestion 30:123

Blair A J, Russell R C G, Cotton P B 1984 Resection for pancreatitis in patients with pancreas divisum. Annals of Surgery 200: 590–594

Bradley J S, Bradley P, McMahon M J 1981 Diagnostic peritoneal lavage in acute pancreatitis, the value of microscopy of the fluid. British Journal of Surgery 68: 245–246

Bradley J W, Vito L, Nugent F W 1978 Total pancreatectomy for end stage chronic pancreatitis. Annals of Surgery 188: 317–322

Frey C F, Child C G, Fry W 1976 Pancreatectomy for chronic pancratitis. Annals fo Surgery 184: 403–414

Hansell D T, Gillespie G, Imrie C W 1986 Effective trans-ampullary extraction of stones in the manageent of chronic pancreatitis. Surgery, Gynecology and Obstetrics (in press)

Imrie C W et al 1974 a pattern of serum amylase results in patients with perforated duodenal ulcer. Journal of the Royal College of Surgeons of Edinburgh

Imrie C W, Benjamin I S, Ferguson J C et al 1978 A single centre double-blind trial of Trasylol therapy in primary acute pancreatitis. British Journal of Surgery 65: 337–341

Imrie C W, Shearer M G 1986 Diagnosis and management of severe acute pancratitis. Recent Advances in Surgery 12: 143–154

Kelly T R 1980 Gallstone pancreatitis: The timing of surgery. Surgery 88: 345–349

Kivilaakso E, Lempinen M, Makelainen A, Nikki P, Schroder T 1984 Pancreatic resection versus peritoneal lavation for acute fulminant pancreatitis. Annals of Surgery 199: 426–428

Leese T, Neoptolemos J P, Carr-Locke D L 1985 Successes, failures, early complications and their management following endoscopic sphincterotomy: Results in 394 consecutive patients from a single centre. British Journal of Surgery 72: 215–219

Leung J W, Bowen-Wright M, Aveling W, Shorvon P J, Cotton P B 1983 Coeliac plexus block for pain in pancreatic cancer and chronic pancreatitis. British Journal of Surgery 70: 730–732

Osborne D H, Imrie C W, Carter D C 1981 Biliary surgery in the same admission for acute pancreatitis. British Journal of Surgery 68: 758–761

Ottinger L W 1978 Occlusion of the superior mesenteric artery. Annals of Surgery 188: 721–731

Ranson J H C, Rifkind K M, Turner K W 1976 Prognostic signs and nonoperative peritoneal lavage in acute pancreatitis. Surger, Gynecology and Obstetrics 143: 209–219

Ranson J H C 1979 The timing of biliary surgery in acute pancreatitis. Annals of Surgery 189: 654–663

Ranson J H C 1984 Acute pancreatitis, pathogenesis, outcome and treatment In: Clinics in Gastroenterology, Saunders, London, p 843–864

Rosseland A R, Solhaug J H 1984 Early or delayed endoscopic papillotomy (EPT) in gallstone pancreatitis. Annals of Surgery 199: 165–167

Russell R C G, Wong N W, Cotton P B 1984 Accessory sphincterotomy (endoscopic and surgical) in patients with pancreas divisum. British Journal of Surgery 71: 954–957

Safrany L, Cotton P B 1981 A preliminary report: Urgent duodenoscopic sphincterotomy for acute gallstone pancreatitis. Surgery 89: 424–428

Shearer M G, Taggart D P, Gray C, Imrie C W 1984 Useful differentiation between pancreatic cancer and chronic pancreatitis by serum testosterone. Digestion 30:106

Stone H H, Fabian T C, Dunlop W E 1981 Gallstone pancreatitis. Biliary tract pathology in relation to time of operation. Annals of Surgery 194: 305–312

Tondelli P, Stutz K, Harder S et al 1982 Acute gallstone pancreatitis: best timing for biliary pancreatitis. British Journal of Surgery 69: 709–710

Trapnell J E, Anderson M C 1964 Role of early laparotomy in acute pancreatitis. Annals of Surger 165: 49–55

Wilson C, Imrie C W 1986 Amylase and gut infarction. British Journal of Surgery (in press)

The management of liver metastases

INTRODUCTION

The development of liver metastases arising from solid tumours are met with feelings of resignation by most surgeons and patients. Treatment is usually limited to alleviating those symptoms which develop in what are usually only a few months remaining in the patients' lives.

Hepatic involvement from most tumours implies more widespread dissemination. However, some tumours may have only spread to the liver at the time of presentation. The majority of these cases are colorectal primaries which enter the mesenteric vein without lymph node involvement. Colorectal carcinoma accounts for 90% of such cases but intestinal leiomyosarcoma and carcinoid tumours may behave in a similar fashion. Much more rarely tumours from a distant site (in terms of circulation) can present with liver metastases only, e.g. mammary carcinoma, ocular melanoma and nephroblastoma.

Although exciting technological advances have been made in the treatment of liver metastases, in only a few patients have they had significant benefit. Early detection and appropriate treatment of the primary are important to prevent metastases. Taylor et al (1985) have shown that adjuvant portal vein infusional chemotherapy to the liver in selected patients with primary colorectal carcinoma may reduce the incidence of liver metastases.

In view of the dual blood supply to the liver, avenues have been explored to determine whether selective therapy by way of one or both of these vessels can control liver metastases without impairment of normal hepatic function and so lessen the marked side effects of systemic chemotherapy.

Any reader making a critical assessment of the literature in terms of liver metastases must be aware of their natural history. Within a group of patients with a single histological type of tumour, there is a spectrum of heterogeneity in terms of behaviour and survival.

NATURAL HISTORY

Liver metastases are the second most common site of spread from tumours

125

after lymph nodes. In a study of 9000 autopsies with metastases by Pikren et al (1982), 50% had liver involvement. The actual frequency of liver metastases were noted in the following tumours, 75% of pancreatic primaries, breast (60%), extrahepatic biliary (60%), colorectal (57%) and stomach (49%).

The natural history of colorectal liver metastases provides the clearest picture and most studies refer to those cases that are synchronous although Cady and Oberfield (1974) showed no difference in terms of survival irrespective of whether they were synchronous or metachronous following treatment. Fifty per cent of patients with colorectal carcinoma will develop liver metastases and in 90% they will present within 2 years of resection. Once they have been diagnosed, the median survival for the whole group is roughly 10 months (Table 8.1). When a mean figure is quoted this is deceptive as there are a few patients who will survive a number of years. However, 90% will be dead within 18 months of diagnosis.

It is important to remember that patients often have local recurrence and extrahepatic spread at time of death (Gilbert, 1983), although Mansfield et al (1969) found that it was the presence of liver metastases which caused the death of patients rather than extrahepatic disease.

Table 8.1   The natural history of liver metastases (survival in months)

Study	Survival mean	(months) median	Primary tumour	Extent of hepatic disease
Pestana et al (1964)	9	—	colorectal	
Jaffe et al (1968)	5.3	—	colorectal	
	2	—	stomach and pancreas	
Cady et al (1970)	13	7		
Nielson et al (1971)	18	—	colorectal	— few
	9	—		— several
	5	—		— multiple
Wood et al (1976)	16.7	—	colorectal	— solitary
	10.6	—		— one lobe
	3.1	—		— both lobes
Bengmark et al (1978)	6	—	colorectal	
	6	—	stomach	
	4	—	pancreatic	
Davis et al (1973)	—	38	carcinoid	symptomatic
Einhorn et al (1974)	—	7	melanoma	

Prognostic factors

It has been found that certain features affect the prognosis of patients with liver metastases (Table 8.2). This is important when considering treatment or matching patients in therapeutic trials.

Solitary liver metastases are associated with a longer survival compared to multiple metastases. Wood et al (1976) found a mean survival of 17 months for patients with solitary liver metastases and only 4.5 months for those with multiple deposits from colorectal carcinoma. Symptomatic

Table 8.2 Factors that help predict survival

Poor prognostic features	Better prognostic features
Multiple metastases	Solitary metastasis
>50% liver replacement	< 25% liver replacement
Extrahepatic disease	Limited to liver
Rapidly enlarging deposits	
Low serum albumin	
Elevated serum bilirubin	
Abnormal clotting	
Ascites	
Primary tumour untreated	Resected primary
Pancreatic and gastric primaries	Carcinoid and Islet-cell primaries

patients, abnormal liver chemistry, the percentage of hepatic replacement (PHR) and whether the disease is confined to liver are the major prognostic factors and these are important when evaluating treatment. Pettavel et al (1984) have recommended a staging system which incorporates all these factors: stage 1 has less than 25% involvement, stage 2 25–75% and stage 3 greater than 75%. This system, known as the Lausanne staging, also takes into account abnormal biochemistry and whether the patient is symptomatic. Low serum albumin, abnormal clotting and elevated bilirubin are indicative of widespread destruction of the liver with end-stage disease although simple mechanical occlusion of a major biliary duct must be excluded.

When Jaffe et al (1968) studied a group of patients with liver metastases from an heterogenous group of primary tumours, the median survival was only 3 months whilst the subgroup of colorectal carcinoma was 5.3 months. The poor prognosis with metastases from gastric or pancreatic tumours is often the result of a longer natural history of the primary tumour prior to symptomatic presentation with liver metastases at a more advanced stage. Liver metastases from intestinal carcinoid tumours and pancreatic islet-cell tumours are unusual in that they are often associated with a natural history of many years (Table 8.1).

PATHOLOGICAL AND ANATOMICAL FACTORS GOVERNING TREATMENT

It has been shown that human liver metastases almost invariably develop a blood supply that is fed by the hepatic artery (Breedis & Young, 1954; Healey, 1965). This is irrespective of whether they have arrived by way of the mesenteric or systemic circulation. As a metastasis grows new vessel formation occurs at the periphery whilst the centre usually becomes progressively necrotic. The portal vein rarely contributes to the tumour blood supply although it can increase following hepatic artery ligation (Taylor et al, 1979).

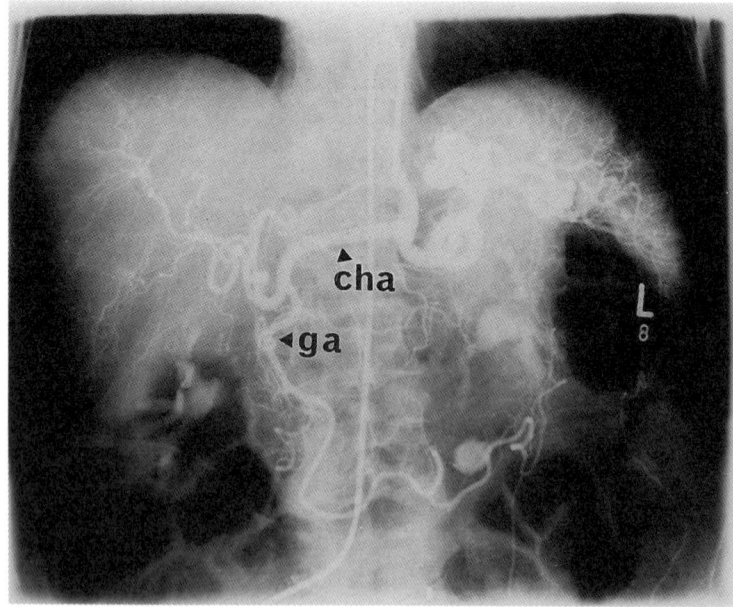

Fig. 8.1 Normal hepatic arterial supply — right and hepatic arteries arising from common hepatic artery (cha = common hepatic artery, rha = right hepatic artery, lha = left hepatic artery, ga = gastroduodenal artery, sma= superior mesenteric artery)

The almost exclusive arterial blood supply to established liver metastases has enabled treatment to be directed at them via this route whilst maintaining sufficient blood flow to normal liver by way of the portal vein. In view of the portal contribution to tumours following dearterialization procedures, this route has also been used for cytotoxic infusion. Portal vein perfusion via a catheter placed in the obliterated umbilical vein has been used as adjuvant chemotherapy to prevent liver metastases from colorectal carcinoma. The reason for this is that micrometastases are thought to still depend on portal flow. When treatment is aimed at liver metastases by interrupting or infusing the hepatic artery, the anatomy must be established by radiological means (Fig. 8.1). Anomalies are frequent with the most common being the right hepatic artery arising from the superior mesenteric and the left hepatic from the left gastric (Figs 8.2, 8.3). There are 26 potential routes of collateral arterial flow to or within the liver (Michels 1953) which can make this modality of treatment complicated.

DIAGNOSIS OF LIVER METASTASES

Diagnosis depends essentially on clinical, haematological and imaging techniques. Biopsy is required for definite confirmation but is not always essential or desirable.

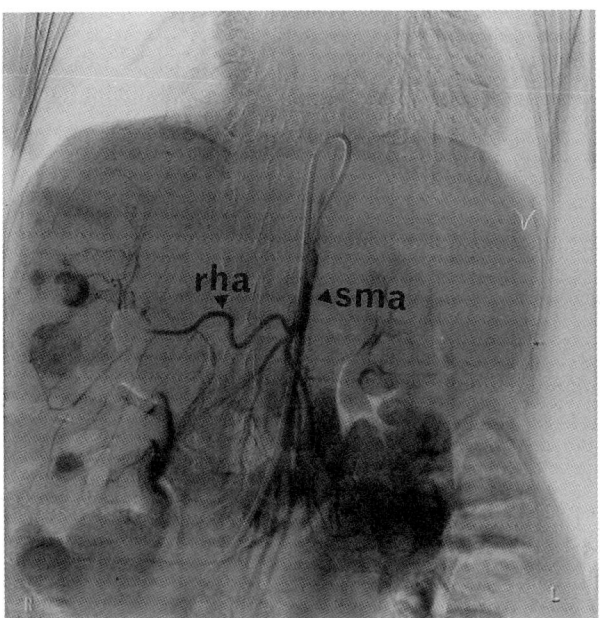

Fig. 8.2 Right hepatic artery arising from superior mesenteric artery (see Fig. 8.1 for abbreviations)

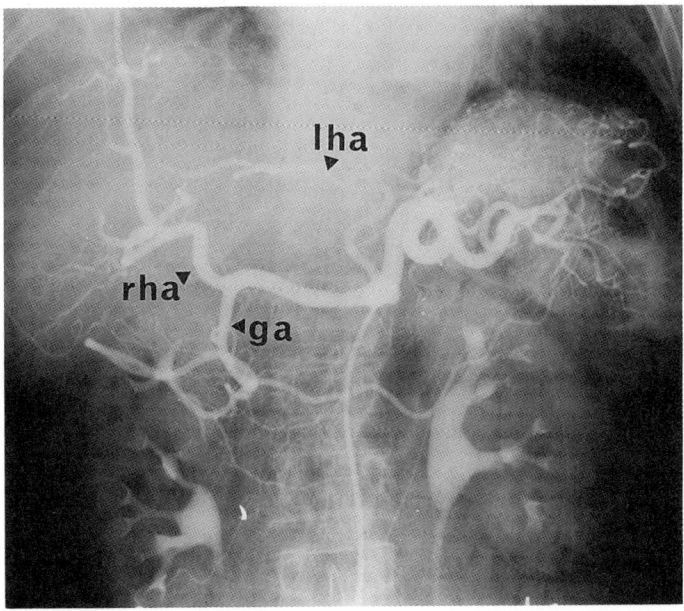

Fig. 8.3 Left hepatic artery arising from left gastric artery (see Fig. 8.1 for abbreviations)

Hepatomegaly

Reflects extensive disease or a large solitary deposit

Liver biochemistry

Liver enzymes may or may not be elevated and often only alkaline phosphatase.

Serum carcino-embryonic antigen (CEA)

This tumour marker is seldom used for diagnostic purposes but is useful as a marker for response to treatment.

Imaging

Scintigraphy

Tc-sulphur colloid was the original form of scanning and is accurate for extensive disease but insensitive for small deposits.

Ultrasound

This is undoubtedly the most useful and cost effective diagnostic non-invasive technique.

CT-scan

This is very useful for visualising the whole liver, staging the extent of disease within the liver, its relation to the structures in the porta hepatis and the presence of extrahepatic spread.

Hepatic angiography

Only used to display vascular anatomy, although a prerequisite prior to resectional surgery, radiological embolization or insertion of a catheter for arterial cytotoxic administration.

Liver biopsy

This is performed either percutaneously under direct vision at time of laparotomy or under imaging control. There is frequently sufficient information to make this unnecessary in many cases.

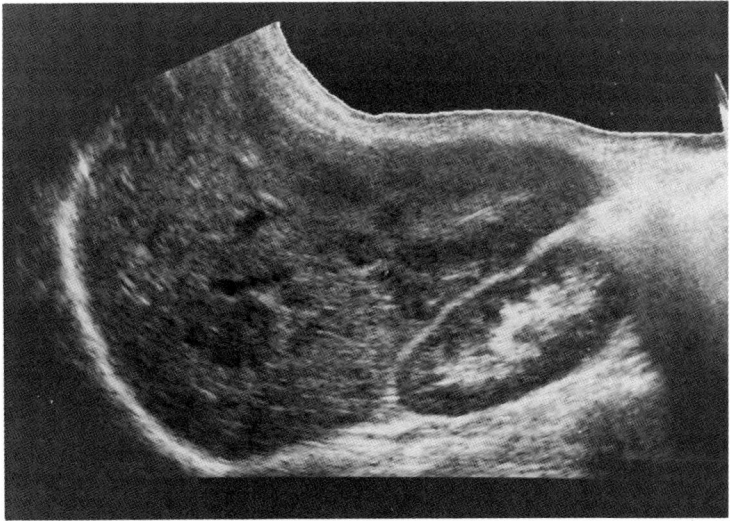

Fig. 8.4 Ultrasound scan showing small metastases (approx. 1 cm in diameter) clearly in centre of liver. The gallbladder is visualised on the right side.

The accuracy and availability of ultrasound has enabled diagnosis to be made at an earlier stage (Fig. 8.4). However in most patients routine scanning is not performed following resections of colorectal carcinoma. Since 90 percent of metachronous liver metastases develop within two years of resection, there is an argument to scan during this time if treatment is to be a viable proposition. This is the current practice in the USA and by diagnosing liver metastases earlier in their natural history may account for the improved survival rates recently reported when compared to historical controls.

Assessment of response to treatment

The response to treatment of liver metastases is measured differently from centre to centre. Subjective, clinical and haematological parameters have been used. The only true index of response is that of increased survival when patients are matched according to the stage of disease. The only reasonable objective measurement is with repeated CT scans. Isotope imaging is too imprecise and ultrasound is poor at reproducing the same 'cut' at subsequent visits. Decrease in clinical hepatomegaly is inaccurate and even a drop in the serum tumour marker, CEA, does not necessarily indicate any true efficacy of the treatment.

THE DIAGNOSTIC AND THERAPEUTIC ROLE OF RADIOLOGY

Imaging plays a vital role in the management of patients with liver metastases. Ultrasound is the method of choice for simple diagnosis and can be used for guidence when biopsy is required. In most cases it is as sensitive as CT in diagnosing deposits greater than 2 cm in diameter. It can be technically difficult in obese patients and in identifying small deposits on the posterior aspect of the liver. CT scanning is more useful in these situations and is also superior at identifying extrahepatic spread in the retroperitoneum (Fig. 8.5). This is particularly important when evaluating a patient for treatment. A patient thought to have only a solitary liver metastases suitable for resection will be spared a laparotomy if imaging shows multiplicity or extrahepatic spread. Enhancement of deposits can be achieved by giving intravenous contrast agents such as urografin with CT examinations. An oil emulsion agent recently developed in the USA called EOE 13 is reputed to be a superior enhancing agent as it is only taken up by normal hepatic parenchyma. Unfortunately, it is not available yet in other countries.

Imaging still has its limitations as the true extent of disease may not be ascertained until a laparotomy has been performed. Thompson et al (1985)

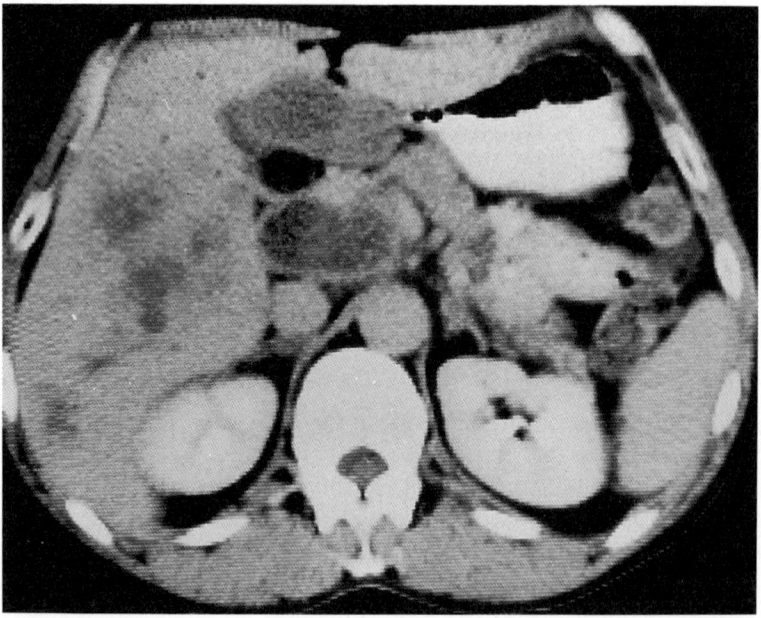

Fig. 8.5 CT scan showing liver metastases and extrahepatic involvement of retroperitoneal lymph nodes

showed in a series of patients being evaluated for hepatic resection for focal liver disease, that 11 percent thought to be resectable on clinical and scanning evidence were not so at the time of laparotomy due to irresectibility or multiple deposits not diagnosed preoperatively.

Angiography is a prerequisite for surgery, embolization or insertion of a catheter for cytotoxic infusion in order to ascertain the arterial anatomy (Fig. 8.6). Late-phase films are taken to establish the presence of portal flow but the hepatic venous distribution can only be shown by retrograde filling by way of the inferior vena cava.

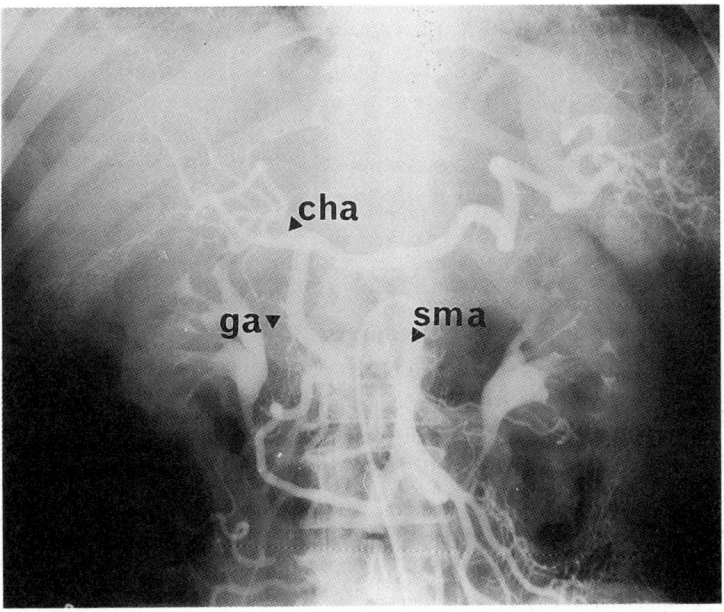

Fig. 8.6 Arteriogram showing a blocked coeliac axis with splenic and hepatic arterial supply collateral flow through the pancreaticoduodenal vessels. This precludes arterial embolization or infusion (see Fig. 8.1 for abbreviations).

Angiography can be performed by using the brachial or femoral arteries as a point of vascular access. Following the procedure the vessels can be embolised or the catheter left in situ for cytotoxic infusion for a few days. This was a popular method of selective infusion in the past but there were frequent complications with the catheter slipping out or thrombosing the hepatic artery (Oberfield et al, 1979). The initial response to short-term infusion was impressive although could not be maintained to significantly improve survival (Watkins et al, 1970; Ansfield et al, 1975). This has led to the current concept of long-term infusion for multiple liver metastases.

Embolization

Radiological embolization is a useful method of alleviating syptoms of the carcinoid syndrome. Lyophilised human dura mater (Lyodura) is used to occlude the small distal vessels which is followed by gelfoam and spring coils for the large proximal branches. Total occlusion will reduce the chances of collateral arterial flow into the tumours. The procedure is often followed by a pyrexia, nausea, vomiting and upper abdominal discomfort and is known as the 'post-embolization syndrome'. This is thought to be due to tumour necrosis. Interestingly, gallbladder infarction is not a complication.

This form of dearterialization has been used for treating liver metastases by Chuang et al (1981) with few complications. It is inadvisable in those patients with portal vein occlusion and in patients with very extensive disease. Chuang's results do not show a major improvement in survival in those patients with liver metastases from colorectal carcinoma. This is partly because of revascualarization due to opening of intrahepatic collaterals. However, its role in treating carcinoid metastases is important. Most patients are relieved of their symptoms almost completely for many months and the procedure can be repeated at later intervals (Maton et al, 1983). It has not been possible to show that survival is improved in this highly selected group of patients because numbers are few and the natural history can extend over many years.

SURGICAL TREATMENT OF LIVER METASTASES

Dearterialization procedures

When liver metastases were discovered to have a blood supply dependent on the hepatic artery, a number of attempts were made at simple surgical ligation (Nilsson, 1966). It was noted as with radiological embolization, that there was often a dramatic diminution in size of the deposits but survival was unaffected. In order to reduce collateral formation, procedures were developed to totally dearterialise the liver by dividing all peritoneal and ligamentous attachments of the liver. Almersjo et al (1972) showed a significant mortality accompanying this procedure and in patients who survived, prolongation of life was not appreciable. As mentioned, one route of collateral flow following these procedures are the tumour vessels which communicate with the portal vein. A recent study of hepatic artery ligation with longterm cytotoxic portal perfusion has reported a median survival of 14 months for patients with liver metastases from colorectal carcinoma (Laufman et al, 1984).

If occlusion of arterial flow is performed radiological embolization is the method of choice, as it is associated with less morbidity and can be repeated with ease on subsequent occasions.

Hepatic resection of metastases

This is the one area where the light shines brightest for treatment of liver metastases. Unfortunately, it is only effective for the small highly selected group of patients with solitary hepatic deposits and no extrahepatic spread. These account for only 5% of all liver metastases from colorectal carcinoma. They are even rarer with other primary sites. Only anecdotal evidence suggests that solitary metastases from nephroblastoma, carcinoid and APUD secreting tumours may benefit from excision.

Relative longevity is not uncommon with solitary liver metastases from colorectal carcinoma in untreated cases. Wood (1984) showed in a prospective study that 16% of patients were still alive 5 years following diagnosis. It appears that sometimes a solitary metastasis has an inherent biological behaviour to remain localised and slow-growing. There is now good evidence that resection of bilobar multiple metastases is of no benefit. Cady & McDermott (1985) have shown that when there is a cluster of up to three in a localised area the results are just as good as for resected solitary metastases. No randomised trial has been carried out due to the rarity of such cases in any one centre but Iwatsuki et al (1983) have shown that 50% 5-year survival can be achieved following surgical excision in this select group. Most series, however, report 30–40% 5-year survival.

Although detailed operative technique cannot be discussed here there is accumulated experience which has enabled post operative mortality to fall below 10% (Foster & Lundy, 1981; Coppa et al, 1985). The following factors are of great importance.

1. Surgery should only be offered to patients with clinically solitary metastases

2. Careful workup and operative assessment is required

3. Resection is aborted if extrahepatic spread is found at laparotomy

4. No serious impairment of hepatic function should be present

5. There is no restriction on size as long as it is operable

6. Resection need only include the liver metastases and a cuff of normal liver

7. Vascular control at the porta and hepatic veins is very valuable

8. Tumours involving the porta and great vessels may often be irresectable

Even though 70% may have some benefit from resection it is important to remember that 30% have undergone a major hepatic procedure with no benefit. In view of the inherent biological ability of some metastases to remain solitary and others not, it may be a reasonable policy to defer surgery for a few months following diagnosis to verify the solitary behaviour of the metastasis. Another approach has been the use of adjuvant chemotherapy at the time of resection either selectively into the hepatic artery, portal vein or even intra-peritoneally. This latter route has been used by August et al (1985) and they report a 4-year survival of 53 percent, which is most encouraging.

CHEMOTHERAPY

A wide variety of chemotherapeutic 'agents have been used to control liver metastases. They have been given as single or multiple regimens in different dosage schedules and by a variety of routes. This multiplicity is a reflection of their limited effect and the search continues to find more efficacious agents.

Cytotoxic agents most commonly used against liver metastases are those which are actively taken up by the liver and/or have a short plasma half-life (Table 8.3).

Table 8.3 Most widely used cytotoxic agents for liver metastases (Engsminger & Gyves 1983)

Drug	Half-life (min)	Hepatic extraction ratio during first pass	Increased hepatic exposure with selective infusion
5-Fluorouracil (5-FU)	10	0.22: 0.45	5–10 times
5-Fluoro-2'-deoxyuridine (5-FUDR)	<10	0.69: 0.92	100–400 times
Mitomycin C	10	—	6–8 times
Bischorethylnitrosurea (BCNU)	<5	—	6–7 times
Cisplatin	10	—	20–30

Even the most active agents against gastrointestinal tumours such as the fluoropyrimidines have only a partial tumoricidal action. Oral agents have very unpredictable pharmacokinetic activities due to their variable intestinal absorption patterns. Systemic therapy which overcomes this problem, has been extensively evaluated with many regimens and these have been reviewed (Kemeny, 1982). Overall, the response rate is around 20% and survival following treatment seldom extends beyond 10 months. As a treatment, it is almost invariably associated with marked side-effects, vomiting, alopecia and, occasionally bone marrow depression. It is hard to believe that patients even get the psychological comfort 'that something is being done' in these circumstances.

Selective hepatic arterial chemotherapy

As a consequence of these findings and with the knowledge that liver metastases almost invariably depend on the hepatic artery, infusion directly into the artery was developed either through a radiologically or surgically placed catheter. Engsminger et al (1978) showed that 5-FU and FUDR are largely removed by the liver during the first pass (Table 8.3). This reduces the systemic side-effects to a minimum whilst delivering a much higher dose to the liver metastases. The only drawback is that it is most suitable for those patients with only liver metastases which is a small proportion of all cases.

Selective arterial infusion was initially given for a few days following radiological catheterization. Problems with catheter migration, occlusion and vascular damage were reported although patients were spared a laparotomy. Short-term infusion was accompanied by an impressive response in 50% of patients with colorectal carcinoma metastases and survival figures of greater than 12 months. In view of the cytotoxic action of the fluoropyrimidines against tumour cells at a specific part of the cell cycle, long-term infusion was hoped to provide the key to longterm responses.

Long-term infusion is not practical through radiologically placed catheters and two alternative systems have been developed over recent years. The first is a simple but ingenious device called the 'Infusaid' pump. The chamber is placed in a subcutaneous pouch and the catheter is positioned in the gastroduodenal artery to lie flush with the common hepatic artery. The chamber is refilled at one or two weekly intervals and there is a separate portal for intermittent bolus injections. It is liable to variation of infusion rates but seldom develops the problems of radiologically placed catheters. However, they are costly (approx. £3000) and this has led to the development of an alternative system where the infusion pump is external and can be transferable between patients. The Cormed pump is one of the first such systems and more recent developments have made the infusion rate more accurate. The infusion reaches the hepatic artery by way of a surgically implanted catheter system which has a subcutaneous chamber with an injectable membrane.

Initial results with longterm infusion for multiple liver metastases are encouraging compared to the short course with survival of 20 months quoted (Table 8.4). Kemeny et al (1985a), however, reported that median

Table 8.4 Review of survival data with long-term cytotoxic infusion

Series	Patients (no.)	From start of infusion (months)	From time of of diagnosis (months)
Balch et al (1983)	81	—	26*
Cohen et al (1983)	10	10	—
Kemeny et al (1985a)			
extrahepatic disease in all	11	12	—
Niederhuber et al (1984)			
liver involvement only	50	18	25
extrahepatic involvement	43	9	14
Weiss et al (1983)	21	13	17
Schwartz et al (1985)	18	10*	21*
Shepard et al (1985)			
liver involvement only	53	17	—
extrahepatic involvement	9	4.5	—

Median survival except * which are mean.

survival was only 12 months when extrahepatic portal nodes were present. There is no doubt that the results can be heavily weighted one way or the other if there is a predominance of stage 1 or stage 3 disease.

Very few complications have arisen with the implantable pumps themselves although there have been frequent reports of chemical hepatitis, gastroduodenitis and peptic ulceration associated with the longterm use of FUDR. These unwanted side-effects are usually reversible but Kemeny et al (1985b) have found that 17.4% of patients develop sclerosing cholangitis which is much more alarming.

The outlook for chemotherapy may look more promising than it did. Technology has developed a system that is very reliable at giving selective treatment to liver metastases but a truely effective agent has yet to be found. Whilst we await this outcome, methods of improving the efficacy of the present generation is all that can be achieved.

For this reason, the use of intra-arterial biodegradable microspheres mixed with chemotherapeutic agents, isolated liver perfusion and selective infusion of monoclonal antibodies are new developments currently being investigated.

RADIOTHERAPY

The use of this modality with the conventional external beam has been used for treating liver metastases with limited success (Turek-Maischeider & Kazem, 1975). It has been claimed to alleviate pain caused by enlarging liver metastases but the dose that would be required to have a significant tumoricidal effect would cause too much radiation damage to surrounding normal tissue. Selective arterial administration of radioactive particles labelled to microspheres in a similar way to chemotherapy was developed as an alternative. Yttrium 90 which is a β-emitter with a short distance of penetration of 2.5 mm was thought to be suitable. Ariel & Padula (1978) gave these microspheres followed by 15 days 5-FU infusion. Mean survival for those patients with colorectal secondaries was 12 months. Grady (1979) gave the radioactive microspheres alone with no appreciable improvement in survival.

One of the reasons that selective arterial infusions of radioactive particles or cytotoxic agents do not have an overwhelming effect is the avascularity at the centre of the deposits which are always likely to contain viable tumour.

CONCLUSION

Liver metastases are often only part of a generalised disseminated tumour process. The more sophisticated means of diagnosis has given a much clearer picture of the natural history and has enabled the formulation of various prognostic factors. The extent of disease can be clearly identified, often without the need for laparotomy. This, in turn, has resulted in successful resection of solitary metastases with a low mortality. The technological advances in selective arterial administration of cytotoxic agents has resulted in reports of significantly increased survival with longterm infusion. These encouraging developments must be tempered by the knowledge that a more effective cytotoxic agent is desperately needed before patients with multiple liver metastases have any chance of surviving 5 years.

REFERENCES

Ansfield F J, Ramirez G, David H L et al 1975 Further clinical studies with intrahepatic arterial infusion with 5-fluorouracil. Cancer 36: 2413–2417

Almersjo O, Bengmark S, Rudenstam C M, Hafstrom L, Nilsson L A V 1972 Evaluation of hepatic dearterialization in primary and secondary cancer of the liver. American Journal of Surgery 124: 5–9

Ariel I M, Padula G 1978 Treatment of symptomatic metastatic cancer to the liver from primary colon and rectal cancer by the intra-arterial administration of chemotherapy and radioactive isotopes. Journal of Surgical Oncology 10: 327–336

August D A, Sugarbaker P H, Ottow R T, Gianola F J, Schneider P D 1985 Hepatic resection of colorectal metastases. Annals of Surgery 201: 210–218

Balch C M, Urist M M, Soong S, Mcgregor M 1983 A prospective phase II clinical trial of continuous FUDR regional chemotherapy for colorectal metastases to the liver using a totally implantable drug infusion pump. Annals of Surgery 198: 567–573

Bengmark S, Hafstrom L 1978 The natural course for liver cancer. In: Ariel I M (ed) Progress in Clinical Cancer, Vol 7, Grune and Stratton, New York, p 195–200

Breedis, C, Young G 1954 The blood supply of neoplasms in the liver. American Journal of Pathology 30: 969–977

Cady B, Monson D O, Swinton N W 1970 Survival of patients after colonic resection for carcinoma with simultaneous liver metastases. Surgery, Gynecology & Obstetrics 131: 697–700

Cady B, McDermott W V 1985 Major Hepatic resection for metachronous metastases from colon cancer. Annals of Surgery 201: 204–209

Cady B, Oberfield R A 1974 Regional infusion chemotherapy of hepatic metastases from carcinoma of the colon. American Journal of Surgery 127: 220–227

Cohen A M, Kaufman S D, Wood W C, Greenfield A J 1983 Regional hepatic chemotherapy using an implantable drug infusion pump. American Journal of Surgery 145: 529–533

Coppa G F, Eng K, Ranson J H C, Gouge T H, Localio S A 1985 Hepatic resection for metastatic colon and rectal cancer. Annals of Surgery 202: 203–208

Chuang V P, Wallace S 1981 Hepatic artery embolization in the treatment of hepatic neoplasms. Radiology 140: 51–58

Davis Z, Moerter C G, McIlrath D C 1973 The malignant carcinoid syndrome. Surgery, Gynecology & Obstetrics 37: 637–644

Engsminger W D, Gyves J W 1983 Clinical pharmacology of hepatic arterial chemotherapy. Seminars in Oncology 10: 176–181

Engsminger W D, Rosowsky A, Raso V et al 1978 A clinical-pharmacological evaluation of hepatic arterial infusions of 5-fluoro-2-deoxyuridine and 5-fluorourcil. Cancer Research 38: 3784–3792

Einhorn L H, Burgess M A, Gottlieb J A 1974 Metastatic patterns of choroidal melanomas. Cancer 34: 1001–1004

Foster J H, Lundy J 1981 Liver metastases. Current Problems in Surgery 18: 161–202

Gilbert J M 1983 Distribution of metastases at necroscopy in colorectal cancer. Clinical and Experimental Metastases 1: 97–101

Grady E D 1979 Internal radiation of hepatic cancer. Diseases of Colon & Rectum 22: 371–375

Healey J E 1965 Vascular patterns in human metastatic liver tumours. Surgery, Gynecology & Obstetrics 120: 1187–1193

Iwatsuki S, Shaw B W, Starzl T E 1983 Experience with 150 liver resections. Annals of Surgery 197: 247–253

Jaffe B M, Donnegan W L, Watson F 1968 Factors influencing survival in patients with untreated hepatic metastases. Surgery, Gynecology & Obstetrics 127: 1–11

Kemeny M 1983 The systemic chemotherapy of hepatic metastases. Seminars in Oncology 10: 148–158

Kemeny M et al 1985a Experience with continuous regional chemotherapy and hepatic resection as treatment of hepatic metastases from colorectal primaries. Cancer 55: 1265–1270

Kemeny M et al 1985b Sclerosing cholangitis after continuous hepatic artery infusion of FUDR. Annals of Surgery 202: 176–181

Laufman L R, Nims T A, Guy J T, Guy J F, Courter S 1984 Hepatic artery ligation and portal vein infusion for liver metastases from colon cancer. Journal of Clinical Oncology: 1382–1389

Mansfield C M, Kramer S, Southard M E, Mandell G 1969 Prognosis in patients with metastatic liver disease diagnosed by liver scan. Radiology 193: 77–84

Maton P, Camilleri H, Griffin G et al 1983 Role of hepatic arterial embolization in the carcinoid syndrome. British Medical Journal 287: 932–934

Michels N A 1953 Collateral arterial pathways to the liver after ligation of the hepatic artery and removal of the celiac axis. Cancer 6: 708–724

Niederhuber E, Engsminger W, Gyves J et al 1984 Regional chemotherapy of colorectal cancer metastatic to the liver. Cancer 53: 1336–1343

Nielson J, Balslev I, Jensen H E 1971 Carcinoma of the colon with liver metastases. Acta Chirugia Scandinavica 137: 463–465

Nilsson L A V 1966 Therapeutic hepatic artery ligation in patients with secondary liver tumours. Review of Surgery 374–376

Oberfield R A, McCaffrey J A, Polio B S et al 1979 Prolonged and continuous percutaneous intra-arterial hepatic infusion chemotherapy in advanced metastatic liver adenocarcinoma from colorectal primary. Cancer 44: 414–423

Pestana C, Reitemeier R J, Moertel C 1964 The natural history of carcinoma of the colon and rectum. American Journal of Surgery 108: 826–829

Pettavel J, Leyvraz S, Douglas P 1984 The necessity for staging liver metastases and standardizing treatment response criteria. The case of secondaries of colorectal origin. In: Van de Velde C J H, Sugarbaker P H (eds) Liver Metastases, Martinus Nijhoff, Amsterdam, ch 15, p 154–168

Pickren J W, Tsukuda Y, Lane W W 1982 Liver Metastasis: Analysis of Autopsy Data. In: Weiss L, Gilbert H A (ed) Liver Metastases, Hall, Boston. ch 1, p 2–18

Schwartz S I, Jones L S, C S McCune 1985 Assessment of treatment of intrahepatic malignancies using chemotherapy via an implantable pump. Annals of Surgery 201: 560–567

Shepard K V, Levin B, Karl R C et al 1985 Therapy for metastatic colorectal cancer with hepatic artery infusion chemotherapy using a subcutaneous implanted pump. Journal of Clinical Oncology 3: 161–169

Taylor I, Bennett R, Sherriff S 1979 The blood supply of colorectal liver metastases. British Journal of Cancer 39: 149–756

Taylor I, Machin D, Mullee M, Trotter G, Cooke T, West C 1985 A randomized controlled trial of adjuvant portal vein cytotoxic perfusion in colorectal cancer. British Journal of Surgery 72: 359–362

Thompson J N, Gibson R, Czerniak A, Blumgart L H 1985 Focal liver lesions: a plan for management. British Medical Journal 290: 1643–1645

Turek-Maischeider M, Kazem I 1975 Palliative irradiation for liver metastases. Journal of American Medical Association 232: 625–628

Watkins E, Khazei A M, Wahra K S 1970 Surgical basis for arterial infusion chemotherapy of disseminated carcinoma of the liver. Surgery, Gynecology & Obstetrics 130: 581–605

Weiss G R, Garnick M B, Osteen R T et al 1983 Long-term hepatic arterial infusion of 5-Fluorodeoxyuridine for liver metastases using an implantable infusion pump. Journal of Clinical Oncology 1: 337–344

Wood C B, Gillis C R, Blumgart L H 1976 A retrospective study of the natural history of patients with liver metastases from colorectal cancer. Clinical Oncology 2: 285–288

Wood C B 1984 Natural history of liver metastases. In: Van de Velde C J H, Sugarbaker P H (eds) Liver metastases, Martinus Nijhoff, Amsterdam, ch 4, p 47–54

Radiation damage to the bowel

INTRODUCTION

Shortly after the discovery of radioactivity it became recognised that certain emissions could have destructive effects upon living tissue. Remarkably rapidly this property was harnessed in the treatment of malignant conditions so that radiotherapy became established. Additionally it was recognised that irradiation may have deleterious effects upon normal tissue. When the radiation was directed towards the abdomen, symptoms were seen to arise from the gastrointestinal tract and remit shortly after exposure ceased. Severe permanent bowel injury was recognised as a complication of radiation for cancer more than 70 years ago (Futh & Ebeler, 1915). Over the years, the greatest number of severe bowel injuries have been after pelvic irradiation especially in the treatment of carcinoma of the uterine cervix and to a lesser extent other gynaecological malignancies and carcinoma of the bladder. In the last few years pelvic radiotherapy has been increasingly used for other types of pelvic malignancy so that we are now seeing reports of radiation bowel disease (RBD) as a consequence of radiotherapy for carcinoma of the rectum (Danjoux & Catton, 1979) and carcinoma of the prostate (Gree et al, 1984). Other parts of the gastrointestinal tract may be injured e.g. stomach and duodenum after abdominal treatment for Hodgkin's disease (Gallez-Marchal et al, 1984) but the rectum and sigmoid colon or the terminal ileum are the areas usually affected after pelvic radiotherapy.

TYPES OF RADIATION DAMAGE

It is possible to recognise at least two types of radiation effect on the bowel — early and late. During or immediately after abdominal or pelvic radiotherapy some minor bowel disturbance is common, particularly after radical radiotherapy for carcinoma of the cervix. In most, this is a passing phase which resolves but in a few patients early bowel reaction may amount to serious life-threatening disease. It is uncertain whether the severity of this reaction predisposes to the later type of irradiation bowel disease though it is denied by many authorities (Rubin, 1984). However, in a recent study, later development of radiation bowel disease seemed to be three times more likely in patients who had severe early reactions (Bourne et al, 1983).

Late onset radiation bowel disease may occur some months or years after the irradiation. We divided this phase into two distinct groups, those that arise between 6 and 18 months which are described as intermediate and those arising after 18 months which are described as late (Schofield et al, 1983). However, the basic pathology underlying these latter two types is similar (Hasleton et al, 1985), so it is perhaps best to describe them as the intermediate and late phase of late radiation bowel disease (Rubin, 1984). The pathology of the early and late disease is discussed more fully later.

CAUSES OF RADIATION DAMAGE

Bowel problems arise because of the relatively narrow therapeutic range for radiotherapy. A dose which will effectively destroy malignant tissue will approach that which may produce damage to metabolically active tissue. From this it will be apparent that the radiotherapy techniques both in targeting the dose as well as in the total dosage are of considerable importance (Hatcher et al, 1985). After pelvic radiotherapy, serious late radiation bowel injury may occur in as little as 1% or as great as 20% of patients treated (Kjorstad et al, 1983). It is a question of balancing cancer control against morbidity.

There are other factors that are known to increase the incidence of irradiation bowel disease such as arteriosclerosis and diabetes but the two most significant non-radiotherapy determinants of morbidity are chemotherapy and previous pelvic surgery (DeCosse et al, 1969). It is well established that chemotherapy reduces the tolerance of normal tissue to radiation. The mechanism is uncertain but in treatment regimes using combined chemotherapy and radiotherapy serious late radiation disease has approached 30% (Danjoux et al, 1979). Previous pelvic surgery is a frequent association in many series of radiation bowel disease (RBD). This is because a loop of ileum or sigmoid colon becomes tethered in the pelvis from post-operative adhesions so that this single loop bears the whole brunt of the treatment dose.

Radiotherapy techniques

In order to appreciate RBD it is important to have some concept of the radiotherapy techniques involved. Treatment for carcinoma of the bladder, rectum or prostate almost invariably involves treatment by external beam radiotherapy. Treatment for carcinoma of the cervix involves an intracavity radionuclide often combined with external beam technique to the more lateral pelvis. Until recents years the intracavity radionuclide has been radium. However, new health and safety regulations for staff protection have led to radium being replaced by the safer artificial radionuclides Caesium 137 and Cobalt 60. At the same time, remote afterloading systems have been introduced where empty applicators may be positioned in the patient and the radioactive source automatically loaded without exposure of any member of staff. These factors have led to considerable changes of well-established techniques in many centres and have been associated with an increase in RBD (Sherrah-Davies, 1985). A final point about intracavity technique that should be noted is that not only are the radiation sources introduced into the cavity of the uterus but also isotope is introduced into the fornices of the vagina in so-called ovoids. The radionuclide is then held in position for a prescribed period of time until the calculated dose is given to the cervix (Fig. 9.1).

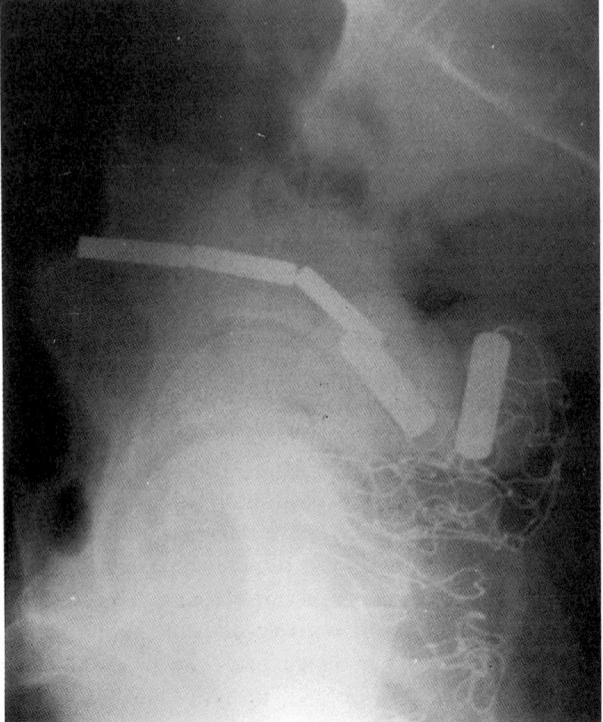

Fig. 9.1 Radiograph of pelvis in patient undergoing intracavity radiotherapy for carcinoma cervix

Consideration of the anatomy of the vagina, anal canal, rectum and pouch of pelvic peritoneum indicates that there are three potential places at which the bowel is at hazard (Fig. 9.2). The mid and upper rectum may suffer from a high dose effect from either intracavity or external beam therapy directly. The Pouch of Douglas descending as it does into the vicinity of the cervix may also receive a high dose from either external beam or intra-

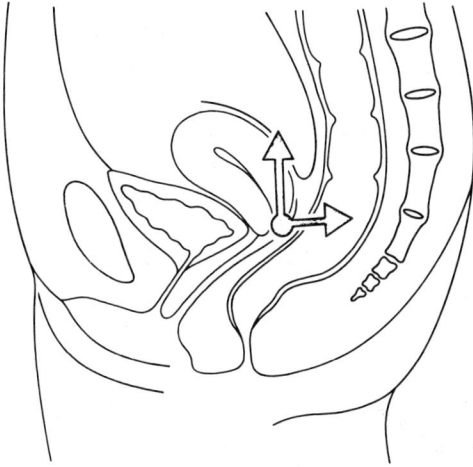

Fig. 9.2 Diagram of lateral pelvis to show close relationship of pelvic peritoneal pouch and rectum to the uterine cervix

cavity treatment. It has been suggested that either long applicators or applicators held rigidly are particularly likely to produce an adverse effect on any bowel within the Pouch of Douglas. It should be noted that the terminal ileum and the sigmoid colon are the regions of the bowel damaged by this mechanism. Finally, and rather rarely, the low rectum or anal canal may be the site of injury and this is probably associated with inadvertent slippage of the vaginal ovoids (Sherrah-Davies, 1985).

PATHOLOGY

Early damage

The changes which occur at the time of radiotherapy have been little studied because most acute reactions settle so that our knowledge of the pathology at this stage largely depends on the gross appearance seen at endoscopy and the microscopic appearance on endoscopic biopsy. Excisional surgery is carried out so rarely at this stage that no group has any large experience and in any event it is an assessment of the most severe and rather atypical type of reaction. At endoscopic examination of the rectum or colon an affected area is recognised by the presence of thickening of the mucosa with loss of vessels and increased friability and on occasions there are small superficial ulcers. Actively-dividing cells are most affected by radiation and for this reason the cells of the gastrointestinal mucosa with their high replication rate are particularly vulnerable and effects are seen within a few days of the radiation. These effects are due to the direct action of the radiation damaging cells of the mucosa. Microscopically there appears to be mucosal necrosis with possibly some inflammation involving the muscle layer and in the more severe cases eosinophilic crypt abscesses can be seen. Recovery takes place by gradual regeneration of epithelium from the deeper layers of the crypts (Rubin, 1984).

Late damage

The later changes do not become manifest until several months or years after radiation and are quite distinct from the early changes. It seems certain that the principal factor in producing these changes is a progressive endarteritis affecting particularly the small mural vessels of the bowel. This leads to relative and localised ischaemia, the degree of which determines the pathology (Carr et al, 1984).

In pelvic radiotherapy the rectum and sigmoid colon are most commonly involved but the ileum is also at risk either together with the recto-sigmoid region or separately. In general, the small bowel is significantly involved in 25–30% of cases (Schofield et al, 1985). Whichever part of the bowel is involved the appearance is similar. The length of bowel involved varies from 2 or 3 cm to lengths as long as 50 cm. The serosa is pale, thick and may have areas of congestion or haemorrhage. The whole of the bowel wall is thick and rigid and may have areas of focal necrosis surrounded by indurated tissue. The mucosal surface is oedematous with some cobble-stoning and ulcers may well be present. These ulcers are usually covered with necrotic slough and penetrate deep into the muscularis and are clearly the basis of the total necrosis of the bowel wall seen in some cases. In patients who present at greater than 18 months, areas of obvious necrosis are rare. There is usually gross thickening of the bowel wall with adhesions between adjacent loops. The serosa is pale but the muscle layer is thick-ened and rigid producing a stricture.

Histology

In the cases that occur some months after treatment there is gross submu-cosal oedema with dilated lymphatics. Similarly the muscularis propria shows massive oedema between the muscle bundles with focal lysis (Hasleton et al, 1985). In some parts there are limited areas of infarction within the wall but in others there is full thickness infarction (Carr et al, 1984). There are bizarre fibroblasts with irregular nuclei and prominent cytoplasm in all layers. Mucosal ulceration and areas of infarction are commonly present. The patients that present after some years show marked fibrosis in the muscularis propria and in the sub-mucosa and thin regener-ative epithelium in the large bowel and villous blunting in the small bowel.

Of particular interest, with regard to pathogenesis, are the chronic vascular changes seen at the site of RBD. The small mural arteries and arterioles show intimal fibrosis which can be occlusive. Additionally sub-

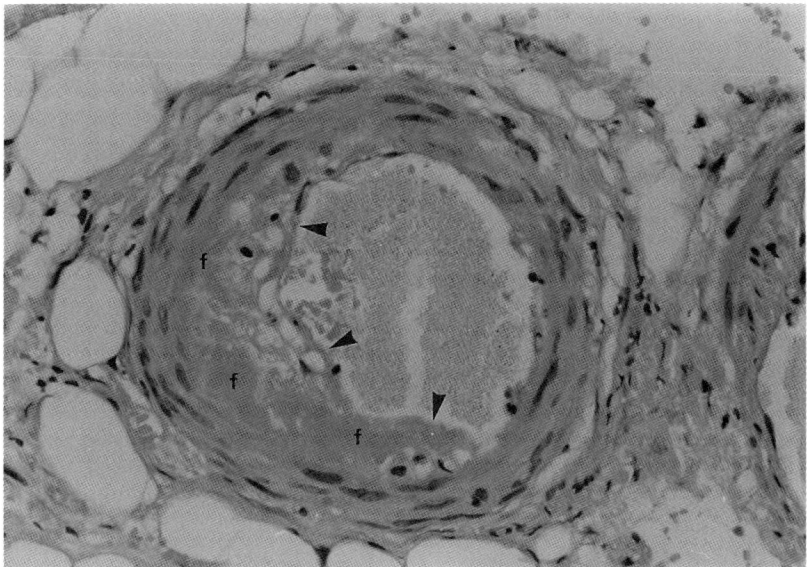

Fig. 9.3 Radiation induced vascular injury:
A small mural blood vessel with subendothelial oedema and fibrin (f).

endothelial deposition of oedema fluid and fibrin will produce marked
intimal thickening (Fig. 9.3). In the more mature cases, the fibrin and
oedema fluid become replaced by fibrous tissue. Similarly, small veins show
intimal fibrosis and thrombosis. A morphometric analysis of the small mural
vessels shows a great increase in the incidence and degree of intimal thickening which is directly related to the dose of radiation. Fibrin thrombi are
commonly found in the small vessels of the gut wall. It seems probable that
these obliterative vascular lesions cause progressive ischaemia leading on to
the other changes observed.

Pathophysiology

Denker et al (1972) used mesenteric angiography to study patients with
bowel symptoms many months or years after pelvic radiation and demonstrated reduced vascularity of the bowel wall in areas affected by RBD.
Microradiography of excised specimens from RBD show marked changes
in the microvasculature. (Fig. 9.4 & 9.5). In cases where there have been
perforations or fistulae there are completely avascular zones in the bowel
wall which may be totally transmural or localised to a part of the wall.
(Fig. 9.5). Fully developed strictures show a reduction in vascularity which
affects all layers of the intestinal wall.

It seems that the early changes occurring at or shortly after the time of
radiotherapy are a direct effect upon the cells whilst later changes are due

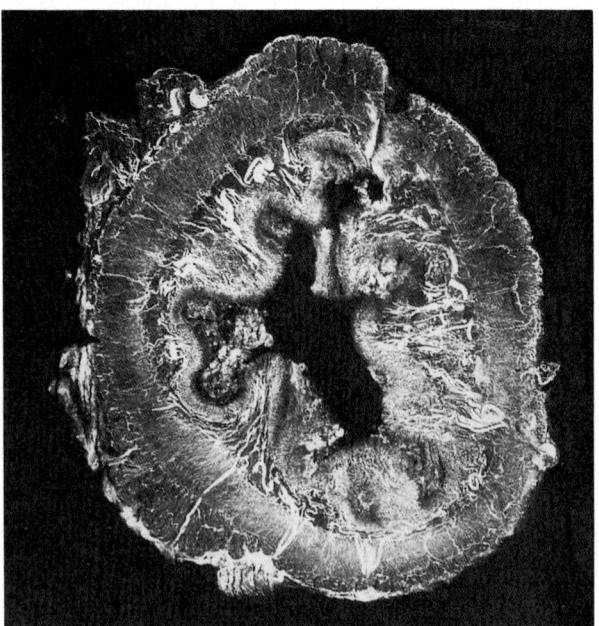

Fig. 9.4 Microradiograph of normal bowel:
A good submucosal plexus and even perfusion of wall are demonstrated

to a progressive vascular occlusion which produces a typical ischaemic bowel disease. As in other types of ischaemic bowel disease one may see mucosal ulceration with bleeding or frank necrosis with abscess formation or fistula. The less severe degrees of ischaemia may be repaired by fibrosis producing a fibrous stricture as a late complication.

CLINICAL PRESENTATION

Early disease

It is common for there to be some bowel reaction after any form of full dosage radiotherapy to the pelvis. Indeed, in treatment of carcinoma of the cervix, diarrhoea with some minor bleeding due to a reactionary proctitis shortly after treatment is almost invariable. This usually settles within a short time and more serious reactions are rare. The serious early reactions include exacerbation of pre-existing inflammatory disease and acute enteritis as well as severe proctitis. Rarely surgery has been reported as necessary for exacerbations of diverticular disease or inflammatory bowel disease (Schofield et al, 1983). Severe diarrhoea occurring during radiotherapy is a cause for grave concern as there may be diffuse small bowel ulceration. Fortunately enteritis presenting with diarrhoea and vomiting usually settles on conservative treatment but occasionally has to be dealt with surgically

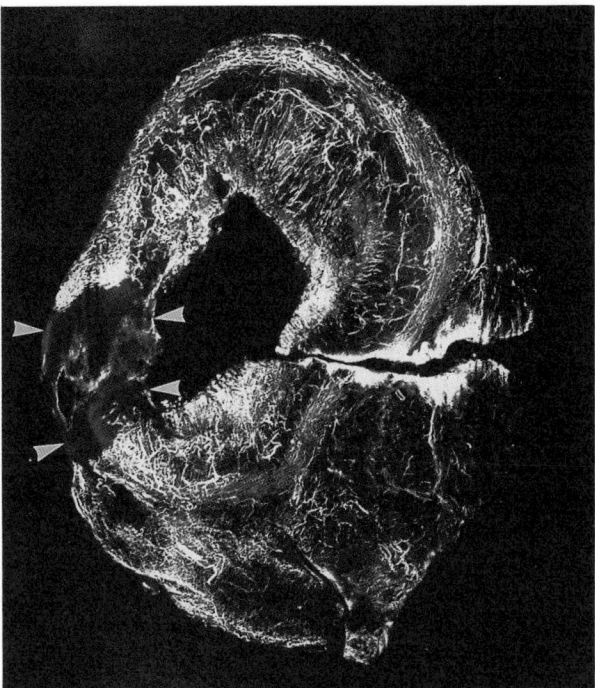

Fig. 9.5 Microradiograph of radiation damaged bowel showing
Poor submucosal plexus with uneven perfusion;
The area arrowed has no vessels and corresponds to full thickness necrosis

when patients develop acute perforation or persistent septicaemia. This is
a very serious situation with a high mortality.

Late disease

There are a number of clinical presentations of late RBD. The presentations
that are seen between 6 and 18 months after treatment (intermediate phase)
are rather different to those seen after 2 or more years (late phase). The
typical presentations in the intermediate phase are rectal bleeding due to
procto-sigmoiditis, incomplete intestinal obstruction with pelvic sepsis
which is due to perforative disease of either the sigmoid colon or the ileum
with local abscess formation; fistula formation from the gut into the vagina.
Most usually this is a recto-vaginal fistula but on rare occasions a fistula may
originate from the sigmoid colon or the ileum. Occasionally the fistula is
at the ano-rectal junction and in these cases it has been preceded by anal
pain due to ulceration. This ulceration presents relatively early (6–9
months) and should have surgical treatment before a fistula develops.

It is relatively rare for the patients with RBD to present as a dramatic
urgency with free perforation or complete intestinal obstruction though this

may occur (Walsh & Schofield, 1984). However, about one-third of the patients present as a semi-urgency and clearly require some form of surgical treatment within a few days. These are the patients with pelvic infection with some signs of intestinal obstruction and the patients with fistulae to the vagina. The commonest presentation is with rectal bleeding and this rarely is so massive as to require great urgency in its treatment. Gilinsky et al (1983) studying a group of patients who presented in this fashion showed that if the bleeding was relatively minor so that the patient did not become anaemic and require blood transfusion and had no other symptoms it was rare for surgical treatment to be necessary and a third of the patients stopped bleeding within 6 months and two-thirds within 18 months. However, if the rectal bleeding was more severe so that the patient required a blood transfusion then at least a quarter of the patients would require surgical treatment. If, in addition, the patients had significant alteration in bowel habit or abdominal pain then spontaneous remission never occurred.

The late phase which occurs more than 2 years after treatment and can be more than 20 years after treatment has somewhat different types of presentation. Most characteristically incomplete intestinal obstruction with abdominal pain, altered bowel habit and distension occurs. At this stage the obstruction is usually due to a stricture without accompanying sepsis. The symptoms tend to be progressive and on occasions patients present with complete obstruction. Other late presentations include ileal disease presenting as malabsorption due to bacterial colonisation above a stricture. Here one may see steatorrhoea or vitamin B12 deficiency. Rarely rectal carcinoma has been reported as developing some years after pelvic radiation and although this may be coincidental such tumours could be irradiation-induced.

Clearly RBD may present in a variety of different ways but it is of importance that clinicians maintain an active awareness of the possibility of bowel disease as a consequence of pelvic radiotherapy. It is only too possible for the symptoms of RBD to be ascribed to recurrent tumour and a potentially curable situation may be overlooked. Of less serious significance but of diagnostic importance is the misdiagnosis of patients with rectal bleeding as due to either ulcerative colitis or even piles due to a lack of appreciation of RBD.

The distinction between RBD and recurrent tumour may still be difficult on examination of the abdomen or pelvis. Abdominal distension, an abdominal mass, or a mass felt on pelvic examination can occur in both conditions. Rectal examination and rigid sigmoidoscopy are often possible in the out patients and may show bleeding, unhealthy mucosa or even narrowing of the rectal lumen in RBD. Flexible endoscopy will help in assessment of the sigmoid colon for evidence of ulceration or narrowing. Examination under anaethesia is often useful particularly for a bimanual examination which may help in the distinction between radiation bowel disease and recurrent tumour.

Haematology

Some anaemia is common especially in the patient with persistent rectal bleeding. Leucocytosis occurs in many patients but is not as marked as one might expect considering the chronic sepsis which is frequently associated with severe RBD. Platelet counts are elevated when there is active RBD present and returns to normal after adequate surgical removal of the diseased bowel (Carr et al, 1985).

Radiology

Plain abdominal films may show some evidence of dilated large or small bowel and may be the only possible investigation when emergency surgery is indicated. Computer tomography has been suggested as a useful investigation but we have not found it valuable in diagnosis of RBD though on occasions it can show undoubted recurrence. Barium contrast studies should be carried out in most patients but tend to underestimate the severity of the disease. Barium enema may show narrowing in the involved sigmoid with irregular mucosa. Small bowel studies may give useful additional information in some patients.

Because of the frequency of coincident or subsequent urinary tract disease, intravenous urography is indicated.

TREATMENT

Prevention

Skilled radiotherapy with an appropriate technique and careful attention to dose, dose distribution, dose rate and number of treatments are vital if RBD is to be minimised. The introduction of after-loading and the new nuclides make it important that the radiotherapist ensures that the design and insertion of the applicators minimises exposure of normal tissue to the source. Further, dangerous applicator movement during treatment must be avoided. Attempts to monitor the dose received by the rectum by intrarectal probes have been tried but rather surprisingly several reports have found that there is not good correlation with later RBD (Bourne et al, 1983). An awareness of the increased risk of postoperative radiotherapy had led to most schedules which combine X-ray therapy and surgery using radiotherapy before operation. When radiotherapy has to be used after surgery, mechanical methods to prevent bowel entering the pelvis can be considered.

Durig et al (1984) described the introduction of a 'spacer' made of dimethyl polyseloxane introduced into the pelvis at an operation which is to be followed by X-ray therapy. Although this was effective in 4 patients it had the disadvantage of requiring a further operation to remove the 'spacer'. Possibly of more practical value is the suggestion that a polyglycolic acid mesh sling can be used to exclude bowel from the pelvis because this material is fully absorbable. Recent animal experiments indicate that it is efficient in excluding small bowel from the pelvis even after it has 'dissolved' (Devereux et al, 1984).

Medical measures

Acute bowel manifestations at the time of radiotherapy have been treated conservatively by symptomatic treatment in the knowledge that they are self-limiting in almost all cases. Prostaglandin E_2 has been shown in rats to protect the mucosal cells from the effects of radiation (Tomus de la Vega et al, 1984) and may have some part to play in human disease in minimising early reactions.

Later developing RBD does not seem to be modified by medical treatment but symptomatic management is useful as the problem may never be sufficiently severe to require surgery. Dietary measures are possibly useful and Donaldson et al (1975) laid down specific criteria for management in children who had total abdominal X-ray therapy for lymphoma or other malignancies and later developed obstructive symptoms. They advocated a low residue, low fat, no milk and no gluten diet and noted 'improvement'. However, in the more usual type of RBD both high and low residue diets have been suggested but no specific diet is known to be of value. Local steroids, sulphasalazine and antifibrinolytic agents have not been shown objectively to alter the disease process. (Gilinsky et al, 1983). Supportive treatment, iron or blood transfusion for anaemia, analgesics for pain and stool softeners may help. Good nutritional support is valuable either enterally or parenterally in severe cases. Parental feeding is usually a preparation for the necessary surgery.

Rarely some symptoms may be arising from bacterial colonisation in the small bowel and if this is confirmed by a breath hydrogen or similar test then a short course of antibiotics may improve the situation.

Operative treatment

There are certain definite indications for operation such as recto-vaginal fistula, abscess formation, complete intestinal obstruction or massive persistent bleeding. Many patients present with abdominal pain and some bowel disturbance but without complete obstruction. In this group operation must be considered but if the symptoms are relatively minor conservatism can be given a trial. Unfortunately symptoms tend to persist or worsen and if this is the case operation should not be delayed overlong.

Suprisingly there is still disagreement about the optimal operative management. Some still maintain that bypass or colostomy is preferable to resection. Recent papers have stressed the greater safety of bypass in ileal RBD (Lillemoe et al, 1983; Wobbes et al, 1984) and of colostomy for diversion away from the involved rectum (Anseline et al, 1981). It is suggested that this will rest the bowel and allow ulceration to heal. It may be significant that the groups who advocate bypass or colostomy do not seem able to close many of the stomata and this accords with the opinion that late disease is progressive even if it is 'allowed to rest'. Most recent experience would favour wide excision of the irradiated bowel (Gazet et al, 1985; De cosse et al, 1969), and this is the author's preference.

Complications

The problems associated with resection are difficulty in distinguishing local recurrence from RBD, poor anastomotic healing leading to fistula or peritonitis, later stricture at the site of anastomosis and coincident or subsequent radiation urinary tract disease. As far as recurrence is concerned, this may co-exist with radiation disease although this is unusual. Distinction between recurrence alone and RBD is usually straightforward at operation but rarely alters the operative management.

The fear of anastomotic leakage is well founded if marginally ischaemic bowel is used for anastomosis (Ormiston et al, 1985). Recently a method has been described in which the microvascular space can be quantitated in excised specimens (Carr et al, 1984). It seems probable that if this space is grossly diminished then the bowel so affected will be potentially ischaemic and would heal poorly. In studies of resected specimens of the ileo-caecal region from patients who had RBD after combined intracavity and external radiotherapy the vascular volume was low and did not attain the normal range in the lower 30–60 cm of the terminal ileum, but only a small amount of the ascending colon had a low microvascular space (Carr et al, 1984). This in part, supports the contention of De Cosse et al (1968) who stressed that radiation damage was more extensive than visual assessment suggested. This has important implications with regard to the extent of excision. Clearly wide excision of the ileum is required and we believe this should be at least 30 cm above obvious disease but only limited resection of the right colon is necessary as the vasculature becomes normal just above the caecum.

RBD appears much more localised if it occurs after intracavity treatment alone and the quantitative studies confirm much shorter lengths of ileum involved in these cases. Using these principles we have no example of anastomotic leakage in 25 resections for RBD of the ileum. In RBD occurring after combined intracavity and external radiotherapy, a reduced microvascular space over an extensive area of bowel on either side of the rectosigmoid junction has been demonstrated by the microvascular studies but a shorter area of abnormality when intracavity treatment alone has been used. The area damaged after beam-directed radiotherapy for carcinoma of the bladder usually appears higher in the sigmoid colon. This is confirmed by our observations where microradiography indicates a much more localised lesion than is seen with combined therapy. It is possible for patients with a sigmoid colon lesion and an apparently normal rectum to have a wide excision with a colo-rectal anastomosis after mobilisation of the splenic flexure. Unfortunately the rectum is usually involved by significant disease so that excision of the rectum with colo-anal anastomosis or abdomino-perineal excision of the rectum are the more usual operations for recto-sigmoid RBD. An assessment of sphincter function as well as the lowest level of the lesion seen at endoscopy are the factors used to decide if a restorative resection is possible. My results with restorative resection are fair in terms of function but some patients have developed late vaginal fistula or anastomotic stenosis. Similar results have been obtained by Gazet (1985) and rather better results come from a large series reported by Barker (1985). We have advocated a protective colostomy but Barker's superior results have been obtained without colostomy.

Although surgery for RBD is difficult the most recent reports of resection indicate that the morbidity is moderate and the operative mortality low. In general the most worrying feature after apparently successful operations has been the development of severe radiation disease involving the urinary tract some months later. The most common problem has been bladder contracture with back pressure leading to a progressive deterioration of renal function. Less common are vesico-vaginal fistula and ureteric stenosis leading to hydroureter and hydronephrosis.

The seriousness of these problems can be seen when it is realised that they are as common a cause of death as recurrent tumour in the patients who have had surgery for RBD.

CONCLUSION

The gastrointestinal tract frequently receives incidental radiation when intra-abdominal malignancy is being treated by radiotherapy. The reaction of the gastrointestinal tract is dose dependent. An immediate reaction is common as the mucosal cells are particularly vulnerable to radiation but later disease is due to a progressive endarteritis. The later changes may be more common than is generally realised but usually do not produce obvious clinical effect so that manifest bowel injury is relatively rare. Radiotherapy directed to the pelvis is particularly prone to cause bowel injury. In the past, 80% of clinically significant RBD was associated with previous treatment for carcinoma of the uterine cervix. Pelvic radiotherapy is now being more widely used for other conditions such as carcinoma of the prostate and carcinoma of the rectum and these are beginning to feature more in reports of RBD.

There are peculiar diagnostic difficulties because the bowel symptoms develop months or years after the radiotherapy and it is all too easy to forget the previous treatment and ascribe symptoms to either recurrence of the malignancy or some totally unassociated condition. Accurate diagnosis is important because many of these patients will require surgery. Provided the operation is based on the correct surgical principle of wide excision, little operative morbidity and good long term results can be expected in a majority of patients. The biggest challenge remains the problems associated with either coincident or subsequent radiation-induced urinary tract injury.

REFERENCES

Anseline P F, Lavery I C, Fazio V W, Jagelman D G, Weakley F L 1981 Radiation Injury of the rectum. Annals of Surgery 194: 716–724
Barker E M 1985 Endo-anal anastomosis without proximal stoma — a safe procedure. British Journal of Surgery 72: S132–S133
Bourne R G, Kearsley J H, Grove W D, Roberts S J 1983 The relationship between early and late gastrointestinal complications of radiation therapy for carcinoma of the cervix. International Journal of Radiation Oncology, Biology and Physics 9: 1445–1450
Carr N D, Holden D, Hasleton P S, Schofield P F, 1985 Platelet Count in radiation bowel disease: an aid to diagnosis. British Journal of Surgery 72: 287–288
Carr N D, Schofield P F, Pullen B R, 1984 A method for the determination of microvascular volume in tissue samples. Clinical Physics and Physiological Measurement 5: 21–27
Carr N D, Pullen B R, Hasleton P S, Schofield P F 1984 Radiation bowel disease. Gut 25: 448–454
Danjoux C E, Catton G E 1979 Delayed complications in Colo-rectal carcinoma treated by combination radiotherapy and 5- Fluorouracil — Eastern Cooperative ONCOLOGY Group (ECOG) Pilot Study. International Journal of Radiation Oncology, Biology and Physics 5: 311–316
De Cosse J J, Rhodes R S, Wentz W B, Raegan J W, Dworken H J, Holden W D 1969 The natural history and management of radiation induced injury of the gastrointestinal tract. Annals of Surgery 170: 369–384
Denker H, Holmdahl K H, Lunerquist A, Olivecrona H, Tyle U 1972 Mesenteric angiography in patients with radiation injury of the bowel after pelvic irradiation. American Journal of Roentgenology 114: 476–481
Devereux D F, Kavanah M I Feldman E, Kondi D, Hull M, O'Brien M Deckers P J, Mozden P J 1984 Small bowel exclusion from the pelvis by a polyglycolic acid mesh sling. Journal of Surgical Oncology 26: 107–112
Donaldson S S, Jundt S, Ricour C et al 1975 Radiation enteritis in children a retrospective review. Clinico-pathological correlation and dietary management. Cancer 35: 1167–1181
Durig M, Steenblock U, Heberer M, Harder I 1984 Prevention of radiation injuries to the small intestine. Surgery, Gynecology and Obstetrics 159: 162–163
Futh H, Ebeler F 1915 Röntgen-und radium therapie des uteruskar. Zinoms Zentralblatt für Gynakologie 39: 217–227
Gallez-Marchal D, Foyolle M, Henry- Amar M, Le Bourgeois J P, Rougier P, Cosset J M 1984 Radiation Injuries of the gastrointestinal tract in Hodgkin's disease. Radiotherapy and Oncology 2: 93–99
Gazet J C 1985 Parks colo-anal pull-through anastomosis for severe complicated radiation proctitis. Disease of the Colon and Rectum 28: 110–114
Gilinsky N H, Burns D G, Barbezat G O, Levin W, Myers H S, Marks I N, 1983 The natural history of radiation induced proctosigmoiditis: An analysis of 88 patients. Quarterly Journal of Medicine 52: 40–53
Gree N, Goldberg H, Goldman H, Lombardo L, Skaist L 1984 Severe rectal injury following radiation for prostatic cancer. Journal of Urology 131: 701–704
Hasleton P S, Carr N D, Schofield P F, 1985 Vascular changes in radiation bowel disease. Histopathology 9: 530–548
Hatcher P A, Thomson H J, Ludgate S N, Small W P, Smith A N 1985 Surgical aspects of intestinal injury due to pelvic radiotherapy. Annals of Surgery 201: 470–475
Kjorstad K E, Martimbeau M D, Iversen T 1983 Stage IB carcinoma of the cervix. The Norwegian Radium Hospital: Results and Complications. Gynaecologic Oncology 15: 42–47

Lillemoe K D, Brigham R A, Harmon J W, Feaster M, Saunders J R, d'Avis J A 1983
Surgical Management of small bowel radiation enteritis. Archives of Surgery
188: 905–907

Ormiston M C E 1985 A study of rat intestinal wound healing in the presence of radiation
injury. British Journal of Surgery 72: 56–58

Rubin P 1984 Late effects of chemotherapy and radiation therapy: A new hypothesis.
International Journal of Radiation Oncology Biology and Physics 10: 5–34

Schofield P F, Holden D, Carr N D, 1983 Bowel disease after radiotherapy. Journal of the
Royal Society of Medicine 76: 463–466

Schofield P F, Carr N D, Holden D 1986 The pathogenesis and treatment of radiation
bowel disease. Journal of the Royal Society of Medicine 79: 30–32

Sherrah-Davies E 1985 Morbidity after selectron therapy for cervical cancer Clinical
Radiology 36: 131–139

Tomas de la Vega J E, Banner B F, Hubbard M, Boston D L, Thomas C W, Straus A K,
Roseman D L 1984 Cytoprotective effect of Prostaglandin E_2 in irradiated rat ileum
Surgery, Gynecology and Obstetrics 158: 39–45

Walsh H P J, Schofield P F 1984 Is laparotomy for small bowel obstruction justified in
patients with previously treated malignancy? British Journal of Surgery 71: 933–935

Wobbes T, Verschueren R C I, Lubbers E-J C, Jansen W, Paping R H L 1984 Surgical
aspects of radiation enteritis of the small bowel. Diseases of the Colon and Rectum
27: 89–92

The management of lower gastrointestinal haemorrhage

DEFINITION

Bleeding from the oesophagus, stomach, and first and second parts of the duodenum accounts for the majority of cases of 'upper gastrointestinal haemorrhage' and can be diagnosed by use of a flexible endoscope. Haemorrhage beyond the range of the gastroscope has empirically been called 'lower gastrointestinal haemorrhage'. Clinically, this definition has merit in that it is often impossible to distinguish between colonic haemorrhage and bleeding from the ileum or jejunum. Assessment of the literature is also confused by the varying volumes of blood transfused to patients before the bleeding is termed 'massive'. Authors refer to 2-unit, 4-unit and even 5-unit transfusions before inclusion into their studies (Eaton, 1981; McGuire & Haynes, 1972; Drapanas et al, 1973)). The identification of 'massive' colonic haemorrhage is important, for these patients have a high rate of recurrent bleeding and an operative mortality up to 50% (Eaton, 1981), unless correctly treated. This group will be discussed in greater depth later in the chapter.

SIZE OF THE PROBLEM

In a review of 7231 consecutive admissions to a Surgical Unit in Southampton from July 1981–1984 (2120 of which were emergencies) 107 patients (1.3%) were admitted with lower gastrointestinal haemorrhage, i.e. 5% of all emergencies. The average age of the 107 patients was 66 (range 19–93). A breakdown of the diagnosis on discharge in each patient is shown in Table 10.1.

The overall mortality in this group was less than 2%. Ninety percent of the subjects stopped bleeding spontaneously. However, of those requiring 4 or more units of blood the mortality rose to 8.6%. In a recent study by Eaton (1981) from Nottingham reviewing 293 cases of rectal bleeding the overall mortality was 15% in those requiring more than 2 units. Furthermore of those undergoing surgery 50% died. These results are by no means unique. Until this decade the surgical treatment of persistent life threat-

Table 10.1   Discharge diagnosis of patients
with lower gastrointestinal haemorrhage,
1981–84; $n = 107$

Diagnosis	Number
Diverticular disease	30*
Carcinoma of colon	28
Inflammatory bowel disease	17
Colonic polyps	10
Vascular ectasia	6
Ischaemic colitis	3
Rectal ulcer	3
Haemorrhoids	2
Anticoagulant treatment	1
Thrombocytopaenia	1
Aorto sigmoid fistula	1*
Malignant histiocytosis	1
Anastomotic bleed	1
Undetermined	1
Total	107

* 2 Deaths (1.8%)

ening haemorrhage from the colon was emergency blind segmental colectomy with a mortality of 30–40% and a rebleed rate of 30–50% (Eaton,
1981; McGuire & Haynes, 1972). The adoption of subtotal colectomy as
the procedure of choice eliminated rebleeding but the mortality rate
remained above 10% (Drapanas et al, 1973) and only after the routine use
of angiography in these patients did it start to fall below this figure (Baum
et al, 1974).

AETIOLOGY

Diverticular disease

Prevailing concepts of the cause of lower gastrointestinal bleeding have been
continually changing during the past fifty years. In the 1920's neoplasms
were considered the most frequent cause of significant bleeding; bleeding
from diverticular disease was thought to be rare (Lockhart-Mummery,
1923). However, by the late 1940's and early 1950's haemorrhage attributed
to diverticular disease was being reported commonly (Young & Young,
1944; Hoar & Bernhard 1954), and Noer (1955) in an elegant piece of work,
clearly showed that colonic diverticular were a major site of massive colonic
haemorrhage and that the complication usually started in an uninflammed
diverticulum (Fig. 10.1).

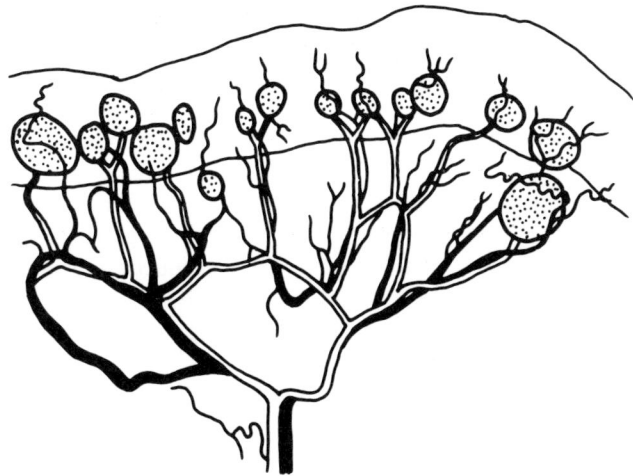

Fig. 10.1 Diagramatic representation of colon showing the distribution of vessels in relation to diverticula; taken from Noer (1955)

In the late 1950's and early 1960's a clear differentiation was made between the frequent occurrence of haemorrhage complicating diverticular disease and the much less common association of bleeding with diverticulitis. It was during this period that the predominant aetiologic role of diverticular disease in massive lower intestinal bleeding was postulated and widely accepted. This role was based upon the acceptance of 'diagnosis by exclusion', that is failure to identify another cause of bleeding in patients with diverticular disease. This approach was exemplified by the criteria established by Quinn & Ochsner (Quinn & Ochsner, 1953; Quinn, 1960), that a diagnosis of diverticular bleeding must have (a) the passage of considerable volumes of bright red or maroon blood via the rectum; (b) radio-graphic evidence of diverticuli; (c) no other demonstrable cause of haemorrhage on barium enema or sigmoidoscopy; (d) no blood in the gastric aspirate and/or no obvious abnormality on gastroscopy; (e) normal blood coagulation studies.

Vascular abnormalities

Margulis, Heinbecker and Bernard in 1960 employed operative angiography to identify a vascular malformation of the caecum which had caused massive bleeding in a 69 year old woman. Since that time and especially after the introduction by Baum et al (1965) of selective angiography for identifying the source of intestinal bleeding there have been numerous reports of bleeding from caecal vascular abnormalities (Baum et al, 1977). Our recent experience and that of others (Richter et al, 1984) suggest that these caecal vascular ectasias or angiodysplasia are as important as or even more important than diverticular disease as a cause of lower gastrointestinal haemorrhage, especially in the elderly.

The condition was described by Margulis in 1960 and the term angio-dysplasia then coined by Galdabini in 1978. The prominent features macros-copically are markedly dilated tortuous submucosal veins. The lesions appear to be ectasias of the normal vascular structures rather that malfor-mations and the pattern of involvement points to dilatation of the submu-cosal veins as the initial morphological change (Fig. 10.2). Partial and intermittent low grade obstruction of the submucosal veins, especially where they pierce the muscle layers of the colon, leads to this high pressure. The obstruction, repeated over many years during muscular contraction and distension of the colon, results in dilatation and tortuosity initially of the submucosal veins and then, in a retrograde fashion, of the venules of the arteriolar-capillary-venular units draining into it. Ultimately the capillary rings surrounding the crypts dilate and the competency of the precapillary sphincter is lost producing a small arterio-venous fistula. Bleeding from angiodysplasia is therefore venous, and that of diverticular disease arterial (Meyers et al, 1973). This has significant clinical implications as venous bleeding tends to result in intermittent large volumes whilst arterial is sudden, and on the whole less in volume. Analysis of the volumes of blood lost in the two conditions bears this out; patients with angiodysplasia require significantly greater volumes of blood than patients with diverticular disease (Wright et al, 1980).

The problem of attributing bleeding to a vascular ectasia or to diver-ticular disease when bleeding from the lesion is not demonstrated endo-scopically or by extravasation of contrast material on angiography is compounded by the frequent occurrence of these disorders without bleeding in people over 60 years of age. Diverticular disease has been estimated to occur in up to 50% of the population — above this age (Hughes, 1969), and in a study by Boley et al (1977), it was suggested that mucosal vascular ectasias of the right colon could be found in over a quarter of the same group without any evidence of bleeding. Therefore, in the absence of a demonstrable site of bleeding, the only basis for determining whether ident-ified angiodysplasia or diverticular disease is responsible for the bleeding is the indirect evidence provided by the course of the patient after resection of the suspected lesion.

MANAGEMENT

The patient is usually admitted as an emergency after having evacuated a huge quantity of blood. The suddeness of the event is surprising as the patient is usually asymptomatic and has no abdominal findings. The symp-toms and signs of hypovolaemia may also be minimal since blood loss often occurs over many hours or days in a colon that can accommodate a litre or more of blood, while plasma volume is partially replenished from the

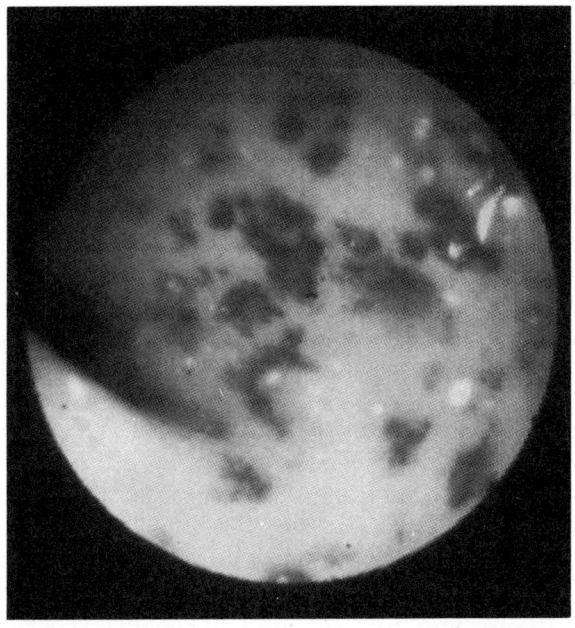

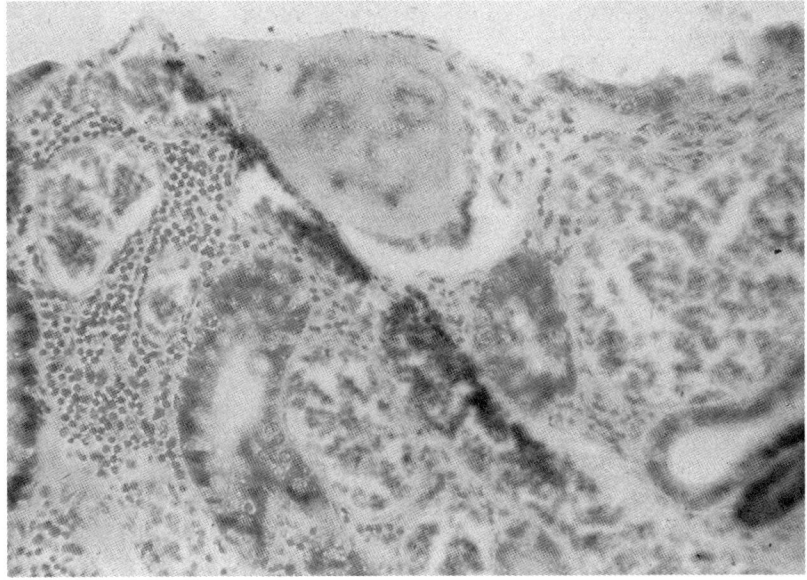

Fig. 10.2 Photograph of (top) macroscpic and (bottom) histological appearance from sections of angiodysplasia illustrating the dilated venules

extracellular fluid. The colon then suddenly empties. Conservative management is indicated at first in all patients. Blood is taken for group and cross match, haemoglobin and coagulation studies and a large bore intravenous cannula inserted (see Fig. 10.3). The patient should then undergo a thorough clinical examination, including rectal examination, proctoscopy and rigid sigmoidoscopy to rule out anal or rectal bleeding sites. Upper gastrointestinal haemorrhage should be excluded by gastroscopy. If these facilities are unavailable the temporary insertion of a naso-gastric tube has been advocated (Wright et al, 1980) but experience has shown this to cause confusion as it may become blocked and gives a false sense of security.

Bleeding will permanently stop in 90% of patients treated conservatively before transfusion requirements exceed 2 units in the first 24 hours. Table 10.2 clearly shows that all 84 individuals receiving less than 2 units of blood stopped bleeding spontaneously. However, if the subject required more than 4 units in the first 24 hours they had a 50% chance of requiring surgery. Although no individuals requiring less than 4 units in the Southampton study required surgery (Table 10.3), most workers label the haemorrhage as 'massive' where more than 3 units of blood are transfused (Wright et al, 1980; Boley et al, 1979). Once 3 units of blood have been given, an aggressive search for the cause of bleeding should be instituted no matter what time of day or night. It is highly likely that surgery will be necessary and highly desirable that such surgery not be done blindly without knowledge of the cause of bleeding.

Table 10.2   Lower gastrointestinal haemorrhage

Volume of blood transfused	Number of individuals	Inviduals requiring surgery
0–2 units minimal)	84	0
2–4 units (moderate)	11	0
4–25 units (severe)	12	7
Total	107	7

The patient who stops bleeding

Some controversy remains about how much further diagnostic work up is necessary in patients who stop bleeding spontaneously on conservative management. Certainly, nothing should be done for several days as bleeding may be started again by a barium enema or colonoscopy, detaching the clot at the bleeding site. It is current practice in Southampton to perform colonoscopy at 10 days. Barium enema is advocated by some workers but there is increasing evidence that the result is inaccurate, especially in the presence of diverticular disease (Farrands et al, 1983).

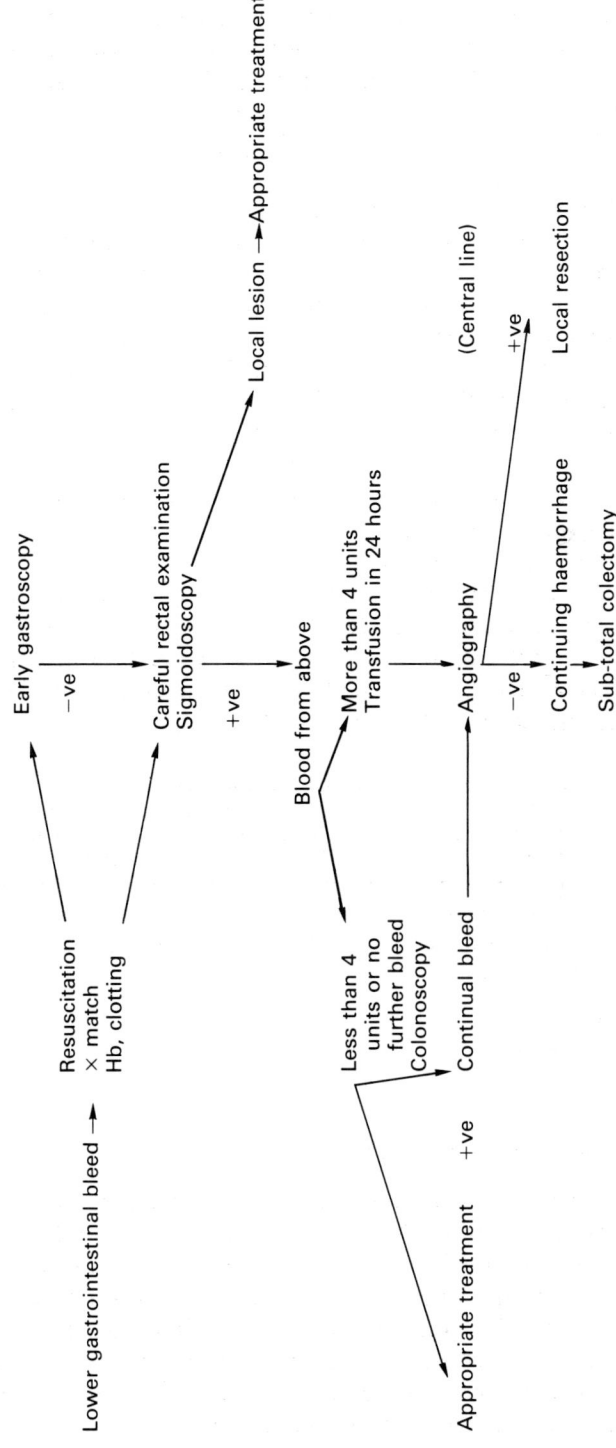

Fig. 10.3 Maagement of lower gastrointestinal haemorrhage

Table 10.3 Lower gastrointestinal haemorrhage requiring more than 2 units of blood

| Diagnosis | Number | Outcome | | |
		Settled	Surgery	Died
Angiodysplasia	6	4	2	–
Diverticular disease	5	4	1	1
Bleeding polyp	4	4	–	–
Crohn's colitis	2	1	1	–
Haemorrhoids	1	–	–	–
Ischaemic colitis	1	1	–	–
No cause found	1	1	–	–
Anastomotic bleed	1	–	1	–
Aorto-sigmoid fistula	1	–	1	1
Malignant histocytosis	1	–	1	–
Total	23	15	7	2

INVESTIGATIONS

A break-down of the investigations undertaken in the 12 individuals requiring more than 4 units of blood is shown in Table 10.4. It can be seen that barium enema was undertaken in all but one of the cases; it was diagnostic in only 2, and in a further 2 it indicated diverticular disease to be present when the patient was in fact bleeding from angiodysplasia.

Adams (1974) studied the usefulness of barium enema as a therapeutic measure. In 49 episodes of massive colonic bleeding (3 unit transfusions or more) 38 patients with known diverticular disease and no other cause of bleeding, stopped following the barium enema. This work has been supported by Wright (1980), who found haemorrhage to be controlled in at least 75% of patients after barium enema examinations. If bleeding recurs the barium is rapidly excreted and no technical problem is created at sugery.

Colonoscopy

If the bleeding rate is less than 0.5 ml per minute, as in patients who require 3–4 units of blood in 48 hours or more and who continue to bleed, colonoscopy may be of value. In 90% of cases it revealed the cause of bleeding (Table 10.4). However, it must be noted that in 3 patients more than 2 examinations were undertaken and in one 3, before the diagnosis was obtained. Wright et al (1980) has found similar results with an 82% accuracy in 11 patients with lower gastrointestinal haemorrhage. Todd & Forde (1979) found colonoscopy to be of value in 43% of 21 studies performed for acute lower gastrointestinal bleeding after barium enema and/or mesen-

Table 10.45 Lower gastrointestinal haemorrhage. *Severe:* (4–25 units) $n = 12$.

Diagnosis	Ba. enema	Colonoscopy	Arteriography	Operation	Outcome
Crohns Colitis	+ve	+ve	NO	Subtotal	
Diverticular disease	+ve	+ve	—	Subtotal	Died
No cause found	—	—	—	NO	
Anastomotic bleed	—	+ve	+ve	Rt. Hemi.	
Aorto-sigmoid fistula	NO	NO	NO	YES	Died
Malignant Histiocytosis	—	NO	NO	Sm. Bowel Resection	
Angiodysplasia 1.	—	+ve	—	Subtotal	
2.	—	+(×3)	—	NO	
3.	—	+(×2)	+ve	NO	
4.	—	+(×2)	+ve	Rt. Hemi.	
5.	DD	+ve	+ve	NO	
6.	DD	+ve	+ve	NO	
Total yield	2/11 (18.8%) 2 false +ve	9/10 (90%)	5/9 (55.5%)	7/12 (58%)	

teric angiographic examinations were inconclusive. Hagihara et al (1977) have had similar results in selected cases and have been able to demonstrate arteriovenous malformations by colonoscopy between massive bleeding episodes. It must be noted that these reports are by experienced colonoscopists and as judged by the number of examinations undertaken in some patients in the Southampton study colonoscopy can be a complicated and difficult procedure. When the patient is actively bleeding, powerful suction and good irrigation are essential. The clinician must exercise extreme caution and be prepared to terminate the procedure if visibility is poor.

Angiography

If transfusion requirements exceed 4 units of blood in the first 24 hours, selective mesenteric angiography is the procedure of choice. Bleeding rates of 1.0 to 1.5 ml a minute are required to demonstrate bleeding by means of angiography. The importance of this is exemplified in Table 10.4. Typical features are recognised in angioplasia and are illustrated in Figure 10.4. Nine patients underwent angiography, in 5 it was diagnostic. All 5 patients had had large bleeds and angiography in all 5 was undertaken within 24 hours of their admission. This point is also emphasised by Bar et al (1980) who in a study of 24 patients were only able to find the bleeding site in 10. Twelve of the 14 examinations providing negative results, having been undertaken after 48 hours despite 'massive' haemorrhages. Nath et al (1981), in a study of 49 patients with massive GI bleeding, found an extravasating lesion in only 12 patients (25%), and a suggested site of bleeding in only a further 12 patients. In 24 (50%) no comment concerning the site of bleeding could be made.

Salem et al (1985) have recently compared the results of selective visceral angiography and colonoscopy in the diagnosis of 34 patients with angiodysplasia. Twenty-three of the colonoscopies were positive, giving a diagnostic yield of 68%. Three colonoscopies were negative and eight were incomplete. Eight patients were found to have coexisting lesions at colonoscopy, four marked diverticular disease, three sigmoid polyps greater than one centimetre in size and one a colonic carcinoma, lesions not identified by angiography.

Technetium labelled red blood cell scintigraphy

The binding of 99 m technetium pertechnetate to red blood cells in patients bleeding into the gastrointestinal tract and then imaging of the patient with a gamma camera has recently been suggested to be superior to both colonoscopy and arteriography in the localisation of the bleeding point (Harvey et al, 1985). Bleeding rates as low as 0.05–0.10 ml/minute can be detected by scintigraphy in experimental animals (Alavi et al, 1977). Harvey et al (1985) studied 16 patients with massive gastrointestinal bleeding. Scintigraphy

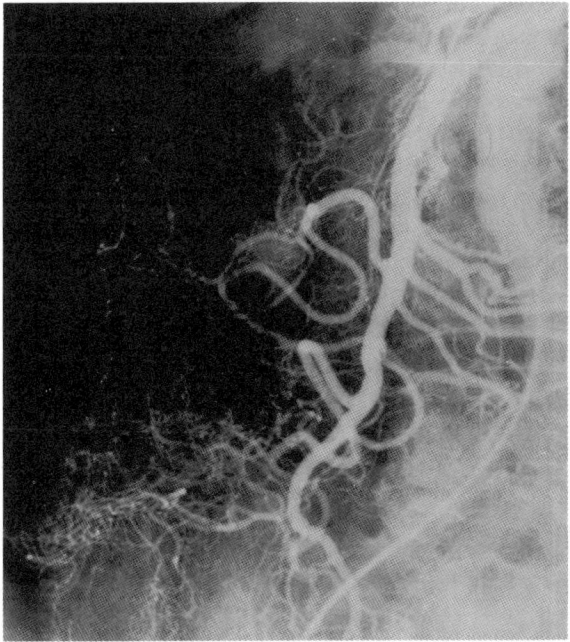

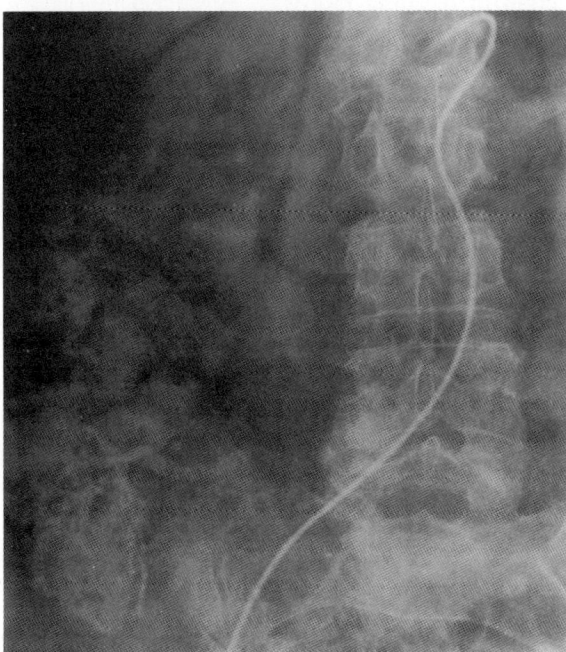

Fig. 10.4 Photograph of two X-ray plates from a patient with angiodysplasia clearly showing (top) the leash of vessels in the right colon and (bottom) the large draining vein diagnostic of this condition

revealed a bleeding site in all 16 patients. Eight patients had positive scans within 30 minutes indicating the ability of the method to detect active bleeding. The other eight patients had delayed positive scans indicating intermittent haemorrhage and suggests a potential advantage over angiography which is so dependent on active bleeding.

TREATMENT

In addition to using colonoscopy for diagnosis, colonoscopy has the added advantage of often being therapeutic. Patients with polyps can undergo polypectomy and areas of angiodysplasia can be elecrocoagulated. Howard et al (1982), in a study of 26 patients with unexplained anaemia or blood loss per rectum, due to angiodysplasia, carried out electrocoagulation in 23 subjects. Six subsequently required surgical intervention, but in 17 no further bleeding occurred. However, follow-up revealed that 11 patients had rebled and in 3 surgical treatment was undertaken without excision of the vascular area.

Rutgeerts et al (1985) have recently published their experience using the Neodymium Yag laser in photocoagulation of vascular malformations of the gastrointestinal tract. In angiodysplasia 82% of 49 patients were successfully treated via the colonoscope. The more numerous the lesions, the less effective the reduction in bleeding rate was. However, this is a most exciting development and may well result in a further reduction in mortality from gastrointestinal haemorrhage.

Surgery

If (despite transfusion) the patient continues to bleed catastrophically surgery is indicated. This is usually apparent after no more than 6 units have been given. Blind segmental resections should *never* be performed. In a review by Eaton (1981) from Nottingham of 28 patients undergoing emergency surgery 2 had right hemicolectomies, 4 left hemicolectomies, 14 sigmoid colectomies with anastomosis, 4 sigmoid colostomies with a mucous fistula, and 4 subtotal colectomies with ileorectal anaestomosis. Sixty-four percent re-bled, 50% required further surgery and 50% died postoperatively. These results mirror all previous results using blind segmental resections (McGuire & Haynes, 1972; Drapanas et al, 1973). If the surgeon is unsure of the site of bleeding a subtotal colectomy with or without an ileorectal anastomosis should be performed. Drapanas (1973) first popularized subtotal colectomy after reviewing 35 patients with massive haemorrhage who had had a subtotal colectomy, only 4, or 11%, of whom had died. Since then other workers have obtained similar results (Wright et al, 1980; Boley et al, 1979).

Despite its popularity the mortality from the subtotal colectomy remains above 10%. If arteriography is available and the site of bleeding is confidently seen, then a segmental resection may be performed. This procedure is less traumatic and carries a lower mortality. Casarella and Welch, using this technique, reported surgical mortality rates of less than 6% (Casarella et al, 1974; Welch et al, 1978). However, it is essential to stress the importance of accurate arteriography before undertaking segmental colectomy.

Surgery for angiodysplasia

When the only demonstrable lesion on angiography has been right sided angiodysplasia, a right hemicolectomy should be performed. Although there is increasing evidence that angiodysplastic lesions are multiple, almost all of them are proximal to the splenic flexure and would be included in a right hemicolectomy. When right-sided angiodysplasia and left sided diverticulosis occur together without a demonstrable bleeding site, a subtotal colectomy should be performed.

Surgery for 'bleeding' diverticular disease

Theoretically ligation of the offending vessel in the wall of a bleeding diverticulum should be curative. However, this procedure is not practical. With a known diverticular bleeding site a limited colectomy, with a concomitant lower mortality, can be performed even when the patient has been known to have universal diverticular disease. If there is any doubt a subtotal colectomy should be performed.

An advance in intraoperative localization of massive colonic bleeding has recently been described by Cambell et al (1985). In a study of four cases, the large bowel was rapidly cleaned at laporotomy by lavage using urological saline. The patient is placed in the Lloyd Davies position and a catheter inserted into the caecum. Fluid is then run into the caecum and allowed to escape from the anus into a bucket until clear. Colonoscopy is then performed. Using this technique, all four patients they describe had identifiable causes of bleeding when previous arteriography and colonoscopy had failed and no patients had a blind resection.

The problem of occult bleeding

Patients bleeding slowly and intermittently may present a difficult problem. If faecal occult blood tests are positive and upper gastrointestinal endoscopy is normal the patient should have a colonoscopy. Barium enema is known to be inaccurate especially in the presence of diverticular disease (Farrands et al, 1983). In a well prepared bowel and with an experienced operator a colonic lesion will be detected by colonoscopy. The problem arises if colonoscopy is normal. Angiography is of limited value if the patient is not actively bleeding. The next step is small bowel studies and then Technetium labelled red blood cell infusions. However, even then there remain a small number of patients who require laparotomy to elucidate the disorder, and ignorant of the source, the surgeon will be forced to take the patient to theatre, attempt to localize the lesion and excise it.

CONCLUSIONS

Ninety percent of patients with colonic haemorrhage stop bleeding spontaneously. Patients with massive gastrointestinal haemorrhage must be identified and if they require more than 4 units of blood in 24 hours should undergo arteriography as soon as possible. For those patients requiring surgery where the source of bleeding is clearly identified segmental resections of the bleeding site should be performed. If the clinician is unsure of the diagnosis, subtotal colectomy with or without an ileorectal anastomosis should be undertaken.

REFERENCES

Adams J T 1974 The barium enema as treatment for massive diverticular bleeding. Diseases of the Colon and Rectum 17: 439–441

Alavi A, Dann R W, Baum S et al 1977 Scintigraphic detection of acute gastrointestinal bleeding. Radiology 124: 753–756

Bar A M, Delaurentis A, Parry C E, Kiohane R B 1980 Angiography in the management of massive lower gastrointestinal tract haemorrhage. Surgery, Gynecology and Obstetrics 150: 226–228

Baum S, Alhanasoulis C A, Waltman A C et al 1977 Angiodysplasia of the right colon: a cause of gastrointestinal bleeding. American Journal of Roentgenology 129: 789–793

Baum S, Alhanasoulis C A, Waltman A C 1974 Angiographic diagnosis and control of large-bowel bleeding. Diseases of the Colon and Rectum 17: 447–453

Baum S, Nusbaum M M, Blakemore W S 1965 The preoperative radiographic demonstration of intraabdominal bleeding from undetermined sites by percutaneous selective coeliac and superior mesenteric arteriography. Surgery 58: 797–805

Boley S J, Dibiase A, Brandt L J, Sammartano R J 1979 Lower intestinal bleeding in the elderly. American Journal of Surgery 137: 57–63

Boley S J, Sammartano R, Adams A et al 1977 On the nature and etiology of vascular eclasias of the colon; degenerative lesions of ageing. Gastroenterology 72: 650–660

Cambell W B, Rhodes M, Kettlewell M G W 1985 Colonoscopy following intra-operative lavage in the mangement of severe colonic bleeding. Annals of the Royal College of Surgeons 67: 290–292

Casarella W J, Galloway S J, Taxin R N et al 1974 Lower gastrointestinal tract haemorrhage. New concepts based on arteriography. American Journal of Roentgenology 121: 357–360

Drapanas T, Pennington D G, Kappelman M et al 1973 Emergency subtotal colectomy. Preferred approach to the mangement of massively bleeding diverticular disease. Annals of Surgery 177: 519–526

Eaton A C 1981 Emergency for acute colonic haemorrhage — a retrospective study. British Journal of Surgery 68: 109–112

Farrands P A, Vellacott K D, Amar S S, Belfour T W, Hardcastle J D 1983 Flexible fibreoptic sigmoidoscopy and double contrast barium-enema examination in the identification of adenomas and carcinomas of the colon. Diseases of the Colon and Rectum 26: 727–729

Galdabini J J, Waltman A C et al 1978 angioplasia of colon. A cause of rectal bleeding. Cardiovascular Radiology 1: 3–13

Hagihara P F, Chuang V P, Griffen W O 1977 Arteriovenous malformations of the colon. American Journal of Surgery 133: 681–687

Harvey M M, Neoptolemos J P, Watkins E M, Cosgriff P, Barrie W W 1985 Technitium labelled red blood cell scintigraphy in the diagnosis of intestinal haemorrhage. Annals of the Royal College of Surgeons of England 67: 89–92

Hoar C S, Bernhard W F 1954 Colonic bleeding and diverticular disease of the colon. Surgery, Gynecology and Obstetrics 99: 101–104

Howard O M, Buchanan J D, Hunt R M 1982 Angiodysplasia of the colon. 26 cases. Lancet ii: 16–19

Hughes L E 1969 Postmortem survey of diverticular disease of the colon. Gut 10: 336–340

Lochkhart-Mummery J P 1923 Diseases of the rectum and colon and their surgical treatment. Bailliere Tindall and Cox, London, p 448

Margulis A R, Heinbecker P, Bernard H R 1960 Operative mesenteric arteriography in the search for the site of bleeding in unexplained gastrointestinal haemorrhage. Surgery 48: 534–539

McGuire M M Jr, Haynes B W Jr 1972 Massive haemorrhage from diverticulululitis of the colon. Annals of Surgery 175: 847–852

Meyers M A, Volberg F, Katzen B et al 1973 Angioarchitecture of colonic diverticular. Radiolaogy 108: 249–260

Nath R L, Sequerira J C, Weitzman A F, Birkett D M, Williams L F 1981 Lower gastrointestinal bleeding: Diagnostic approach and management conclusions. American Journal of Surgery 141: 478–481

Noer J N 1955 Harmorrhage as a complication of diverticulities. Annals of Surgery 141: 674–683

Quinn W C 1960 Diverticular disease of the colon with haemorrhage: A study of 78 cases. American Journal of Surgery 26: 171–174

Quinn W C, Ochsner A 1953 Bleeding as a complication of diverticulitis. American Journal of Surgery 1: 397–401

Richter J M, Medberg S E, Alhanasoulis C A, Schapiro R M 1984 Angiodysplasia, clinical presentation and colonoscopic diagnosis. Digestive Diseases and Sciences 2: 481–485

Rutgeert, Van Gampel F, Geboes K et al 1985 Long term results of treatment of vascular malformations of the gastrointestinal tract by neodymium Yag Laser Photocoagulation. Gut 26: 586–593

Salem R R, Wood C B, Rees M C, Kheshavarzian A, Hemingway A P, Allison D J 1985 A comparison of colonoscopy and arteriography in the diagnosis of colonic angiodysplasia. Annals of the Royal College of Surgeons 67: 225–226

Todd G J, Forde K A 1979 Lower gastrointestinal bleeding with negative or inconclusive radiographic studies: the role of colonoscopy. American Journal of Surgery 138: 627–628

Welch C E, Alhanasoulis C A, Galdabini J J 1978 Haemorrhage from the large bowel with special reference to angiodysplasia with diverticular disease. World Journal of Surgery 2: 73–76

Wright M K, Pelliccia O, Higgins E F, Sreenivas V, Gupta A 1980 Controlled semielective, segmental resection for massive colon haemorrhage. American Journal of Surgery 1980; 139: 535–537

Young E L, Young E L 1944 Diverticulitis of the colon: a review of the literature and an analysis of ninety one cases. New England Journal of Medicine 230:33

SUGGESTED FURTHER READING

Veidenheimer M C, Corman M L, Coller J A 1978 Colonic Haemorrhage. Surgical Clinics of North America 58 (3)

Best E B, Teaford A K, Rader F H 1979 Angiography in chronic/recurrent gastrointestinal bleeding: A nine year study. Surgical Clinics of North America 59 (5)

Surgical aspects of constipation, anal incontinence and anorectal pathophysiology

Any patient presenting with a complaint of constipation or of anal incontinence should be fully investigated to detect organic disease. This includes a full history, physical examination and the appropriate investigations, including radiology and endoscopy. In this review it is proposed to concentrate on the problems involved in patients with constipation who do not have a clear organic explanation for their symptom on routine examination; on the aspects of both constipation and incontinence that are related to the changes in the functions of the anus and rectum, and on the techniques in use specifically to assess these functions. These techniques will be considered first followed by a discussion of their place in the elucidation of the causes of the two main symptoms.

ASSESSMENT OF ANORECTAL FUNCTION

History

It is important to have as exact a quantitation of the presenting complaint as possible in order to be able to assess its severity when considering the possible side effects of any therapy, and in order to be in a position to document any improvement. Counts of the number of stools or the incidents of soiling must be made meticulously with the help of a diary card. Many of these patients have psychological features to their illness and it is worthwhile considering an objective personality profile. Other aspects to be noted especially are urinary symptoms, abdominal symptoms, history of trauma, of childbirth (with any difficulties) and of drugs because so many have a tendency to cause constipation.

Clinical examination

The extent of faecal loading should be looked for both in the abdomen and in the rectum. Inspection of the perineum will detect evidence of soiling and scarring and should include the effects of straining, of voluntary sphincter contraction and of stretching the perineum. The anal reflex should be elicited. Digital examination of the rectum will give information about the anal sphincteric tone, the puborectalis sling and their responses; althouth only the extremes of power can be detected with accuracy. If the anus remains gaping after pulling posteriorly with the examining finger and withdrawing it, clear evidence is provided of weakness of the control mechanism.

Radiology

Anorectal angle

The angle between the axis of the rectal lumen and the axis of the anal canal which is about 80° in normal subjects (Tagart, 1966) can be measured by several techniques. With a lateral X-ray projection the rectum can be outlined with barium and the anal canal with barium powder or with a string of radio-opaque beads (Read et al, 1984). A balloon filled with barium can be placed in the rectum with a tube attached so it can visualise the axes of the anal canal and rectum. (Preston et al, 1984).

Pelvic floor

The above techniques can show the level of the pelvic floor relative to the ischial tuberosities when the patient strains down although a more clinically useful method is described below.

Colonic transit

Twenty ingested radio-opaque markers are used both to estimate total gastrointestinal transit time and relative colonic transit: the first requires daily collection of stools which are X-rayed so obviating any radiation to the patient (Hinton et al, 1969): the second requires daily abdominal radiographs for seven days or until the markers have all been passed, whichever is the shorter (Corazziari et al, 1975; Martelli et al, 1978).

Examination with simple apparatus

Rectal sensation

A balloon on a tube placed in the rectum will give a measure of the sensation to distension when it is inflated with air. It is important that the balloon should be spherical and of high compliance. The lower end of the balloon should be at least 5 cm from the anus to stimulate the lower rectum. Threshold of sensation can be recorded when sensation is only felt fleetingly (normally about 20 ml) as well as the levels at which the sensation becomes patients (about 100 ml) and then just tolerable (about 350 ml): the lower rectum is more sensitive than the upper rectum and sigmoid (Ihre, 1974).

Artificial faecal bolus

The capacity to expel a balloon placed in the rectum and filled with variable amounts of fluid can help to assess the explusive forces (Barnes & Lennard-Jones, 1985) as can the introduction of plastic spheres of varying sizes which are attached to tapes for retrieval should the subject be unable to pass them. More difficulty is encountered in passing the smaller boluses — less than 50 ml in a balloon or spheres smaller than 1.0 cm in diameter. In cases where continence is being examined warm saline can be run into the rectum at a fixed rate (60 ml/min) up to a maximum of 1500 ml to detect any leakage, ie an escape of 10 ml of fluid or more (Read et al, 1985).

Descent of the pelvic floor

Objective measurements of the movement of the pelvic floor can be made with a frame consisting of two rods which rest on the ischial tuberosities joined by a crossbar containing a hole through which a freely moveable graduated perspex rod is placed against the anus. The position of the anus relative to the tuberosities can then be measured with and without the subject straining. The anus in normal subjects is 2.5 cm above the tuberosities at rest and descends 1.5 cm on straining. (Henry et al, 1982)

Examination with complex apparatus

Anorectal manometry

Strain gauges, amplifiers and suitable recording apparatus are needed for accurate measurement of the force exerted in the anal canal and rectum by the action of the muscles — smooth and striated. Fluid-filled fine tubes 0.5 to 1.0 mm in diameter with small side openings and having a low compliance perfusion system or small balloons 2 to 5 mm in diameter mounted on fine tubes are connected to strain gauges and are the most frequently used methods. Alternatives are to use a 'sleeve' on an obturator or to place the strain gauges themselves on the probe (Duthie, 1971). The precise measurements obtained with any system should be checked for reproducibility by each group of workers before establishing their own range of normal. We utilise a triple lumen tube 4 mm in diameter with side openings 1 cm apart. By inserting the measuring device into the rectum and withdrawing it through the anal canal either in steps or in one continuous movement the relative strength of the sphincter barrier is recorded. The stepwise procedure also indicates the length of the functional sphincter from the first rise in pressure above that in the rectal ampulla which the measuring device encounters on entering the orad part of the anal canal to its exit from the anus when it records atmospheric pressure. The maximal resting pressure and the maximal pressure in response to voluntary squeeze are usually noted. A balloon for distension of the rectum is also frequently used in order to document relaxation of the pressure in the orad part of the anal canal (so-called rectoanal reflex RAR) which follows upon inflation of the rectal balloon, both as to the extent of the relaxation and the volume required in the rectal balloon. In adults 20 to 30 ml is the threshold volume for RAR, that is, slightly smaller than the volume for conscious appreciation of balloon inflation. In addition, if the recording sites are kept steady a regular pattern of oscillations is seen in the orad part of the anal canal usually 6 to 16 cycles per minute — very occasionally a wave form lasting 1 to 1.5 minutes may be observed (ultraslow waves).

Electromyography of striated muscle

Concentric needle electrodes connected to amplifiers and analysing recorders are used to detect electrical activity in the external anal sphincter (EAS) and in puborectalis (PR). Both exhibit an unusual feature for striated muscles in that they have a continuous tonic activity, which is increased on coughing, on Valsalva and at the commencement of balloon distension of the rectum. However a diminution occurs on straining and when a bolus is withdrawn through the anal canal. Inhibition results when the rectal balloon is maintained sufficiently distended (Porter, 1962). A more sophisticated analysis of the signals results in a capacity to measure nerve conduction times from electrodes placed on the skin over the sacral cord or placed on the pudendal nerve by attaching the electrodes to a finger stall and directing them onto the nerve no insertion through the anal canal.

If suitable expertise is available single fibre electromyography is possible. This can indicate the density of muscle fibres in the area sampled and hence the extent of any motor denervation (Swash, 1986). The measurement of the latency in an evoked response from perianal skin (Bartolo et al, 1983) was also used as an indication of denervation but has been overtaken by the more precise single fibre electromyography (Swash 1986).

Electromyography of smooth muscle

The electrical activity of smooth muscle in vivo is best detected by two electrodes 3 to 5 mm apart and such have been placed in the internal anal sphincter by means of needle introducers or on an obturator in the anal canal. Wave forms have been detected but their role in relation to the maintenance of internal anal sphincter function is not clear (Wienbeck & Altaparmacov, 1980).

CONSTIPATION

It is not proposed to make a list of the causes of constipation, but rather to concentrate on those with clear anorectal pathophysiological changes at three periods in the lifecycle in children, in adults and in the elderly.

CHRONIC IDIOPATHIC CONSTIPATION IN CHILDREN

History

The majority of children brought for medical consultation because of constipation have encopresis and have some problems with their relationships within the family. In distinction to adults most children with constipation are males. A history lasting from birth leads to suspicion of Hirschprung's disease.

Pathophysiology

Over 90% of children with idiopathic constipation are found to have an enlarged rectum although it does not necessarily relate directly to findings when rectal compliance is measured, but in general there is a greater volume of air required in a rectal balloon to reach the maximum tolerable volume; almost twice that in controls. (Meunier et al, 1984) There is some conflict of evidence on the threshold for reflex inhibition of the anal canal pressure with some workers finding it to be significantly raised (Cucchiara et al, 1984) and others finding it raised but not significantly (Loening-Baucke, 1984). Similarly, the resting pressure in the anal canal has been found to be increased in a proportion of children in some studies (Ahran et al, 1983) while others indicate a reduction (Loening-Baucke & Younoszai, 1982), which may be explained on the possible presence of faeces in the rectum. Agreement does exist that all constipated children have a diminished rectal sensation and that this indicates damage to the rectal wall. An abnormal response of the pelvic floor muscles studied by electromyography has also been found in about 40% of children with encopresis (Meunier et al, 1984). Total gastrointestinal transit time is significantly increased in children with chronic constipation and decreases with successful treatment.

Thus it would seem that children with idiopathic constipation have abnormalities in the rectum, with diminished sensation, and in the anal sphincteric mechanism, either a hypertensive sphincter or one which relaxes poorly to rectal distension.

It should be mentioned that one of the best methods of diagnosing Hirschprung's disease is by manometry when there is no reduction of the pressure in the anal canal in response to the inflation of a balloon in the rectum, ie the rectoanal inhibitory response is lost.

Management

These children are usually treated with a medical and dietary regime but in cases with an overactive sphincter formal internal sphincterotomy has been used with good effect.

CHRONIC IDIOPATHIC CONSTIPATION IN ADULTS (Fig. 11.1)

History

Much has been written on the difficulties of defining constipation, as what can seem a normal bowel habit to one individual may seem constipation to another. Most agree that a prospective record of stool frequency is the most reliable method of assessment (Manning et al, 1976) and that three stools per week is the lower limit of normal. (Paese et al, 1985) This symptom must have lasted for several years and organic causes excluded before it can be classed as chronic idiopathic constipation. Associated symptoms of difficulty in expelling stools and of a feeling of incomplete emptying of the rectum are common. Abdominal pain may be a feature and raises the question of the irritable bowel syndrome in which many patients are constipated. Almost all patients with chronic idiopathic constipation are women.

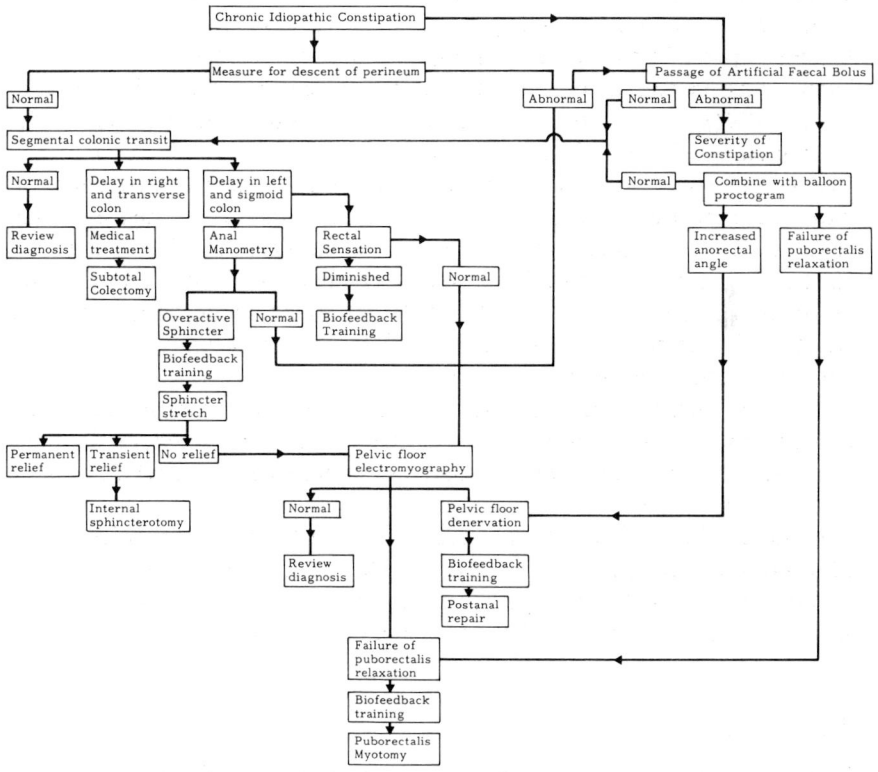

Fig. 11.1 Algorithm of investigation and management of idiopathic constipation

Those who have to resort to digital evacuation of faeces are amongst the most difficult to treat. Psychological factors are important in this complaint as in many others but patients who have no positive findings on examination are rare in practice and no patient should be labelled as having psychogenic constipation without a full investigation. The group of patients we shall be considering are those who have failed to respond to dietetic measures, addition of fibre to the diet and the use of laxatives. Some of this hard core of resistant cases respond to biofeedback training and others to surgical treatment, but the use of these methods is ill-defined and by no means generally accepted.

Pathophysiology

Testing the capability of expelling a balloon or solid spheres introduced into the rectum can indicate the severity of the difficulty in defaecation. In some patients who are unable to pass a balloon filled with barium, lateral radiography has shown a failure of the normal increase in the anorectal angle on straining, indicating an inability of the puborectalis to relax (Preston et al, 1984). The failure to pass a balloon is found both in patients with a normal barium enema and in those with megarectum and has been attributed to failure of inhibition of the voluntary component of the anal canal high pressure zone (Barnes & Lennard-Jones, 1985)

Study of transit times is most useful in that it provides an objective measure of the symptoms and if the technique of sequential abdominal radiographs is used it may give information about the site of hold up. (It may also detect that the initial complaint is not valid.) The markers may accumulate in the rectum, in the rectum and left colon or ascending and/or transverse colon. It has been suggested that when they are held up in the rectum that some form of outlet obstruction exists and that when held up more proximally the term slow transit constipation should be used. In young women with severe slow transit constipation about 75% have urinary symptoms and a lack of sensitivity can be detected on bladder distension and on rectal distension, indicating a possibility of a similar type of sensory abnormality involving both organs (Bannister et al, 1985). Patients who have painless constipation are found to have slow colonic transit whereas those with pain tend to have abnormalities in the anorectal manometry findings similar to those mentioned below (Lanfranchi et al, 1984).

When anorectal manometry is performed on patients with colonic transit studies suggestive of outlet obstruction some abnormalities indicative of an overactive internal anal sphincter may be found: an increased resting sphincter pressure: a diminution in the relaxation response to balloon distension of the rectum: an overswing of pressure in the sphincter after the above relaxation in response to rectal distension: the presence of ultraslow waves in the sphincteric pressure tracing (Martelli et al, 1978; Orr & Robinson, 1981).

Patients with the descending perineum syndrome may have constipation at an early stage before developing incontinence with or without a prolapse of the rectum and will be considered when anal incontinence is discussed.

Management

Biofeedback training

Patients can be taught to change the pattern of action of the muscles of the pelvic floor and anal sphincter complex by watching the effects of their efforts on a monitor or a chart recorder (Schuster, 1986). The technique is used more often in anal incontinence and has been successful in North America (Engel et al, 1974; Cerulli et al, 1979) but is largely neglected in the United Kingdom. In cases with constipation for example, it is possible to teach a patient to relax the puborectalis sling on straining and so alleviate one of the mechanisms of outlet obstruction leading to constipation. A patient with an overactive internal sphincter is more difficult to manage and efforts have to be directed to encourage them to increase the amount of relaxation in the sphincters when they feel the balloon in the rectum being inflated. Where possible biofeedback training should be tried before resorting to surgery. In cases with slow transit constipation biofeedback training has not yet found a place.

Surgery

It cannot be overemphasised that surgical treatment for chronic constipation is used for a small minority and that great care must be taken to have a full psychological assessment of these patients as well as having established as far as possible the nature of the defects leading to constipation.

Slow colonic transit

When slow transit in the colon is found it is useful to distinguish between those who have a great deal of abdominal pain and those who are not troubled by this symptom: the latter tend to have more successful results from surgery. Other information which may help to detect those likely to respond comes from measuring the motor response to local instillation of bisacodyl into the colon by manometry: those with no effective response should benefit from resection. The procedure undertaken for slow transit constipation without evidence of outlet obstruction is subtotal colectomy with either ileorectal or caecorectal anastomosis. The former is said to give more effective results at the expense of more frequent bowel actions. Relief can be expected in about two-thirds of cases (Preston et al, 1984).

Outlet obstruction

An overactive internal anal sphincter found on manometry may be treated by stretching or by sphincterotomy. However, great care must be taken to ensure that there are no features suggestive of pelvic floor neuropathy (see later) because interference with the sphincters will most likely lead to symptoms of incontinence which can occur after anal dilation done for other conditions (Snooks et al, 1984). It seems logical to perform a sphincter stretch first. This abolishes the manometric changes and gives symptomatic relief. Should the effect be transient, internal sphincterotomy can then be performed in which a strip 1 cm wide and 5–6 cm long is removed from the midline posterior part of the muscle beginning at its inferior edge. When the overactive anal sphincter is associated with adult megacolon, anal dilatation has proved an effective treatment (Taylor, 1984).

In those patients in whom a failure of the puborectalis sling to relax has been detected it has been advocated that this muscle should be divided in the midline posteriorly through an intersphincteric approach. This gives relief in a proportion of subjects but more have problems with incontinence (Barnes et al, 1985) and the procedure cannot yet be said to be established.

CHRONIC IDIOPATHIC CONSTIPATION IN THE AGED

History

The majority of aged patients with severe constipation present with faecal impaction and with overflow incontinence and constitute about a fifth of patients admitted to geriatric hospital units. Many of these patients have been taking laxatives for years which may have induced damage to the myenteric plexus: other medicaments include analgesics. In addition, most have associated prolapsed haemorrhoids which may be exacerbated by straining to pass the faecal bolus in contrast to a frequently-advanced explanation for their constipation, namely that they ignore the urge to pass faeces because of the confusion and depression which is common in the elderly. Other features include lack of mobility, general muscular weakness and lack of readily available toilet facilities.

Pathophysiology

Studies of intestinal transit time in geriatric patients with constipation have shown delay mainly in the rectosigmoid but there is an overlap with both subjects of the same age and with younger patients (Melkersson et al, 1983).

Tests of simulated defaecation indicate that, while almost all such patients can pass a balloon containing fluid, only about one third are able to pass solid spheres of 1.8 cm diameter. Sensation in the anal canal and the awareness of the inflation of a balloon in the rectum are blunted. The maximum volume tolerable on the stepwise inflation of the rectal balloon is greatly increased and is often so large that the balloon is expelled spontaneously before the patient finds it intolerable. Anal manometry reveals no difference from normal in maximal resting pressure or squeeze pressure, but patients with impaction of faeces show an increase in the amount of air required in the rectal balloon to initiate inhibition of the anal sphincteric pressure (Read et al, 1985).

Thus in distinction to younger patients the elderly show few manometric changes and no indication of overactivity of the sphincters but rather a blunting of sensation in the anal canal and rectum, which could be contributed to by straining at stool over a long period with consequent neurological changes (see under descending perineum syndrome).

Management

Surgery has little if any place in the treatment of elderly patients with chronic idiopathic constipation and reliance is placed on attempting to re-educate them to awareness of rectal contents and to bulking agents and osmotic laxatives.

ANAL INCONTINENCE

History

The most important aspect of anal incontinence is the extent to which frank faecal soiling occurs because this complaint is truly disabling and can lead to the patient leading a hermit-like existence. Careful documentation of its occurrence and relationship to the consistency of the stools is required. The severity of incontinence has a descending scale of priorities: leakage of solid stool, soft stool, liquid stool and then flatus: the last alone needs no treatment.

Some indication of which of the two anal sphincters is mainly at fault may be found from the symptoms: leakage of mucus between soiling episodes when the internal sphincter is weak: urgency and frequent small stools passed spontaneously when the external sphincter is weak: lack of awareness that soiling has occurred in idiopathic (neurogenic) incontinence.

Known causes

The majority of patients suffering from anal incontinence have had some form of trauma — direct injury to the perineum as in a road traffic accident, injury during childbirth or following surgery to the anal canal or rectum (Keighley & Fielding, 1983). In the postsurgical group operations for fistula, stretching of the sphincters, haemorrhoidectomy and coloanal anastomosis following rectal excision are the most frequently encountered procedures.

Patients with diarrhoeal diseases may have soiling at the height of their symptoms and, as observed above, patients with constipation and rectal impaction may have overflow incontinence.

Idiopathic anal incontinence

The gradual onset of faecal incontinence occurs in patients, the majority being women, most of whom have been straining excessively to pass their stools for many years. The symptoms progress from occasional soiling when the faeces are fluid to frank daily incontinence which demands treatment. Occasionally, urinary incontinence is also found, and uterine prolapse may be present. While this complaint has been entitled idiopathic, a sufficent body of evidence has been accumulated for it to be more correctly called neurogenic.

Descending perineum syndrome

A subgroup of patients with neurogenic incontinence has been defined by the fact that they have an abnormal degree of descent of the pelvic floor on straining coming to below the level of the ischial tuberosities, as measured with the apparatus described previously. They have the typical long history of straining at stool, eventually having incontinence. In addition, they experience a persistent dull aching pain in the anal region or the perineum in general which is not related to defaecation but can be made worse by long periods of standing and can be relieved by lying down. Mucus discharge and bleeding from the anus can occur if the anterior rectal wall becomes inflamed or ulcerated. These patients may also complain of rectal prolapse.

Examination

Inspection of the perineum may show soiling and scarring in and around the anal canal. The anus may be patulous, gape on stretching the surrounding skin or gape when the examining finger is removed after pulling posteriorly on the anal canal muscles. A rectal or vaginal prolapse may be evident on straining. Measurement of the amount of descent of the perineal floor on straining should be made as outlined previously. Digital assessment of the puborectalis sling and anal canal with and without voluntary contraction of the muscles will give an indication of their strength. Endoscopy may reveal an ulcerated area on the anterior rectal wall and should be extended to detect any inflammatory or neoplastic disease.

Pathophysiology of anal incontinence

Objective measurement of the capability of the sphincteric mechanism to hold up to 1500 ml fluid run in through a rectal tube shows the extent of the deficiency, and similarly anorectal manometry will show a low pressure in the anal canal. However, neither can indicate the reason for the weakness. In patients with known causes the history usually indicates damage to the external anal sphincter — trauma, surgery or childbirth — and electromyography can be used to pinpoint the extent of a gap in the external anal sphincter. Electromyography of the smooth muscle of the internal anal sphincter has not been clinically useful to indicate the extent of damage, as for example after forcible sphincter stretching.

Pathophysiology of neurogenic incontinence and the descending perineum syndrome

The voluntary muscles of the pelvic floor and the anal canal have been found to have changes indicating partial denervation. Histological studies have shown an increase in the diameter of both Type 1 and Type 2 fibres along with an increased variability of fibre size. In some cases there is severe loss of muscle fibres and fibrosis. (Type 1 fibres are capable of sustained contraction and are responsible for the continuous activity found in the pelvic floor and anal canal striated muscles. Type 2 fibres are more short-acting and are recruited with voluntary action.) These changes are compatible with denervation. Further supporting evidence has come from electromyographic and neurological investigations which have been mainly of two forms — single fibre electromyography and nerve conduction studies. Single fibre electromyography shows a great increase in fibre density, indicating marked re-innervation from collaterals in the damaged muscles. The terminal latency in the pudendal nerves, innervating the external anal sphincter, is significantly increased in patients with incontinence, and the conduction in spinal roots S_3 and S_4, innervating puborectalis is also slower than normal: this would indicate that both muscles are involved in these patients with incontinence, some of whom had a rectal prolapse (Snooks et al, 1985). In patients in whom denervation is found only in the external anal sphincter there is less likelihood of severe incontinence than when the puborectalis is also affected (Bartolo et al, 1983). It is not clear whether the neurological changes are primary or secondary. One hypothesis which has been advanced is that the continual straining leads to stretch damage to the pudendal nerves with an increase in the anorectal angle, so that the anterior rectal mucosa can prolapse into the proximal anal canal with consequent increased difficulty in emptying the rectum. Further stress on the pudendal nerves produces increasing denervation of the pelvic floor which weakens and descends further, so further reducing the effectiveness of the puborectalis in maintaining continence and gives rise to the descending perineum syndrome with incontinence and the possibility of rectal prolapse. Also associated is a solitary rectal ulcer found on the anterior rectal wall in the area of mucosa that recurrently prolapses into the anal canal on straining.

Although most attention has been concentrated on the motor aspects of denervation some evidence is available that the sensory innervation of the pelvic floor may also be impaired (Womack et al, 1986).

Management of anal incontinence

In patients with traumatic damage to the external anal sphincter, electromyography permits accurate localisation of the retracted ends of the muscle which can then be dissected out of the fibrous scar tissue and sutured together with an overlap which prevents disruption of the repair when the muscle retracts. Four out of five patients treated by this method regain continence for solid and liquid stools, but not for flatus and a further one in ten can control solid stools only. Best results are in young patients with direct injury: obstetrical damage and surgical treatment of fistulae do not respond so well (Browning & Motson, 1984).

Incontinence in diarrhoeal disease in managed as part of the overall treatment but a specific effect of the antidiarrhoeal loperamide (Read et al, 1982) has been observed in increasing the resting pressure in the anal canal. Constipation with overflow similarly falls under the management of constipation.

Biofeedback training When traumatic defects in the striated muscles are imcomplete, biofeedback training has been most useful in restoring confidence (Schuster, 1986). Some patients have also responded to the use of biofeedback techniques when electromyography and anal mamometry indicate that the deficiency is in the internal anal sphincter, a situation where no surgical manoeuvre is available.

Neurogenic constipation and the descending perineum syndrome

In the phase of constipation and straining before incontinence occurs, conservative management of the constipation with dietary measures, bulking agents and enemas may halt the progress of the disorder. When incontinence has occurred recourse may be had to biofeedback techniques to augment the strength of the muscles (Schuster, 1986). With an intensive regime good responses may be achieved in 60% of cases (Cerulli et al, 1979). Electrical stimulation of the striated muscles has also been used by means of an intra-anal plug bearing electrodes (Hopkinson & Lightwood, 1967) or by implanting electrodes on the puborectalis, but the longterm results have not lived up to initial expectations in some groups (Collins et al, 1969) whereas others have been more successful (Glen, 1971). This method has not gained general popularity.

In the fully developed descending perineum syndrome post anal repair of the puborectalis and external anal sphincters restores continence in four out of five patients (Browning & Parks, 1983). Through a postanal incision an approach is made between the internal and external anal sphincters and a three layer repair of the pelvic floor posterior to the rectum is combined with a repair of the external anal sphincter. To maintain the result patients must be managed to avoid straining at stool to prevent further nerve damage.

When a full thickness rectal prolapse is present and the patient is incontinent, abdominal rectopexy, though successful in curing the prolapse, seldom benefits the incontinence and so a second procedure, namely postanal repair, is required at a later date (Keighley & Matheson, 1981). It is usual to perform the operations in that order. However, it has been suggested that in young patients a postanal repair should be used first as it may also control the prolapse and it avoids deep pelvic dissection which may compromise fertility (Browning et al, 1983).

CONCLUSION

Considerable advances have been made in the management of constipation and anal incontinence so that less and less recourse has been made to the ultimate surgical intervention of a colostomy.

REFERENCES

Ahran P et al 1983 Idiopathic disorders of fecal continence in children. Pediatrics 71: 774–779
Bannister J J, Lawrence W T, Thomas D G, Read N W 1985 Urological abnormalities in patients with slow transit constipation. Gut 26 (in press)
Barnes P R H, Hawley P R, Preston D M, Lennard-Jones J E 1985 Experience of posterior division of the puborectalis muscle in the management of chronic constipation. British Journal of Surgery 72: 475–477
Barnes P R H, Lennard-Jones J E 1986 Balloon expulsion from the rectum in constipation of different types. Gut 26: 1049–1052
Bartolo D C C, Jarratt J A, Read M G, Donnelly T C, Read N W 1983 The role of partial denervation of the puborectalis in idiopathic faecal incontinence. British Journal of Surgery 70: 664–667
Bartolo D C C, Jarratt J A, Read N W 1983 The cutaneo-anal reflex: a useful index of neuropathy? British Journal of Surgery 70: 660–663
Browning G G P, Parks A G 1983 Postanal repair for neuropathic faecal incontinence: correlation of clinical results and anal canal pressures. British Journal of Surgery 70: 101–104
Browning G G P, Rutter K R P, Motson R W, Neill M E 1983 Postanal repair for idiopathic faecal incontinence. Proceedings of Sir Alan Parks Memorial Symposium, Annals of Royal College of Surgeons, London
Browning G G P, Motson R W 1984 Anal sphincter injury: management and results of Parks sphincter repair. Annals of Surgery 199: 351–357
Cerulli M A, Nikoomanesh P, Schuster M M 1979 Progress in biofeedback conditioning for fecal incontinence. Gastroenterology 76: 742–746
Collins C D, Brown B H, Duthie H L (1969) An assessment of intraluminal electrical stimulation for anal incontinence. British Journal of Surgery 56: 542–546
Corazziari E, Dani S, Pozzessere C, Anzini F, Torsoli A 1975 Colonic segmental transit times in non-organic constipation. Rendiconti di Gastroenterologia 7: 67–69
Cucchiara S et al 1984 Gastrointestinal transit time and anorectal manometry in children with fecal soiling. Journal of Pediatric Gastroenterology and Nutrition 3: 545–550
Duthie H L 1971 Anal continence. Gut 12: 844–849

Engel B T, Nikoomanesh P, Schuster M M 1974 Operant conditioning of rectosphincteric responses in the treatment of fecal incontinence. New England Journal of Medicine 290: 646–649

Glen E S 9171 Effective and safe control of incontinence by the intra-anal plug electrode. British Journal of Surgery 58: 249–252

Henry M M, Parks A G, Swash M 1982 The pelvic floor musculature in the descending perineum syndrome. British Journal of Surgery 69: 470–472

Hinton J M, Lennard-Jones J E, Young A C 1969 A new method for studying gut transit times using radio opaque markers. Gut 10: 842–847

Hopkinson B R, Lightwood R 1967 Electrical treatment of incontinence. British Journal of Surgery 54: 802–806

Ihre T 1974 Studies on anal function in continent and incontinent patients. Scandinavian Journal of Gastroenterology 9: Supplement 25

Keighley M R B, Fielding J W L 1983 Management of faecal incontinence and results of surgical treatment. British Journal of Surgery 70: 463–468

Keighley M R B, Matheson D M 1981 Results of treatment for rectal prolapse and fecal incontinence. Diseases of the Colon and Rectum 24: 449–453

Lanfranchi G A, Bazzochi G, Brignola, C, Campieri M, Labo G 1984 Different patterns of intestinal transit times and anorectal motility in painful and painless chronic constipation. Gut 25: 1352–1357

Loening-Baucke V A 1984 Abnormal rectoanal function in children recovering from chronic constipation and encopresis. Gastroenterology 87: 1299–1304

Loening-Baucke V A, Younoszai M K 1982 Abnormal anal sphincter response in chronically constipated children. Journal of Pediatrics 100: 213–218

Manning A P, Wyman J B, Heaton K W 1976 How trustworthy are bowel histories? Comparison of recalled and recorded information. British Medical Journal 2: 213–214

Martelli H, Devroede G, Arhan P, Dugay C 1978 Mechanisms of idiopathic constipation: outlet obstruction. Gastroenterology 75: 623–631

Melkersson M, Andersson H, Bosaeus I, Falkheden T 1983 Intestinal transit time in constipated and non-constipated geriatric patients. Scandinavian Journal of Gastroenterology 18: 593–597

Meunier P, Louis D, Jaubert de Beajeu M 1984 Physiologic investigation of primary chronic constipation in children: comparison with the barium enema study. Gastroenterology 87: 1351–1357

Orr W C, Robinson M G 1981 Motor activity of the rectosigmoid in patients with chronic constipation. Gastroenterology 80:1244

Paese P, Staiano A, Bausano G, Cucchiara S, Corrazziari E 1985 Bowel frequency in healthy subjects. Italian Journal of Gastroenterology 17: 133–135

Porter N H 1962 A physiological study of the pelvic floor in rectal prolapse. Annals of the Royal College of Surgeons 31: 379–404

Preston D M, Hawley P R, Lennard-Jones J E, Todd I P 1984 Results of colectomy for severe idiopathic constipation in women (Arbuthnot Lane's Disease). British Journal of Surgery 71: 547–552

Preston D M, Lennard-Jones J E, Thomas B M 1984 The balloon proctogram. British Journal of Surgery 71: 29–32

Read M, Read N W, Barber D C, Duthie H L 1982 Effects of loperamide on anal sphincter function in patients complaining of chronic diarrhea with fecal incontinence. Digestive Diseases and Sciences 27: 807–814

Read N W, Abouzekry L, Read M D, Howell P, Ottewell D, Donnelly T C 1985 Anorectal function in elderly patients with faecal impaction. Gastroenterology 89: 959–966

Read N W, Bartolo D C C, Read M G 1984 differences in anal function in patients with incontinence to solids and in patients with incontinence to liquids. British Journal of Surgery 71: 39–42

Schuster M M 1986 Anorectal motility in health and disease. In: Szurszewski J (ed) Proceedings of the 10th International Symposium on Gastrointestinal Motility, Elsevier, Amsterdam (in press)

Snooks S J Henry M M, Swash M 1984 Faecal incontinence after anal dilation. British Journal of Surgery 71: 617–618

Snooks S J, Henry M M, Swash M 1985 Anorectal incontinence and rectal prolapse: differential assessment of the innervation to puborectalis and external anal sphincter muscles. Gut 26: 470–476

Swash M 1986 Faecal continence: role of the levator ani and external anal sphincter. In: Szurszewski J (ed) Proceedings of the 10th International Symposium on Gastrointestinal Motility, Elsevier, Amsterdam (in press)

Tagart R E B 1966 The anal canal and rectum. Their varying relationship and its effect on anal continence. Diseases of the Colon and Rectum 9: 449–452

Taylor I 1984 Assessment of anorectal motility measurements in the management of adult mega colon. Scandinavian Journal of Gastroenterology 19: Supplement 96 61–68

Wienbeck M, Altaparmacov I 1980 Is the internal anal sphincter controlled by a myoelectrical mechanism? In: Christensen J (ed) Gastrointestinal Motility, Raven Press, New York, P 487

Womack N R, Morrison J F B, Williams N S 1986 Impaired recruitment of the pelvic floor musculature by intra-abdominal pressure in faecal incontinence. Gut 27 (in press)

Adjuvant systemic therapy for carcinoma of the breast

BACKGROUND

For the most part of this century the management of loco-regional disease has dominated discussion of breast cancer treatment. At the centre of these arguments have been the principles of therapy laid down almost a century ago by Halstead in the United States and Sampson Hadley in this country. Breast cancer was conceived as spreading from the primary tumour along lymphatics to its regional lymph nodes which acted as a type of filter. Eventually as these nodes became exhausted the cancer would migrate via its afferent channels to the next group of nodes and eventually through the fascial planes to the viscera and skeleton.

On the basis of this mechanistic model Halstead developed his radical en bloc operation which became the standard management in Europe and North America for more than 50 years (Halstead, 1907). Such was the domination of these ideas that there was little serious criticism of them until after the Second World War. Disillusion with radical surgery had in actual fact been first voiced as early as 1937 by Sir Geoffrey Keynes when he published the results of a consecutive series of patients treated by wide local excision supplemented with radium needles (Keynes, 1937). Results for this approach matched those for radical mastectomy both for early and more advanced cases. Whether it was the advent of the war or the post-war concern with the controlled trial that the impact of Keynes' work was ignored for nearly 40 years and is only now receiving more widespread significance.

Carefully controlled studies from both the United States and Britain have clearly exposed the fallacy of the Halstead and Sampson Hadley approach (Fisher, 1977; CRC, 1980). The American National Surgical Adjuvant Breast Project and the Cancer Research Campaign early breast cancer trials both demonstrate that survival after conservative surgery is no different from that after Halstead mastectomy, and morbidity is considerably reduced. Indeed recent controlled trials of tumour excision combined with radiotherapy have confirmed Keynes' results that this is as effective a therapy as mastectomy (Fisher, 1985).

One further point that these and similar clinical experiments have highlighted has lead to a new concept of breast cancer biology. Evidence that 20% of patients without axillary node metastases would relapse after radical mastectomy (Fisher, 1977) would seem to disprove the Halstead model of an orderly progressive spread via the lymphatics. Even the extension of the radical operation to include the lymphatics of the supraclavicular fossa and internal mammary nodes did not improve survival (Veronesi, 1967). From this Fisher has concluded that breast cancers commonly spread systematically and this probably occurs at a very early stage in the tumour's natural history before it is clinically detectable.

This concept of early systemic spread of disease has become widely accepted and has enormously influence the thinking about breast cancer over the last 15 years. Despite recent controversy over conservative surgery, emphasis in the management of breast cancer has switched to the treatment of its occult systemic spread, the so-called micrometastases, which are undetectable by our current screening procedures. From this has resulted a determined effort by clinicians to develop a systemic therapy capable of dealing with micrometastatic disease, that is adjuvant systemic therapy.

RATIONALE FOR ADJUVANT THERAPY

Further substantiation for systemic spread comes from those studies of the long-term natural history of the disease which reveal that about 70% of patients die of their disease (Brinkley, 1975; Mueller, 1975). More recent data from Brinkley and Haybittle who have been observing a cohort of patients in the Cambridge area suggest that this is probably an underestimate (Brinkley, 1984). Even our clinical appreciation of early diagnosis does not fit with biological reality; a one centimetre tumour has already been through 30 of the 40 doublings that are going to be lethal to the patient (De Vita, 1975). It is therefore not surprising that it has been shown that more than half the patients with apparently localised disease at diagnosis have micrometastases (De Vita, 1979).

TUMOUR CELL KINETICS

It has been suggested that micrometastatic disease may respond differently to chemotherapeutic agents than the primary tumour or advanced disease and that excision of the main bulk of disease alters the kinetics of the residual tumour. Data to support these hypotheses have come from Mendlesohn and Skipper who have defined the concept of a growth faction in tumour cell populations (Mendlesohn, 1960; Skipper, 1971). They regard tumours as consisting of three cell compartments. One compartment consists of actively proliferating cells responsible for tumour growth and susceptible to cell cycle specific chemotherapeutic agents. The cells of the second compartment are not actively proliferating but maintain the potential to do so if there is depletion of proliferating cells. These cells are consequently more resistant to cell cycle specific drugs and only become sensitive to these agents when the proliferative compartment is being destroyed. Cells in the third compartment are permanently non-proliferating and only contribute to tumour volume.

The growth fraction of a tumour is the ratio of proliferations to non-proliferating cells and the greater it is the more sensitive is the tumour to chemotherapy. Growth fraction changes with tumour growth, initial exponential growth becomes inhibited with increasing tumour size and sensitivity to chemotherapy consequently decreases. Micrometastases, however, have smaller populations of cells, often less than 10^6 cells which will approach exponential long-phase growth and these cells should theoretically be more sensitive to chemotherapy than their primary tumours.

Cell kill by cytotoxic drugs follows first order kinetics which means that a consistent proportion of the total tumour population is killed by a constant dose of drugs regardless of the size of the population (Skipper, 1971) This only applies to cell populations growing exponetically with constant growth fractions and tumour doubling times. This further increases the sensitivity of micrometastases over primary tumour or clinically detectable metastases to the same cytostatic therapy. Accordingly in a micrometastasis exhibiting exponential growth a drug may kill 99.9% of tumour cells no matter how many there are. In a micrometastasis of 100 cells there is a high statistical probability that all would be destroyed by a given dose of chemotherapy and that the patient would be cured. However in a metastasis consisting of 10^{10} cells the same chemotherapy would leave 10^6 viable cells with a potential of regrowth.

Skipper's experimental work suggests that the optimal time to eradicate all residual cells by chemotherapy is immediately after tumour reductive surgery when the number of remaining cells is smallest. In agreement with these observations a large number of experimental studies of adjuvant cytotoxic therapy have shown that the smaller the number of residual tumour cells, the greater the chemotherapeutic cure rate (Martin, 1981). These same studies have also shown that multiple drug chemotherapy is superior to single agent therapy. As the doubling times of breast cancers range from 20 to 200 days, it would be expected that to be effective adjuvant chemotherapy would have to be sustained for long periods at a time (Spratt, 1977).

Some of these theoretical considerations have been confirmed by the clinical trials of adjuvant chemotherapy although there are some contradictions which will be discussed below. There are now many such trials in the literature although few of these are mature enough to draw any conclusions from. It is not the intention to review all these trials comprehensively but to draw conclusions from more significant studies. Mainly cytotoxic and hormonal therapy have been used in the adjuvant setting and will be discussed separately. The main trials are summarised in Table 12.1.

Table 12.1 Summary of chemotherapy trials

Trial	Therapy and duration	Effect of treatment on relapse free survival		
		All patients	Subgroups	
Bonadonna 1984 (Italy	CMF (6 cycles)	12% improvement $P < 0.001$	23% improvement in pre- but not in postmenopausal patients	
Fisher 1981 (USA)	Melphalan (2 years)	No significant difference	Small improvement in premenopausal patients	
Howell 1984 (UK)	CMF (6 cycles)	17.4% improvement $P < 0.005$	Main difference in premenopausal patients	
Howell 1984 (UK)	Melphalan (16 cycles)	No significant difference	No difference	
Nissen-Meyer 1982 (Scandinavia)	peri-operative cyclophosphamide (5 days)	12.8% improvement $P < 0.02$		
Baum 1983 (UK)	Tamoxifen (2 years)	Significant improvement $P < 0.013$	No difference	

CYTOTOXIC CHEMOTHERAPY TRIALS

Early results

The earliest trials to test the hypothesis that chemotherapy given as an adjuvant to surgery might improve survival were initiated more than a quarter of a century ago (Fisher, 1968). It was not until the mid-1970s that widespread interest was aroused by the publication of the initial results of randomised, prospective controlled trials. These studies have had a profound effect on the treatment in the United States although they were treated with more scepticism in Britain. In these original trials entry was mainly restricted to patients with a poor prognosis, with Stage II carcinomas.

The first of these studies instituted by the National Surgical Adjuvant Breast Project (NSABP) in North America used a two-year course of melphalan (L-PAM) in patients with histologically positive axillary nodes. The preliminary results published in 1975 based on a total of 125 patients with an average follow-up of only 9 months. Recurrence-free survival was 22% in the placebo group compared with 9.7% for the patients receiving melphalan (Fisher, 1975).

The Milan trial started in June 1972 had identical entry criteria to the NSABP with the patients being stratified by age, (below 50 and 50–75 years) and nodal status (1–3 and more than 4 nodes). Randomisation was to 12 monthly cycles of cyclophosphamide, methotrexate and 5-Fluorouracil (CMF) or to no further treatment. Preliminary results after an equally short follow-up period to the melphalan trial were published in 1976. In 386 evaluable patients relapse-free survival was found to be significantly improved in those receiving CMF compared to controls (Bonadonna, 1976).

These trials were seen as a major advance in the treatment of breast cancer and immediately resulted in the indiscriminate use of this form of therapy outside of clinical trials, especially in the United States. The consequence of this has been to set back progress in the treatment of the disease. It has become impossible, because of medico-legal reasons, for randomised trials which contain a no further treatment arm to be carried out in North America, although most British and European experts would think this was mandatory. This insistance on proper controls by surgeons and oncologists in this country has been borne out by the longer-term follow-up data from these two studies.

Long term results

The melphalan trial, with longer follow-up, has failed to show any advantage in survival for the patients receiving chemotherapy. Any effect of the melphalan is to delay the appearance of clinically detectable metastases without having any effect on subsequent survival (Fisher, 1981). This was confirmed by a British study of the same design, which combined results from South Manchester and Guy's Hospital, and likewise showed no advantage for chemotherapy in terms of both survival and prolongation of the disease free period (Rubens, 1983). The most important lesson to be derived from these trials is the danger of too early publication of results. In many cases as Skipper suggested in his hypothesis chemotherapy may have the effect of retarding tumour growth without completely eradicating it. Therefore only survival data after long-term follow-up rather than the extension of the disease-free period should be accepted in the evaluation of these trials.

The Milan CMF trial does continue to give some encouragement after longer follow-up (Rossi, 1981). At 5 years the predicted survival for treated patients is 78% compared with 68% for controls and this is significantly better ($P < 0.04$). The difference appears to be mainly due to the effects of chemotherapy in premenopausal women which was also seen in the melphalan trial. Exactly similar results in this country for CMF therapy were found by the Manchester-Guy's group (Howell, 1984).

Overview of clinical trials

The euphoria of the 1970s has given way to a more pessimistic attitude. Contradictory claims have been made from the results of the many published studies, most of which have major defects in their design. In an attempt to get over these problems all trial organisations who have conducted randomised trials were asked to submit their data to be combined in one central analysis. It was hoped that an overview of the results from many studies might yield an estimate of the effect of the treatment that was more accurate than that provided by any single study (Review of mortality results in randomised trials in early breast cancer, 1984).

An analysis of over 10 000 women randomised into chemotherapy trials indicated that among women with early breast cancer there was a clearly significant reduction in short-term morbidity in those receiving adjuvant therapy ($P < 0.001$). These survival benefits were seen to be mainly confined to women under the age of 50 years confirming the result of the CMF studies and it has been suggested that some of this effect may be due to cytotoxic suppression of ovarian function. However some workers now feel that the data is strong enough to consider treating premenopausal women with adjuvant chemotherapy.

Other chemotherapy trials

Of interest is one other chemotherapy trial from Scandinavia. Patients were randomised to a six-day course of intravenous cyclophosphanide immediately after operation. This study has shown a survival advantage of more than 10% for treated patients which is still apparent at 15 years of follow-up (Nissen-Meyer, 1982). The difference between treatment groups did not become apparent until 4 years after treatment, and this trial would seem to fulfill Skipper's concept that early treatment is most effective. Given the clinical course of breast cancer a delay in the appearance of treatment effects would be expected if adjuvant therapy really were curing minimal metastatic disease rather than slowing tumour growth and lengthening the disease-free period.

Toxicity of chemotherapy

The proponents of adjuvant chemotherapy in their enthusiasm for the positive benefits often overlook its adverse effects. It is often claimed that these regimes are well tolerated but this is not the universal experience. A British self-assessment study found that 79% of patients reported side-effects severe enough to interfere with their lifestyle and almost one third of them said that they could not go through the experience again (Palmer, 1980). Similar experiences have been documented in America. In one report 78% of patients treated with CMF suffered severe nausea and vomiting and more than half had anticipatory vomiting. More worrying was that 30% of the patients could not continue treatment because of side-effects presumably, despite being told that it might prolong life (Wilcox; 1982). Psychiatric morbidity also increased and is also more apparent in these patients receiving chemotherapy (Maguire, 1980).

These side effects cannot be ignored. If the effect of present adjuvant chemotherapy is mainly to prolong disease-free survival that is to only delay recurrence, without any impact on actual survival, then its toxicity may outweigh this benefit. Balanced against this is the severe psychological impact that recurrence of disease has on women who think that they have undergone curative treatment. It may be for this reason that the single agent low toxicity regimen as seen in Nissen-Meyer's Scandinavian study may be the approach that should be adopted. Some of these problems may also be overcome with the use of hormonal therapy.

ADJUVANT HORMONE THERAPY

Early studies

Hormone therapy was first considered as an adjuvant to surgery as early as 1948. At that time a randomised centre trial was instituted at the Christie Hospital, Manchester, comparing oophorotomy to no further treatment in 596 premenopausal patients (Cole, 1975). Similar studies were set up in Oslo and Toronto differing only by the addition of predinisilone to some of the treatment groups (Nissen-Meyer, 1975; Meakin, 1969). The results of these trials are similar in that castration lengthens the disease-free survival without affecting overall survival, although a survival benefit almost reaches statistical significance in the Toronto study. These results are analogous with those achieved with chemotherapy although side-effects are considerably less.

Interest in the use of hormonal agents fell away in the 1970s because of the preliminary results of the chemotherapy studies. This is now increasing again following the disillusion with chemotherapy and the reported benefits of the use of the anti-oestrogen tamoxifen.

Adjuvant anti-oestrogens

In 1977 a British multicentre trial was set up to evaluate tamoxifen as an adjunct to local treatment in patients with operable breast cancer. The 1131 patients were randomised to receive tamoxifen 10 mg twice daily or no further treatment. After an average follow-up period of 35 months, 218 deaths were reported, 91 in the treated group and 127 in controls. This difference in survival was statistically significant ($P < 0.008$). After stratification by nodal, menopausal and by oestrogen receptor status, no difference in response rate was found for these sub-groups (Baum, 1983).

These results are encouraging and have been confirmed by other studies. Follow-up periods are still relatively short and we may still be observing the delay in recurrence seen in other hormonal and chemotherapy trials. The major difference between this drug regime and the cytotoxic chemotherapy is the almost complete lack of unwanted side-effects. It could therefore be argued that if in a subsequent analysis tamoxifen only appears to delay the onset of recurrence this effect may be worthwhile in itself. The same could obviously not be said for adjuvant chemotherapy with its very much greater toxicity.

There are still some questions that have not been answered by these trials. For instance there appears to be no relationship in response to the oestrogen receptor content of the primary tumour. It is difficult to explain how tamoxifen is effective in its action on receptor negative cancers. A second point that arises from this study is whether there will be any difficulty in treating patients when they relapse if they have already received a course of tamoxifen, as tamoxifen would normally be the first line of therapy in advanced disease. There is no clear evidence that these relapses will be amenable to a second course of anti-oestrogen. With these minor reservations adjuvant tamoxifen appears to be a significant contribution to breast cancer therapy.

CONCLUSION

So far adjuvant chemotherapy has had little effect on the prognosis of breast cancer except in some subgroups of patients, particularly pre-menopausal women. There is also evidence that this treatment may actually have adverse effects on the patient. This is not to say that the concept of adjuvant chemotherapy to deal with occult disease after surgery is wrong; it may imply that we do not yet have completely effective drugs.

Evidence is accruing that short courses of peri-operative single agent chemotherapy and hormonal therapy may be achieving some improvements in disease-free periods if not survival. This is being accomplished without the toxicity of multi-nodal chemotherapy.

These regimes still require evaluation and the role of adjuvant therapy should continue to be tested in controlled prospective trials.

REFERENCES

Baum M, Brinkley D M et al 1984 Improved survival amongst patients treated with adjuvant tamoxifen after mastectomy for early breast cancer. Lancet ii: 450

Bonadonna G, Brusamolinu E, Valagussa P et al 0000 Combination chemotherapy as an adjuvant treatment in operable breast cancer. 55: 405–410

Bonadonna G, Rossi A, Tancini G, Valagussa P, Veronesi U 1984 CMF adjuvant programs at the Milan Cancer Institute. In: Senn H J (ed) Recent Results in Cancer Research, Springer-Verlag, Berlin, p 66–73

Brinkley D, Haybittle J L 1975 The curability of breast cancer. Lancet i: 95–99

Brinkley D, Haybittle D L 1984 Long-term survival of women with breast cancer. Lancet i: 1118

Cole M P 1975 A clinical trial of an artificial menopause in carcinoma of the breast. In: Namer M, Lalanne C M (eds) Hormones and Breast Cancer, Paris INSERM, Vol 55, p 143–140

Cancer Research Campaign Working Party 1980 Cancer Research Campaign (Kings/Cambridge) Trial for early breast cancer. Lancet ii: 55

De Vita V T, Young R C, Canellos G P 1975 Combination versus single agent chemotherapy: a review of the basis for selection of drug treatment of cancer. Cancer 35: 98–110

De Vita V T, Henney J E, Storehill E 1979 Cancer mortality: the good news. In: Jones S E, Salmon S E (eds) Adjuvant therapy of cancer II, Grune & Stratton, New York, 212–216

Fisher B, Carbone P, Economou S G 1975 I-Phenylalanine mustard (L-PAM) in the management of primary breast cancer. New England Journal of Medicine 292: 117–122

Fisher B, Montague E, Redmond C, Barton B et al 1977 Comparison of radical mastectomy with alternative treatments for primary breast cancer. Cancer 39: 2827

Fisher B, Redmond C, Wolmark N, Wieland H S 1981 Disease-free survival at intervals during and following completion of adjuvant chemotherapy: the NSABP experience from three breast cancer protocols. Cancer 48: 1273–1280

Fisher B, Bauer M, Margolese R, Poisson R et al 1985 Five year results of a randomised clinical trial comparing the total mastectomy and segmental mastectomy with or without radiation in the treatment of breast cancer. New England Journal of Medicine 312: 665–673

Halstead W S 1907 The results of radical operations for the cure of cancer of the breast. Annals of Surgery 46: 1–9

Howell A, Rubens R D, Bush H, George W D et al 1984 A controlled trial of adjuvant chemotherapy with Melphalan versus cyclophosphamide, Methotrexaate and Fluorouracil for breast cancer. In: Senn H-J (ed) Recent Results in Cancer Research, Springer-Verlag, Berlin, p 74–89

Howell A, Bush H, George W D, Howat J M T et al 1984 Controlled trial of adjuvant chemotherqpy with cyclophosphamide, theotrexate and flurouracil for breast cancer. Lancet ii: 307–311

Keynes G. Conservative treatment of cancer of the breast. British Medical Journal ii: 643

Maguire G P, Tait A, Brooke M et al 1980 Psychiatric morbidity and physical toxicity associated with adjuvant chemotherapy after mastectomy. British Medical Journal 281: 1179–1180

Martin D S 1981 The scientific basis for adjuvant chemotherapy. Cancer Treatment Reviews 8: 169–189

Meakin J W, Allt W E C, Beale F A et al 1979 Ovarian irradiation and prednisilone following surgery and radiotherapy for carcinoma of the breast. In: Mouridsen H T, Polshof T (eds). Breast cancer: experimental and clinical aspects. Pergamon Press, Oxford, p 179–181

Mendelsohn M L 1960 The growth fraction: a new concept applied to tumours. Science 132: 1496

Mueller C B, Jeffries W 1975 Cancer of the breast: is outcome as measured by the rate of dying and causes of death. Annals of Surgery 182: 334–341

Nissen-Meyer R 1975 Ovarian irradiation and its supplement by additive hormonal treatment. In: Namer M, Lalanne C M (eds) Hormones and Breast Cancer, Paris INSERM, Vol 55, p 151–158

Nissen-Meyer R, Kjellgren K, Mansson B 1982 Adjuvant chemotherapy in breast cancer. Cancer Research 80: 142–148

Palmer B V, Walsh G A, McKinna J A, Greening W P 1980 Adjuvant chemotherapy for breast cancer: side effects and quality of life. British Medical Journal 281: 1594–1597

Review of mortality results in randomised trials in breast cancer. 1984 Lancet ii: 1205

Rossi A, Bonnadonna G, Valagussa P, Veronesi U 1981 Multinodal treatment inoperable breast cancer: five-year results of the CMF programme. British Medical Journal 282: 1427–1431

Rubens R O, Hayward J L, Knight R K et al 1983 Controlled trial of adjuvant chemotherapy with melphalan for breast cancer. Lancet i: 839–843

Skipper H E 1971 Kinetics of mammary tumour cell growth and implications for therapy. Cancer 28: 1479–1499

Spratt J S, Kaltenbach M L, Spratt J A 1977 Cytokinetic definition of acute and chronic breast cancer. Cancer Research 37: 226–230

Wilcox P M, Felting J H, Nettersheim K M, Abeloff M O 1982 Anticipatory vomiting in women receiving cyclophosphamide, methotrexate and 5-FU (CMF) adjuvant chemotherapy for breast carcinoma. Cancer Treatment Reports 66: 1601–1604

Veronesi U, Zung L 1967 Extended mastectomy for cancer of the breast. Cancer 20: 677–680

Progress in tumour biology of interest to the surgeon

During the last few years, exciting developments in tumour biology have occurred which are providing great interest and are beginning to suggest important implications for clinical practice. It is likely, however, that any benefit or 'spin-off' from these developments will take many years to affect patient management.

In this chapter two of the more intriguing innovations, monoclonal antibodies and oncogenes, will be reviewed, with particular emphasis on diagnostic, prognostic and therapeutic implications for surgical practice in the future.

MONOCLONAL ANTIBODIES

The localisation of tumours with radiolabelled antibodies is dependent upon the antigen specificity for cancer and antibody. In the absence of human cancer-specific markers, tumour associated antigens have been utilised. Unfortunately such antigens, e.g. carcinoembryonic antigen (CEA) are by no means specific. They are chemically and immunologically polymorphic and conventional immunization results in a spectrum of antibodies with diverse specificities.

The production of monoclonal antibodies by Kohler & Milstein (1975) has stimulated much interest in both biology and medicine. The actual technique of producing monoclonal antibodies has changed little since the original report. The technique is based on the principle of fusing stimulated B cells from the spleen of a mouse immunised with the appropriate antigen, with a myeloma line in vitro. The cells to be fused are each deficient in either hypoxanthine guanine phosphoribosyl transferase (HHPT) or thymidine kinase (TK) which are enzymes required for the salvage pathway of nucleotide synthesis for DNA. Hybrid cells can then be selected by their growth in specific medium (HAT) which blocks the major pathway of nucleotide synthesis. This enables fused cells to grow whilst all other cells die. The hybrids are cloned and propagated either in vitro or as an ascites. The antibodies in the monoclonal antiserum are of uniform specificity and are chemically homogenous. Monoclonal antibodes are thus monospecific and discriminate between variations in a complex antigen. Whole cells are a complex mixture of antigens, the hybridoma technique can be used to specifically recognise antigens associated with the cell.

Specific monoclonal antibodies will be considered with particular reference to breast and colon cancer.

Breast cancer

A wide range of antigens associated with breast cancer have been identified for many years. These antigens can be conveniently divided into 3 categories.

Oncofoetal products

The presence and clinical significance of pregnancy specific and associated proteins have been demonstrated in tissue and sera of patients with breast cancer. Examples of these are; pregnancy specific glycoprotein, pregnancy associated glycoprotein and placental alkaline phosphatase.

In addition, carcinoembryonic antigen (CEA) — a glycoprotein bearing several antigenic determinants — has been demonsdtrated in breast carcinoma. It is distributed on the luminal border of the acini in well differentiated tumours and in the cytoplasm of poorly differentiated tumours.

Membrane molecules of transformed or neoplastic cells

Of the many antigens associated with breast carcinoma most are glycoprotein or glycolipid in nature. These antigens have been recognised by antisera raised against:

(a) breast cell lines
(b) metastastic breast cancer cells or
(c) breast cancer cell membrane extracts.

Antigens in normal differentiated breast cells

The milk fat globule (MFG) is a glycoprotein present in the membrane of differentiated breast cells. In lactation the milk fat is secreted from the apical region of the mammary epithelial cell into the mammary ducts by pinocytosis. In the milk, the fat, surrounded by the membranous envelope is called the MFG.

However, in addition to these, monoclonal antibodies are now available. The prominent ones are:

HMFG1 & HMFG2 — formed from the fusion of female mice immunised against delipidated HMFG with the myeloma cell line (Taylor-Papadimitrou et al, 1981, Berry et al, 1985).

M8 — raised against human milk fat globule membrane (HMFGM) (Foster et al, 1982).

3E1.2 — reacts strongly with membrane and cytoplasm of breast carcinomas and with the luminal membrane of normal breast (Thompson et al, 1984).

NCRC11 — raised against human mammary carcinoma cells. The antigen it recognises has a specific distribution in normal tissues similar to that of antibodies raised to human milk fat globule membrane and is expressed on the luminal surface of exocrine gland epithelium (Ellis et al, 1985).

Colon cancer

Monoclonal antibodies

79IT/36 — (Farrands et al, 1982). This monoclonal antibody reacts with human malignant colorectal cells (Embleton et al, 1981). It has been shown to localise in human tumour xenografts growing in immunodeprived mice.

YPC2/12.1 — This monoclonal antibody binds strongly to colorectal cancer but binds weakly to normal colon (Smedley et al, 1981).

Immunohistochemical staining

The localisation of antigens in histological sections relies on a specific antigen-antibody reaction. The antibodies are used to locate the antigen in the tissue. The problem is how to locate the antibody. Coons et al (1941) visualised antibodies in a tissue by labelling them with a fluorescent molecule and observed them under ultra-violet light. However, the staining is not permanent and the technique involves an U–V light microscope. Another technique, which overcomes these problems, was devised by Graham and Karnovsky (1966). They labelled the antibody with an enzyme which reacts with a reagent to give a coloured product. Using peroxidase as the enzyme and 3–3′ Diaminobenzidine (DAB) as the reagent, antigens are localised by the brown colour of the reaction product. This stain gives a permanent record and can be observed by the light microscope (Fig. 13.1).

A major problem of immuno-histochemical techniques is background staining. There are many causes for this but rapid advances in immuno-histochemistry in the last 10 years have made it a major tool in modern histology.

Radioimmunolocalisation

The ability to detect the extent of primary tumour involvement and metastatic spread at an early stage is a desirable aim. Moreover, the recognition of pre-symptomatic recurrence would have therapeutic implications.

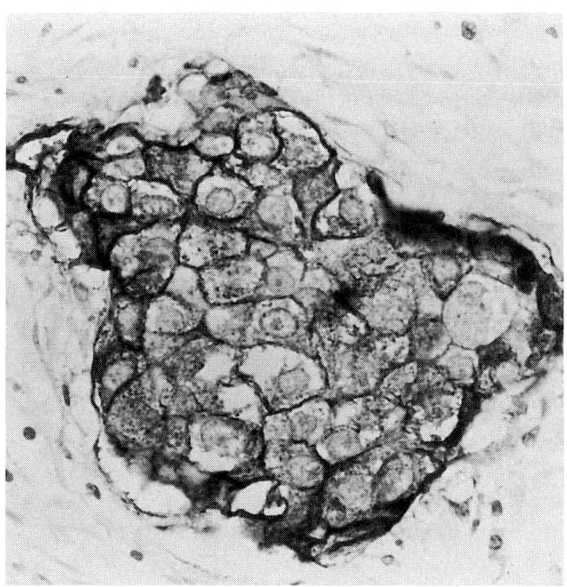

Fig. 13.1 Intracellular staining of breast cancer with HMFGl using immunohistochemical staining

Attempts to radiolabel antibodies and detect their localisation in vivo have not been entirely successful.

Goldenberg et al(1978) initially studied this problem using antibodies to CEA, α fetoprotein and human gonadotrophin. A total of 142 patients were scanned at 24 hrs and 48 hrs with a gamma camera to detect the localisation of polyclonal goat anticarcinoembryonic antigen antibodies. They accurately located 85% of colorectal cancers, 88% of ovarian cancers, 40% of primary breast cancers and 78% of metastatic breast cancer. Other groups have had difficulty in matching these results.

Monoclonal antibodies should have distinct advantage in radioimmunol-ocalisation because of their specificity and purity. However, unexpected cross reactions may occur between monoclonals and normal tissue resulting in poor imaging. Begent (1983) found no advantage of monoclonal over polyclonal anti CEA antibodies in patients with cancer of the colon and rectum.

Circulating antigen in the blood will bind with the antibody to form immune complexes which interfere with radiolocalisation especially over the liver because of the uptake of the complexes by the reticuloendothelial system. The blood flow and vascular permeability of the tumour affect the delivery of antibody to available binding sites. Indeed, antibody tends to bind more avidly to viable tissue then to areas of necrosis.

Subtraction techniques

Interpretation of the scans taken after injection of a radiolabelled antibody can be difficult because of background radioactivity due to the presence of labelled antibody outside the areas affected by tumour. The technique used to avoid this problem is a subtraction method. This involves giving technetium labelled albumen and free technetium pertechnetate before the scanning procedure. Technetium identifies blood pool radioactivity and non-specific accummulation of labelled protein in the stomach, bladder and thyroid and this image is subtracted, using a computer, from the image due to ^{131}I to give pictures identifying only tumour specific localisation.

Clinical uses of monoclonal antibodies

Diagnosis

(1) *Aspiration cytology.* This is becoming an accepted diagnostic technique for solid lumps in various organs, e.g. breast, thyroid, pancreas, prostate. With regard to cytology of breast lumps, when evaluable smears are obtained the diagnostic accuracy of needle aspirates is around 90% (Gardecki et al, 1980; Smallwood et al, 1984). The frequency, however, of technically unsatisfactory aspirates due to the presence of too few or no cells ranges from 5% to 34% but decreases with experience. In addition, incorrect diagnoses can result when the distinctive characteristics of a particular condition are not sufficient for a definitive diagnosis. Also, cell characteristics can be misleading, e.g. in well-differentiated carcinomas or small cell carcinomas whose cells can be confused with those of a benign tumour (Duguid et al, 1979).

Immunocytochemical staining of needle aspirates for an antigen which distinguishes normal and benign cells from malignant breast cells could be a most valuable technique. Unfortunately this ideal cannot be achieved at present since there is no antibody which distinguishes completely between benign and malignant cells. We have investigated the use of HMFG1 and HMFG2 antigens as possible candidates for distinguishing between benign and malignant breast cells in needle aspirates. Immunoperoxidase staining of normal, benign and malignant breast tissue sections show that HMFG2 antigens can be found extracellularly on the luminal surface of epithelial cells and in the secretions in the ducts and tubules of normal, benign and well-differentiated breast carcinoma. Intracellular staining was rarely observed in normal and benign breast tissue, whilst 95% of breast carcinoma stained intracellularly to some extent (Fig. 13.2). Unfortunately no difference in staining characteristics between benign and malignant breast cells were recognised.

However, other workers have achieved some success in distinguishing benign and malignant pleural and peritoneal effusions using immunocytochemical staining. This success is due to the differential

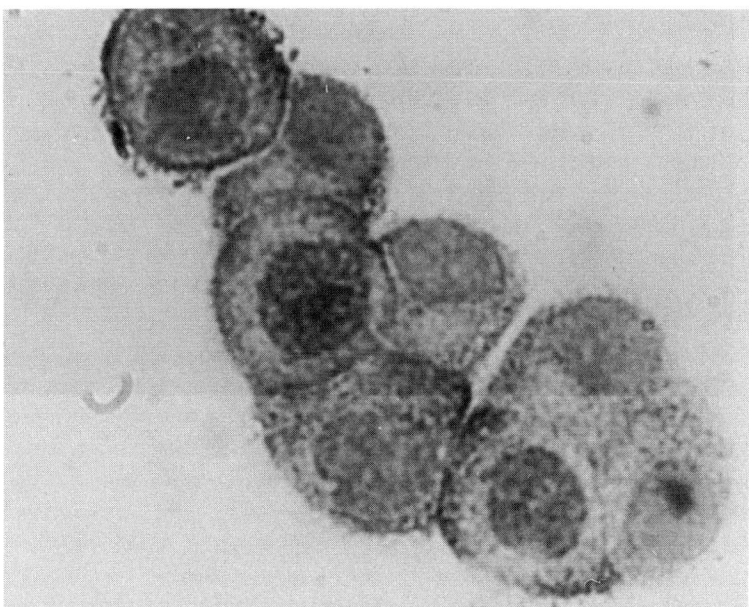

Fig. 13.2 Malignant cells obtained from breast cancer by aspiration and stained with HMFG1

staining characteristics of reactive mesothelial cells and malignant epithelial cells (Epenetos et al, 1982).

(2) *Recognition of metastases in lymph nodes.* Using a range of monoclonal antibodies and immunocytochemical staining of lymph nodes removed at mastectomy with axillary clearance in 50 women, there was a 17% increase in detection of metastases in lymph nodes (Berry et al, 1985). Since lymph node involvement is an important prognostic indicator in breast cancer this increased detection rate using monoclonal antibodies could have important implications in prognosis and treatment.

(3) *Monoclonal antibodies for radioimmunodetection of tumours.* Several reports have described the utilisation of radioimmunodetection for the diagnosis of tumours — both primary and metastatic. Some examples of these relating to breast and colon cancers are as follows:

(i) *^{123}I labelled HMFG1 and HMFG2 (Epenetos et al, 1982).* Six patients with breast and two with colon carcinomas were studied. The mean tumour uptake of radiolabel was 0.6% of the injected amount.

(ii) *^{131}I-labelled 79IT/36 (Farrands et al, 1982).* In 10 of 11 patients with colorectal cancer radiolabelled antitumour monoclonal antibody (79IT/36) was localised to the tumour. The mean tumour to non-tumour uptake ratio was 4.4/1 after subtraction of background radioactivity. In addition metastases were also localised by this technique (Fig. 13.3).

(iii) *Indium-III labelled DTPA-M8 (Rainsbury, 1984).* All 10 patients with skeletal metastases from breast cancer had positive scans (labelled with I-III

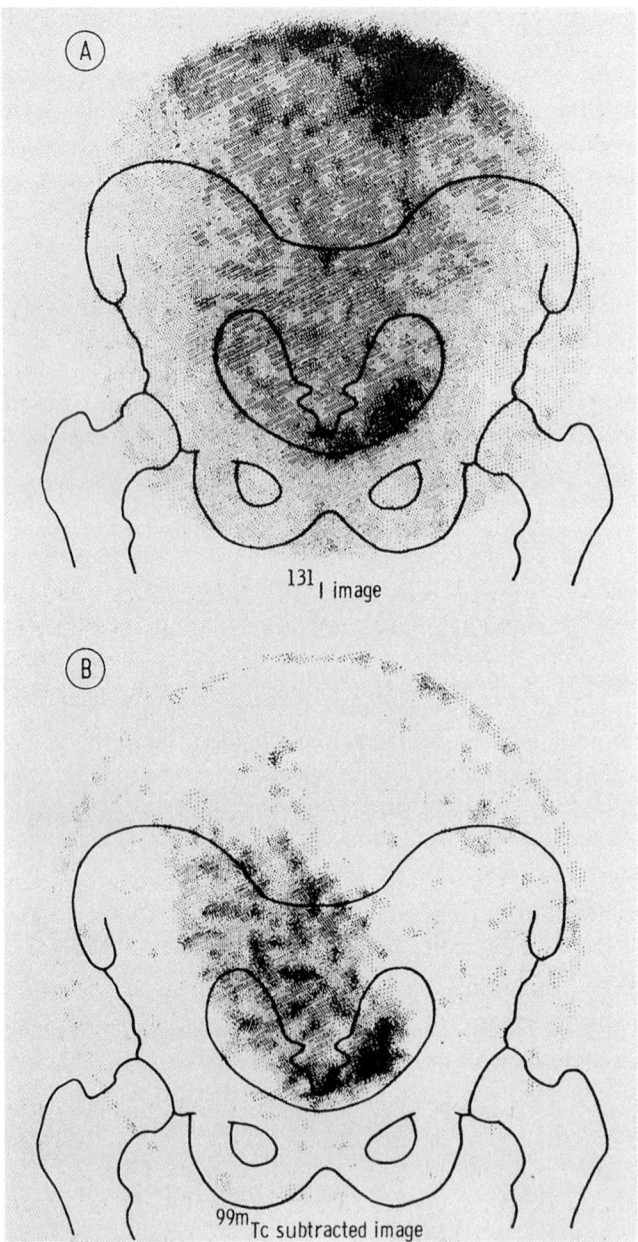

Fig. 13.3 Localisation of monoclonal antibody (79IT/36) in colorectal recurrence in pelvis before and after enhancement (Farrands et al, 1982)

DTPA-M8). The greatest tumour to non-tumour ratio was 5:1 in one patient with pelvic bone metastases.

(iv) ^{131}I labelled 3E 1.2 (Thompson et al, 1984). This has been used for the detection of lymph node metastases from breast cancer. Eight women with breast cancer were scanned following injection into the web space of each hand. Scans were positive in 7 axillae with palpable lymph nodes and in 2 axillae with inpalpable lymph nodes.

(v) ^{131}I labelled YPC2/12.1 (Smedley et al, 1983). Computerised subtraction revealed localised areas of uptake corresponding with areas of known disease in 13 of 16 patients with colorectal carcinoma and in 3 of 4 patients with breast cancer.

(vi) Indium-III labelled H17E2 (Epenetos et al, 1985). This monoclonal antibody is labelled against placental alkaline phosphatase (PCAP) and testicular placental-like alkaline phosphatase. It has been used in 15 patients with germ-cell carcinoma of testis or carcinoma of ovary or cervix. Good images have been obtained. It has been suggested that this method may be useful in diagnosis, staging and monitoring of PCAP positive tumours of testis, ovary or cervical origin.

Monoclonal antibodies as prognostic indicators

Controversy exists with regard to the different immunohistochemical staining patterns particularly in breast cancer. Using HMFG1 and HMFG2 it has been suggested that the absence of staining in breast cancer tissue is associated with a poor prognosis. However, this has not been confirmed by other groups (Berry et al, 1985). The majority of breast cancers have variable staining patterns and are often intracellular. Ellis et al (1985) have suggested a strong relationship between intensity of staining with NCRC11 and patient survival. Intense staining being associated with improved survival.

However, it should be recognised that with the present methods available for grading staining patterns, although of diagnostic value, monoclonal antibodies are unlikely to assist in determining either the degree of tumour differentiation or prognosis.

Monoclonal antibodies for treatment

The ultimate use for monoclonal antibodies would be in targetting effective drugs to tumours in a selective fashion. This aim has not yet been realised but much work is directed to this goal. A phase I trial of treatment of gastrointestinal tumours with a monoclonal antibody has been reported (Sears et al, 1982) and others are awaited. In another preliminary study arterial infusion of radioactive monoclonal antibody against epidermal growth factor receptor and blood group A antigen has been used in a patient with a grade IV brain glioma (Epenetos et al, 1985).

Conclusions

Monoclonal antibody technology has been extremely productive in recent years. Specific antibodies are now available but their role in clinical practice is still being evaluated. Undoubtedly they can be of value as diagnostic tools and in the recognition of small quantities of malignant cells. Immunocytochemical staining has enabled different patterns to be recognised but these do not appear to correlate closely with prognosis. Immunolocalisation of recurrent tumours holds promise but at present the specificity is poor and the tumour to non-tumour ratios are not sufficiently high to enable this technique to be clinically valuable.

Specific targeting of drugs (the 'magic bullet') is still a long way away. This would be an ultimate aim for monoclonal antibody technology and hopefully will prove effective.

ONCOGENES

A good deal of interest has surrounded the possible role of cellular oncogenes in the development of human cancer.

DNA is of paramount importance in the understanding and treatment of cancer. Work on carcinogenesis has involved interactions of carcinogens with DNA since most carcinogens are able to produce mutations and in addition, both radiotherapy and cancer chemotherapy (e.g. alkylating agents) act by either damaging or interfering with the synthesis of DNA.

What are oncogenes?

In 1910 Rous isolated the first RNA virus capable of causing tumours in animals (Rous, 1910). Recent studies utilising recombinant DNA technology have demonstrated how this virus interacts with the cell. The virus genome is a single-stranded RNA molecule and on entering the cell is converted into a double-stranded DNA copy; hence the term 'retroviruses' since the gene is transcribed backwards from RNA to DNA.

The viruses have few genes and it is possible to identify the stretch of DNA required to transform cells, known as the viral oncogene (v-onc). Hence when the oncogenic virus infects a cell its RNA genome is converted into DNA with an enzyme, reverse transcriptase (Gerard et al, 1980). The DNA becomes integrated with the hosts chromosomal DNA and the viral genes are transcribed, in other words, mRNA copies are made. When the host cell translates these mRNAs into protein, viral proteins appear in the cell. How these proteins, some of which include the protein coded for the viral oncogene, affect the cell has been studied using a number of retroviruses. The avian sarcoma virus (ASV) is one of the most thoroughly studied. Its oncogene, V-src, codes for a phosphoprotein which because of its phosphokinase activity is able to add phosphate groups to tyrosine residues of other proteins. This phosphorylation of enzymes controls for the metabolic activity of a cell and hence could have wide ranging effects on cell behaviour and growth (Collett et al, 1978).

At present there are some 18 different v-oncs described.

The proteins that are encoded for by the oncogene sequences fall into several classes. The largest group typified by V-src are cytoplasmic protein kinases. Another group are known to be nuclear proteins, e.g. v-myc. How these influence the cell is not known. Recent evidence has suggested that the product of the oncogene v-sis (simian sarcoma virus) might belong to a third class of proteins, namely growth factors, which are commonly produced by tumour cells. Finally, a group of oncogene products exist for which no activity has yet been described. This includes the two viral ras genes which are gaining importance and interest because of recent observations in human cancer.

Cellular oncogenes

It has now been shown that for each of the 18 viral oncogenes there are closely related sequences present in the genomes of all vertebrate cells, including man. These have been called cellular oncogenes (c-oncs) or proto-oncogenes. They are not cancer-causing but with appropriate 'signals' or modifications can be converted into true oncogenes. A number of examples of activation of the C-oncs in animals have been observed. For example, v-myc is carried by a chicken virus. Mc29, the chicken c-myc gene can also be activated by another virus, avian leucosis virus (ALV). This virus does not carry an oncogene but can insert itself into the chicken chromosome next to the c-myc gene. This results in over-production of the c-myc product and this apparently is the initiating event in the development of chicken B-cell lymphomas.

Hence cellular oncogenes probably play an important role in converting normal cells to tumour cells. There is increasing evidence that these genes are important in human cancer.

Human oncogenes

V-onc

There is no known human RNA-tumour virus that contains an oncogene.

Alterations in c-onc genes

There is circumstantial evidence for an involvement of some cellular oncogenes in human cancer, e.g. Burkitts lymphoma, chronic myeloid leukaemia and human promyelocytic leukaemia. Amplification of the c-myc gene has been reported in a colon carcinoma line (Hall, 1984).

Alteration in the expression of c-onc genes

Several workers have been exploring the possibility of abnormal expressions of transcripts from the human c-onc genes in different kinds of tumours. However, in order to show that a particular c-onc is over-expressed in a tumour cell it is necessary to compare values with a normal cell. In one study 3 out of 5 gliomas contained high levels of the c-sis transcript (Hall, 1984).

More recent evidence has suggested that anti-oncogenes may exist and their dysfunction within the cell allows abnormal expression of the proto-oncogenes (Green & Wyke, 1985).

Transfection

Certain mouse fibroblasts (NIH 3T3 cells) have the ability to take up foreign DNA, incorporate it into their own DNA and express its genes (Weinberg, RA 1981). This technique of gene transfer is called transfection.

The DNA of certain human tumour cell lines and some solid tumours can transform 3T3 cells. These show loss of contact inhibition and are able to grow as tumours when injected into immunosuppressed mice. This provides a method for studying the part of the DNA of the donor cell that is responsible for converting the 3T3 cells to tumour cells (Hamlyn & Sikora, 1983).

The DNA from a human bladder carcinoma was studied in this way. When the DNA that caused the 3T3 cells to become tumourigenic was reduced by successive rounds of transfection to a piece small enough for study, it was found to be very similar to a cellular oncogene belonging to the ras family — c-ras (Der et al, 1982).

It appears that human oncogenes detected by transfection almost always belong to the ras family.

Clinical significance

It is likely that studies on oncogenes will lead, within the next few years, to more detailed knowledge of some of the molecular alterations that contribute to neoplastic transformation. This knowledge should provide insight into the control of cell proliferation (Weiss & Marshall, 1984).

Clearly, oncogene products may provide specific sites for interference with tumour growth without affecting normal cells. Recent work has indicated that c-ras oncogene situated on chromosome 12 is specifically expressed in colorectal carcinomas. An anti-ras monoclonal antibody has been developed which appears to inhibit RNA synthesis by human colorectal cancer cells in vitro (Habib et al, 1985).

It is also becoming likely that the different patterns of oncogene activation will have clinical significance. For example, its interactions with other cells and ability to metastasise. Hence the patterns of oncogene activation in a particular tumour may allow predictions of the course of disease and of the response of that tumour to therapy.

In addition, it may well be that with our increasing knowledge of oncogenes and oncogene products chemotherapy and radiotherapy could become more exactly applied against the DNA of cells especially if targetted against the excess of oncogene protein products.

These exciting and novel technologies are progressing at a rapid rate and the clinical implications are becoming increasingly apparent. Hopefully in the not too distant future this will be translated into very real therapeutic benefit for our patients with cancer.

REFERENCES

Begent R H J 1983 radioimmunolocalisation. Cancer Topics 4: 41–47

Berry N, Jones D B, Smallwood J, Taylor I et al 1985 The prognostic value of the monoclonal antibodies HMFG1 and HMFG2 in breast cancer. British Journal of Cancer 51: 179–186

Berry N, Jones D B, Marshall R, Smallwood J, Taylor I 1985 Increased detection of axillary lymph node metastases from primary breast cancer by immunohistochemical staining with monoclonal antibodies. British Journal of Surgery 72:1035

Collett M S, Erickson C, Purchio A F et al 1978 A normal cell protein similar in structure and function to the avian sarcoma virus transforming gene product. Proceedings of the National Academy of Sciences USA 76: 3159–3163

Coons A M, Creech H J, Jones R N 1941 Immunological properties of an antibody containing a fluorescent group. Proceedings of the Society for Experimental Biology and Medicine 47: 200–202

Der C J, Kronitiris T G, Cooper G M 1982 Transforming genes of human bladder and lung carcinoma cell lines are nomologous to the ras gene of Harvey and Kirsten sarcoma viruses. Proceedings of the National Academy of Sciences USA 79: 3637–3640

Duguid H L D, Wood R A B, Irving A D et al 1979 Needle aspiration of the breast with immediate reporting of material. British Medical Journal II:185

Ellis I O, Hinton C P, Macnay J et al 1985 Immunocytochemical staining of breast carcinoma with the monoclonal antibody NCRC II: a new prognostic indicator. British Medical Journal 290: 881–883

Embleton M J, Gunn B et al 1981 Anti-tumour reactions of monoclonal antibody against a human osteogenic sarcoma line. British Journal of Cancer 43: 582–587

Epenetos A A, Canti G et al 1982 Use of two epithelium specific monoclonal antibodies for diagnosis of malignancy in serious effusions. Lancet ii: 1004–1006

Epenetos A A, Mather S, Granowska M et al 1982 Targetting of Iodine-123-labelled tumour associated monoclonal antibodies to ovarian, breast, and gastrointestinal tumours. Lancet II: 999–1004

Epenetos A A, Courtney-Luck N, Pickering D et al 1985 Antibody guided irradiation of brain glioma by arterial infusion of radioactive monoclonal antibody against EGF receptor and blood group A antigen. British Medical Journal 290: 1463–1466

Epenetos A A, Snook B, Hooker G et al 1985 Indium-III labelled monoclonal antibody to placental alkaline phosphatase in the detection of neoplasms of testis, ovary and cervix. Lancet II: 350–353

Farrands P A, Pimm C V et al 1982 Radioimmunodetection of human colorectal cancers by an anti-tumour monoclonal antibody. Lancet II: 397–400

Foster C S, Edwards P A W, Dinsdale E A et al 1982 Monoclonal antibodies to the human mammary gland. Distribution of determinants in non-neoplastic mammary and extra-mammary tissues. Virchows Arch (Pathol Anat) 394: 279–294

Gardecki T, Hogbin B M, Melcher D M et al 1980 Aspiration cytology in the pre-operative management of breast cancer. Lancet ii: 790–792

Gerard G F, Grandgenett D P 1980 Retrovirus reverse transcriptase. In: Stephenson J R (ed) Molecular biology of RNA tumour viruses, Academic Press, New York, p 346–381

Green A R, Wyke J A 1985 Anti-oncogenes. Lancet II: 475–477

Goldenberg D M, Deland F M, Kim E et al 1978 Use of radiolabelled antibodies to CEA for the detection and localization of diverse cancers by external photoscanning. New England Journal of Medicine 298: 1384–1388

Graham R C, Karnovsky M J 1966 The early stages of absorption of injected horse radish peroxidase in the proximal tubules of mouse kidney; ultrastructural cytochemistry by a new technique. Journal of Histochemistry and Cytochemistry 14: 291–302

Habib N A, Niman H C et al (1985) Directed monoclonal antibodies against ras-oncogene products in the therapy of in-vitro human colorectal cancer cells. British Journal of Surgery 72:1025

Hall A 1984 Oncogenes — implications for human cancer. Journal of the Royal Society of Medicine 77: 410–416

Hamlyn P, Sikora K 1983 Oncogenes. Lancet II: 326–330

Kohler G, Milstein C 1975 Continuous culture of fused cells secreting antibody of predefined specificity. Nature 256: 495–497

Rainsbury R M 1984 The localization of human breast-carcinomas by radiolabelled monoclonal antibodies. British Journal of Surgery 71: 805–812

Sears H F, Atkinson B, Mattis J et al 1982 Phase-1 clinical trial of monoclonal antibody in treatment of gastrointestinal tumours. Lancet I: 762–765

Smallwood J, Herbert A, Guyer P, Taylor I 1985 Accuracy of aspiration cytology in the diagnosis of breast disease. British Journal of Surgery 72: 841–843

Smedley H M, Finana P, Lennox E S et al 1983 Localisation of metastatic carcinoma by a radiolabelled monoclonal antibody. British Journal of Cancer 47: 253–259

Taylor-Papadimitrou J, Pedterson J A, Arklie J et al 1981 Monoclonal antibodies to epithelium specific components of the milk fat globule membrane: production and reaction with cells in culture. International Journal of Cancer 28:17

Thompson C H, Jones S L, Whitehead R H et al 1983 A human breast tissue-associated antigen detected by a monoclonal antibody. Journal of the National Cancer Institute 70: 409–419

Thompson C H, Lichtenstein M, Stacker S A et al 1984 Immunoscintigraphy for detection of lymph node metastases from breast cancer. Lancet II: 1245–1247

Weinberg R A 1981 Use of transfection to analyse genetic information and malignant transformation. Biochimica et Biophysica Acta 651: 25–35

Weiss R A, Marshall C J 1984 Oncogenes. Lancet II: 1138–1142

Carotid endarterectomy for transient ischaemic attacks

Transient cerebral ischaemic attacks (TIAs) are the principle indication for carotid endarterectomy in the United Kingdom. Carotid endarterectomy accounts for some 100 000 operations per annum in the USA but a variable percentage of these are prophylactic in asymptomatic patients. In a TIA an area of the brain is rendered ischaemic for a short period of time — usually minutes but maximally 24 hours. The cause of these attacks may be haemodynamic as the result of a tight carotid arterial stenosis or the result of embolism from an ulcerated atheromatous plaque. Repetitive episodes are often similar in character but this may be because only motor and sensory symptoms affecting the face, limbs and speech are easily recognised by the patient. However computerised tomography (CT) has demonstrated that silent infarcts are not uncommon and may be found in areas of the brain remote from the symptomatic areas. Another frequent symptom of carotid artery disease and a manifestation of transient ischaemia is transient monocular blindness or amaurosis fugax. The embolus is sometimes seen in the retina and so the aetiology here is more apparent.

Disease of the carotid artery is the subject of this chapter but it should not allow one to forget the other causes of these symptoms such as cardiac arrhythmias, hypertension, cardiac sources of embolism, diseases in the arch and great vessels and cerebral tumours. Hence a careful medical history and examination are essential preliminaries to the consideration of a carotid aetiology. These important differential diagnoses will not be considered further here.

HISTORY

The typical history is of a sudden onset of a mono or hemiplegia with complete resolution. In order to qualify as a TIA it should have resolved completely in 24 hours and the majority do so in a far shorter time. Some neurological deficits although resolving completely take longer and have been labelled by some as PRINDS — prolonged but reversible ischaemic neurological deficits. These episodes require the same diagnostic considerations as the true TIAs but the management may be different. Other episodes fail to resolve and must be considered as strokes.

Transient ischaemic attacks are often repetitive and frequently identical. They are a well recognised risk factor for stroke but there is no means of identifying accurately in one individual how high that risk is. Nor can the frequency of these attacks be considered as a guide. In some patients, one TIA may be followed by a permanent stroke and in others frequent attacks may occur without permanent deficit.

Episodes of transient monocular blindness are frequently described as similar to a blind or curtain descending and later clearing with restoration of vision. The blindness may not be complete and the direction of the curtain may vary. Bilateral attacks are virtually never of extracranial carotid origin.

SIGNS

As already stressed a general examination of the patient is essential. When turning to the vascular tree this examination must include the heart and all accessible vessels. Palpation and auscultation will often indicate the presence of degenerative vascular disease elsewhere even when examination of the neck is negative.

In the neck it should be possible to palpate both carotids and both subclavian arteries. The carotid usually bifurcates close to the angle of the mandible and auscultation should begin at the aortic valve and work up to that level so as not to misinterpret a murmur transmitted from the aortic valve or brachiocephalic artery.

Too much stress should not be placed on the finding of a murmur over the carotid bifurcation. If present it is a most valuable sign of disease in this area. If absent it must not lull one into a sense of false security. A bruit may not be audible over an ulcerated atheromotous plaque which reduces the lumen only to a minor degree but is nevertheless capable of embolism. Also when a stenosis has progressed to 90–95% the murmur may disappear as is the case with complete occlusion of the internal carotid. It must be remembered that the murmur may be arising from a stenosis of the external carotid.

Murmurs in the base of the neck are also important and if not transmitted along the subclavian artery may well indicate a stenosis of the vertebral artery. The presence of the superficial temporal pulse should be noted as an indicator of the patency of the external carotid artery.

Full neurological examination, looking for asymptomatic neurological deficits is essential hence the need for close cooperation between vascular surgeon and neurologist. All my patients are seen by and discussed with a consultant neurologist.

Even when a cardiac cause of embolism of arrhythmia has been excluded the heart should not be forgotten because in the follow up of patients with transient ischaemic attacks the commonest cause of death is myocardial infarction and preventive measures may sometimes be possible. In a series of 329 patients followed for 10 years after carotid endarterectomy, myocardial infarction accounted for 37% and strokes for 15% of the late deaths (Hertzer & Arison, 1985). With careful medical supervision in postoperative cases Lord (1984) observed a mean postoperative survival rate comparable with a matched population when the only risk factor was cardiac. It should be noted that this group received aorto-coronary bypass grafting when indicated.

DIAGNOSTIC INVESTIGATIONS

The major consideration in the patient suspected of having carotid artery disease is the prevention of stroke. The more invasive the investigation, however the greater the potential hazard.

The final diagnostic step remains angiography and most vascular surgeons remain committed to the need for radiographic visualisation prior to surgery. However it is possible to exclude some patients from angiography by various non-invasive investigations.

Undoubtedly the leader in the field of non invasive investigations is the duplex doppler scan. This enables a B-mode real time ultrasound image to be obtained along with a doppler probe to sample velocity and measure flow. Baird (1985) has described the technique as a safe and rapid screening method which enables selection for contrast radiology.

In addition to screening of symptomatic patients it enables follow up of asymptomatic patients and the progression of stenoses. Postoperative follow up and detection of restenosis without risk will improve our knowledge of the results of surgery. Strandness has contributed largely to the accurate assessment of the degree of stenosis and in a recent paper has drawn our attention to the risk of occlusion in those with stenosis of greater than 80% (Roederer et al, 1984).

CT scanning

A CT scan of the brain is now considered by many to be an essential prerequisite to carotid surgery. The availability of such information has added a great deal to our understanding of carotid disease.

With the advent of less invasive angiography has come the reduction in detailed intracranial studies. CT scanning will ensure that a tumour mimicking or coincidental with carotid disease is not overlooked.

In addition it has taught us several important lessons about carotid disease. Firstly transient ischaemic attacks may or may not be associated with infarction. Secondly, apparently asymptomatic carotid disease may be associated with infarcts on CT scanning and thirdly the repetitive nature of TIAs does not indicate that emboli always arrive in the same area of the brain since multiple silent infarcts may be seen in other areas. Finally it has enabled clinicians to demonstrate what they had long suspected — ulcerated atheromatous plaques are associated with cerebral infarcts (Zukowski, 1984).

Other abnormalities such as cerebral atrophy extensive infarction and haemorrhagic events may influence decision making. Knowledge of the latter may be life-saving by preventing the use of anticoagulants.

Positron tomography

An esoteric development of CT scanning is the positron emission tomogram. This is certainly not part of the routine work up but Gibbs et al (1984) have extended our understanding of cerebral perfusion in critical circumstances. An excellent review by Frackowiak (1985) outlines the advances in knowledge brought about by this new technique. It includes the physiology of cerebral perfusion and the pathological changes associated with ischaemia.

ANGIOGRAPHY

Contrast studies remain the final step in the process of diagnosis. Percutaneous puncture of the carotid artery is rarely needed now and conventional studies are usually based on selective catheterisation using the Seldinger technique. High quality images are obtained but there is a small risk of neurological complications even in the most experienced hands (Fraught et al, 1979; Eisenberg et al, 1980). This may explain in part the wide variation in the use of angiography by neurologists involved in the UK — TIA aspirin trial. Of the 959 patients in the trial by 1983 only 32% had angiography and the rate per neurologist varied from 3 to 100%.

Digital subtraction angiography has reduced the risk considerably. It can be carried out by the intravenous route usually employing a catheter in a central vein and large volumes of contrast (a disadvantage). Or it may be employed by the intraarterial route whereby a catheter is placed in the arch of the aorta and using a small quantity of dilute contrast gives good views of carotid and vertebral arteries. Both of these methods avoid the risks associated with a catheter placed into the affected artery.

Inevitably there are some disadvantages and even using the intra-arterial route the fact that all the vessels in the neck contain contrast will result in some difficulties in interpretation due to overlapping vessels. These can largely be overcome by a series of oblique views but may never achieve the precise definition of a selectively placed catheter.

In addition the intracranial views are largely confined to the major vessels and precise knowledge of the state of the intracranial carotid and its branches may be lacking. The presence of an intracranial aneurysm may also influence decision making and is not always well seen.

In spite of these reservations digital subtraction angiography is an important advance because of its greater freedom fom complications.

THE DECISION TO OPERATE

This will be based on the clinicians interpretation of the risk of a stroke for the individual patient and will be balanced against the 'track record' of the surgeon. The decision will be based on the knowledge that the risk of stroke after TIA is at least 5% per annum and in some circumstances is much higher. I can only recommend the joint consultation process enjoyed by myself and colleagues at St Mary's whereby all such decisions are made with a neurologist. There are cases where there is doubt about the correct course to pursue and at the present time patients in this 'grey area' are entered into the UK-TIA surgery trial being conducted by the MRC.

PREPARATION FOR OPERATION

Hypertension

A stable blood pressure is desirable during and after surgery. Hypertension may be discovered when the patient presents with TIAs and if the carotid is tightly stenosed it may be unwise to lower the blood pressure too rapidly until the stenosis has been dealt with.

Blood

Transfusion is rarely required but the patient should be grouped and screened for antibodies. Most teams will prepare at least one unit for immediate use because if an unexpected haemorrhage were to occur the rapid restoration of blood volume would be vital in a patient with a tight stenosis.

Aspirin

Many patients are started on treatment with aspirin by their physician when TIAs occur. My personal preference is to discontinue this one week prior to surgery but this is often not possible and one must tolerate the very real discomfort of operating on a patient whose platelet function is deranged. This does not apply to the patient taking warfarin where the drug has little noticeable effect at operation.

Informed consent

This must include a true statement of the risk of stroke from the audit of the operating team.

THE OPERATION

Anaesthesia

In my own practice general anaesthesia is used but it is still the preference of a small number of surgeons to carry out carotid endarterectomy under local anaesthesia or more elegantly cervical plexus block so that cerebral function can be monitored during carotid clamping. Various methods of protecting cerebral function have been employed by anaesthetists in the past and the whole subject is well reviewed by McMeniman & Kam (1983). The methods include hypothermia to 30°C in order to reduce cerebral oxygen requirements. Hypercapnia induced by increasing the inspired carbon dioxide was also employed but has now been discredited as it probably worsens blood supply to the ischaemic brain by a steal phenomenon whereby the normal brain is overperfused at the expense of the ischaemic. At one time pressure agents were used to induce hypertension but we now appreciate that this increases the risk of myocardial infarction or arrhythmias in those patients with coronary artery disease.

At the present time the emphasis is on the maintenence of a stable and normal (for that individual) blood pressure. This is required both during the induction of anaesthesia and throughout the operative and postoperative course. For this reason an arterial line is inserted, usually into the radial artery and continuous pressure monitoring carried out throughout.

Light general anaesthesia with controlled ventilation via an endotracheal tube is employed and a capnograph may be used to measure end tidal CO_2 in order to maintain normocapnia.

During the operation the blood pressure is most likely to be disturbed by dissection around the carotid bifurcation and if this cannot be corrected in any other way, such as by fluid infusion or atropine, then it may occasionally be necessary to infuse the carotid sinus nerve with local anaesthetic in order to control the blood pressure. My own preference is to use a short acting local anaesthetic such as lignocaine. It becomes essential to warn those caring for the patient post operatively of the likely time that this effect will cease so that they can be especially vigilant for the possible change of blood pressure at that time.

Postoperative monitoring is ideally carried out in an intensive care unit where swings of blood pressure can immediately be corrected. Hypotension usually responds to volume expansion with Dextran 70 in saline or haemaccel. Hypertensive swings can best be treated by a drug such as Labetolol or Hydralazine or by a Tridil infusion. The management must always be directed both to the prevention of stroke and to the prevention of myocardial infarction.

Position on the table

The patient is placed supine with both arms by the side. A litre bag of fluid is placed with its long axis parallel with and under the upper thoracic spine. The neck is extended and the head rotated. The patient is level without elevation of the head.

Incision

The incision is placed along the anterior border of the sternomastoid and centered over the position of the bifurcation of the carotid.

The platysma is divided and the sternomastoid freed and retracted posteriorly. The internal jugular vein is exposed and the tributaries ligated. The main one is the common facial vein and the division of this vein usually reveals the bifurcation of the carotid.

In the groove between the internal jugular vein and the common carotid artery lies the vagus nerve and this must be preserved and not disturbed. The hypoglossal nerve usually crosses the carotid above the level of the bifurcation and it is normally possible to identify the descendens hypoglossi and to preserve it.

Control of the artery

Slings are placed around the common carotid artery, internal and external carotid arteries. The superior thyroid artery is identified. Manipulation of the artery is minimised to prevent loose debris from becoming dislodged. 5000 units of Heparin is administered by the anaesthetist.

Measurement of stump pressure

A needle is placed in the common carotid artery and the arterial pressure is measured with a transducer. The common carotid and external carotid and its branches are clamped and the pressure change is observed. If this stump pressure is less than one third of the pre clamp pressure then a shunt is indicated. If the pressure is above one third of the systemic pressure then the operation proceeds without a shunt. This method is one of several ways of assessing the cerebral circulatory reserve when the clamp has been applied. An arbitrary cut off of 40 or 50 mm Hg is the more usual criterion for shunting but I find it is more reliable to relate this to the patients blood pressure just as one would normally do in the assessment of the ischaemic limb. Other surgeons use EEG monitoring during the proceedure to determine cerebral ischaemia. Baker (1984) reported a series of 940 carotid endarterectomies carried out without shunt and concluded that the risks were related to a stump pressure below 50 mmHg and particularly if this was combined with occlusion of the opposite carotid. With this combination of risk factors and without the use of a shunt he reported a stroke risk of 11%. In my opinion this risk can virtually be eliminated by the selective use of a shunt.

Carotid endarterectomy without a shunt

After clamping an arteriotomy is made beginning in the common carotid and extended with Potts scissors towards the origin of the internal carotid keeping to the lateral aspect. Adequate back flow from the internal carotid is confirmed visually. The endarterectomy is commenced in the common carotid and I use a MacDonalds dissector to develop the plane of the endarterectomy. At the lower end the plaque is usually transected with a knife but at the upper end the whole tail of atheroma must be dissected cleanly from the wall so that there is no loose flap at the upper end. If a clean end point cannot be achieved then it is occasionally necessary to tack down a residual rim of atheroma to prevent its dissection when blood flow is restored. Similar care is taken to free the external carotid of atheroma as it is a valuable cerebral collateral.

A meticulous search for loose or partially attached particles of atheroma is made and these are made more obvious by an occasional wash with saline.

No time limit is imposed and the emphasis is on meticulous technique. The cross-clamp time in my own series varies between 10 and 30 minutes. The artery is repaired with 6/0 Prolene in a continuous suture line. I do not routinely employ a patch although other surgeons may do so. Towards the completion of the suture line each clamp is removed in turn to flush out any debris. Finally just as the last suture is being tightened the artery is filled with blood by releasing the external carotid clamp in order to expell any air in its lumen. This is most easily completed with the patient lying flat. The final order of clamp removal is external carotid, then common carotid and finally internal carotid so that blood first flows up the external carotid in case any tiny particle has been overlooked. A check is made for suture line bleeding and the wound closed employing a closed suction drain.

Carotid endarterectomy with a shunt

When the stump pressure to systemic pressure ratio is less than one third then it is assumed that the brain would be rendered ischaemic if the flow ceased. Hence the perod of continuous interuption of flow must be iminimised to less than 3 minutes.

The steps are similar but following the arteriotomy the lower end of a Brenner shunt is inserted into the common carotid and held in place with a shunt clamp. The shunt and its side arm are flushed through to expell air or debris and the upper end is inserted and flow reestablished. There are several alternative shunts available of which the Javid is probably the most commonly used in this country (Jarvid et al, 1979). It is longer and can be looped outside the arteriotomy. The endarterectomy is completed in an unhurried fashion and finally the arteriotomy is closed leaving a gap just large enough for the removal of the shunt. A further period of cross clamping then follows while the closure of the arteriotomy is completed and the flow reestablished as above.

Vascular surgeons are divided about the advisability of the routine use of a shunt. The shunt itself can cause problems such as injury to the arterial wall or embolism and as the operation can be performed quite safely without it in over 80% of cases I favour the selective policy.

Postoperative care

This is as important as the peroperative care and involves monitoring of pulse and blood pressure as indicated in the section on anaesthesia. Informed medical staff must be immediately available to correct any marked changes.

RESULTS

Most of the published series report a post operative neurological complication rate of 2 to 3%. In a recent survey of the risk of carotid endarterectomy carried out by 36 surgeons in NE Ohio, Hertzer et al (1984) found a neurological complication rate of 2.7% in those patients having preoperative neurological symptoms and 2% in the asymptomatic patients. This gives a overall deficit rate of 2.5% in 2646 patients. There was an overall mortality rate in the same group of patients of 1.2%.

In the series already refered to by Hertzer & Arison a 10 year follow up of 329 patients revealed a cumulative incidence of stroke of 24% but only 10% of patients suffered strokes from the ipsilateral hemisphere. This draws attention to the contralateral vessel. When this was stenosed greater than 50% and not corrected the stroke rate was 36%. However when the stenosed second side was electively corrected the stroke rate was only 8%.

The second side therefore needs careful observation and there may be a case for correction of a stenosis.

Roederer et al (1984) following up the non operated side in 134 patients employing duplex doppler also drew attention to the tight stenosis of over 80%. In this series the incidence of symptoms was 5% per annum and all were TIAs. There was a close relationship between symptoms and a greater than 80% stenosis.

THE ASYMPTOMATIC CAROTID BRUIT

Much has been written and spoken about the advisability or otherwise of carotid surgery for the asymptomatic bruit. There has never been a controlled trial of sufficient magnitude to resolve the dilemma. The title itself implies woolly thinking as there is no direct correlation between what is heard and the pathology existing in the artery. The murmur may well be arising from the external carotid artery or elsewhere. While it quite correctly identifies that patient as being at risk of cardiovascular disease (Wolf, 1981) it is no more precise than that.

More accurate information is now being collected from several centres both here and in the USA based on duplex doppler and it may soon be possible to identify a patient with an asymptomatic bruit who because of the nature of its cause is at great risk of stroke. Then provided that surgery is a lesser hazard we may be in a position to recommend an operation. At present the majority view in the UK is a cautious one.

Prophylactic surgery for the asymptomatic patient with a well defined and tight stenosis of the internal carotid who requires cardiac surgery (usually aortocoronary bypass grafting) is being carried out in some centres (including my own) but even here evidence of the necessity for such intervention is unsatisfactory.

THE EXTERNAL CAROTID ARTERY

The importance of the external carotid artery as a cerebral collateral is well established and attention has already been drawn to the need to include this artery when carrying out surgery for internal carotid stenosis. As an isolated procedure, when the internal carotid is occluded it may be expected to improve cerebral circulation in its own right or as a preliminary to extracranial to intracranial by pass grafting. In view of the results of the Canadian multicentre trial (1985) this latter operation is likely to decline in frequency and caution needs to be expressed about the former. Two recently published series (Halstruk, 1984; O'Hara, 1985) described the unexpectedly high neurological complication rate especially in the more extended proceedures. 162 patients in 21 collected series had a 2% mortality and a 14% neurological complication rate. Contrary to widely held views it may be just as important to measure stump pressure here and to shunt when indicated. These facts are probably further evidence of the importance of this artery as a collateral.

RESTENOSIS

Two types of recurrent stenosis are recognised. There is the early neointimal hyperplasia appearing usually within the first two years and the later redevelopment of atherosclerosis.

Assessment of the incidence of recurrent disease is difficult but Strandness' group (Nichols et al, 1985) have suggested that at 4 years the rate may be as high as 17%. This is higher than other workers have reported but probably relates to the method of detection used, in this case Duplex Doppler. Several series however recognise that women are at greater risk of recurrence than men. Surgical correction of recurrent stenosis is hazardous

TIMING OF OPERATION AFTER STROKE

If the event which preceeds carotid surgery is a stroke (i.e. deficit persisting for longer than 24 hours) then timing of the operation is difficult. In Giordano's series (1985) there were no postoperative strokes in those operated on after an interval of at least 5 weeks but in the early group of 27 patients operated on within 5 weeks there were five strokes i.e. 18.5%. Cautious interpretation is needed as this was not a randomly allocated series.

CAROTID AND CORONARY SURGERY

When patients require both carotid and coronary surgery it is my usual practice to carry out carotid surgery first and about one week later the coronary surgery. However when there is left mainstem disease or unstable angina, I would deal with both lesions together. Perler et al (1985) reported on the reslts in 37 patients having combined surgery for these indications with only one transient neurological problem postoperatively. There were three cardiac deaths.

SUMMARY

Carotid endarterectomy is a well established operation for the symptomatic patient with carotid artery disease. In spite of the fact that it has been part of surgical management for almost 30 years there remain a number of questions about its place. Some of these will be answered by current trials comparing surgical treatment with the best available medical treatment.

ACKNOWLEDGEMENT

I wish to thank Dr Peter Knight with his help in preparing the section on anaesthesia.

REFERENCES

Baird R N 1985 Recognition of carotid artery disease. Annals of the Royal College of Surgeons 67: 284–287
Baker W H, Littooy F N, Hayes A C, Dorner D B, Stubbs D 1984 Carotid endarterectomy without a shunt: The control series. Journal of Vascular Surgery 1: 50–61
EC/IC Bypass Study Group 1985 Failure of extracranial to intracranial bypass to reduce the risk of ischaemic stroke. Results of an international randomised trial. New England Journal of Medicine 313: 191–200
Eisenberg R L, Bank W O, Hedgcock M W 1980 Neurological complications of angiography for cerebrovascular disease. Neurology 30: 895–897
Faught E, Trader S D, Hanna G R 1979 Cerebral complications of angiography for transient ischaemia and stroke: prediction of risk. Neurology 29: 4–15
Frackowiak R S J 1985 The pathophysiology of human cerebral ischaemia: a new perspective obtained with positron tomography. Quarterly Journal of Medicine New Series 57: 713–727
Gibbs J M, Wise R J S, Leenders K L, Jones T 1984 Evaluation of cerebral perfusion reserve in patients with carotid artery occlusion. Lancet 1: 310–314
Giordano J M, TroutIII H H, Kozloff L, Depalma R G 1985 Timing of carotid artery endarterectomy after stroke. Journal of Vascular Surgery 2: 250–254

Halstuk K S 1984 External carotid endarterectomy. Journal of Vascular Surgery 1: 398–402

Hertzer N R, Avellone J C, Farrell C J, Plecha F R, Rhodes R S, Sharp W V, Wright G F 1984 The risk of vascular surgery in a metropolitan community: with observations on surgeon experience and hospital size. Journal of Vascular Surgery 1: 13–21

Hertzer N R, Arison R 1985 Cumulative stroke and survival ten years after carotid endarterectomy. Journal of Vascular Surgery 2: 661–668

Javid H, Julian O C, Dyne W S et al 1979 Seventeen years experience with routine shunting in carotid artery surgery. World Journal of Surgery 3: 167–177

Lord R S A 1984 Late survival after carotid endarterectomy for transient ischaemic attacks. Journal of Vascular Surgery 1: 512–519

McMeniman W J, Kam P C A 1983 Cerebral perfusion and cerebral protection during carotid endarterectomy. Anaesthesia and Intensive Care 11: 228–236

Nicholls S C, Phillips D J, Berdgelin R O, Beach K W, Primozich J F, Strandness D E 1985 Carotid endarterectomy. Relationship of outcome to early restenosis. Journal of Vascular Surgery 2: 375–382

O'Hara P J, Hertzer N R, Beven E G 1985 External carotid revascularisation: review of a ten year experience. Journal of Vascular 2: 709–14

Perler B A, Burdick J F, Melville Williams G 1985 The safety of carotid endarterectomy at the time of coronary artery by pass: analysis of results in a high risk patient population. Journal of Vascular Surgery 2: 558–563

Roederer G O, Langloin Y E, Jager K A, Primozich J F, Beach K W, Phillips D J, Strandness D E 1984 The natural history of carotid arter disease in asymptomatic patients with cervical bruits. Stroke 15: 605–613

Roederer G O, Langlois Y E, Lusiani L, Jager K A, Primozich J F, Lawrence R J, Phillips D J, Strandness D E 1984 Natural history of carotid artery disease on the side contralateral to endarterectomy. Journal of Vascular Surgery 1: 62–72

UK-TIA Study Group 1983 Variation in the use of angiography and carotid endarterectomy by neurologists in the UK-TIA aspirin trial. British Medical Journal 286: 514–517

Wolf P A, Kannel W B, Sorlie P, McNamara P 1981 Asymptomatic carotid bruit and risk of stroke. The Framingham study. Journal of the American Medical Association 245: 1442–1445

Zukowski A J, Nicolaides A N, Lewis R T, Mansfield A O Williams M A, Helmis E, et al 1984 The correlation between carotid plaque ulceration and cerebral infarction seen on CT scan. Journal of Vascular Surgery 1: 782–786

Brain tumours — recent advances in diagnosis and treatment

INTRODUCTION

As a group brain tumours constitute one of the most lethal and therapeutically challenging types of neoplasm. Whilst most benign tumours can now be safely resected, malignant tumours continue to present major problems. Of all primary tumours about 8% arise in the brain. Intracranial tumours are the sixth most common neoplasm in adults and are the commonest solid tumour occurring in children, being second to leukaemia. The annual incidence of primary brain tumours is approximately 4.5 per hundred thousand and for childhood brain tumours is about 3 per hundred thousand.

Precise figures for involvement of the brain by metastatic tumours do not exist but the incidence of secondary deposits almost certainly exceeds that of primary lesions.

The principal types of primary intracranial tumours occuring in children and adults are summarised in Table 15.1 which show frequencies, common sites, radiosensitivities and average survivals.

The last decade has seen the development of new imaging techniques which have resulted in greater surgical accuracy and also improvements in the technology of tumour resection. Advances in pathology using marker techniques have achieved an improvement in the final diagnosis of the tumour. Finally the present revolution in molecular biology is already having a clinical impact. Monoclonal antibodies are already being used to enhance tumour diagnosis, and are being considered as agents for targeted therapy when labelled with suitable isotopes or toxins. Molecular probes for oncogenes are being developed and might soon have a similar application. This chapter will describe these new technical advances, rather than attempt a systematic review of each type of brain tumour, which can be found in some of the references for further reading.

IMAGING TECHNIQUES

CT scanning

Since the original introduction of CT scanning 10 years ago, there has been

Table 15.1 Primary intracranial tumours — frequency, site, radiosensitivity and survival

	Frequency (%)	Common site	Radiosensitivity	Survival*
Neuroectodermal				
Malignant astrocytoma	30	Hemisphere	+	40% at 1 year
Differentiated astrocytoma	10	Hemisphere	+	50% at 5 years
Oligodendroglioma	3	Hemisphere	+	50% at 5 years
Ependymoma	3	Hemisphere/posterior fossa	+	40% at 5 years
Medulloblastoma	3	Posterior fossa	+ +	50% at 5 years
Choroid plexus tumour	1	Ventricle	−	50% at 10 years
Colloid cyst	1	Ventricle	−	potentially curable†
Meninges				
Meningioma	18	Hemisphere	−	potentially curable
Nerve sheath				
Schwannoma	10	VIII nerve	−	potentially curable
Pituitary				
Adenoma	10	Pituitary	+ +	potentially curable
Craniopharyngioma	3	Suprasellar	+	70% at 10 years
Pineal				
Germinoma			+ +	80% at 5 years
Pineocytoma	<1	pineal	+ +	50% at 5 years
Others			+ −	variable
Lymphocytes				
Primary brain lymphoma	<1	Hemisphere	+ +	20% at 2 years
Blood vessels				
Haemangioblastoma	5	Hemisphere/posterior fossa	−	potentially curable
Others	<1			

* Survival data taken from recent series of radical therapy which usually include surgical resection and radiotherapy.
† Recurrences related to incomplete removal.

a dramatic improvement in image quality. CT scanning remains the single most important investigation for brain tumour cases and has largely replaced angiography and air-encephalography. Computer reconstruction of images in coronal and sagittal planes can allow the surgeon to visualise the anatomical relations of the tumour more clearly and help in planning a surgical approach.

It is now possible to transfer clear CT images via telephone lines. Since CT scanners are now being more widely deployed in district general hospitals this means that clinical management decisions can be made by image transfer and telephone consultation with regional neurosurgical centres.

CT scanning to assist tumour biopsy will be described below.

Magnetic resonance imaging

The clinical application of magnetic resonance imaging (MRI) was pioneered in Britain and is rapidly becoming an increasingly important neuro-diagnostic tool. The technique is non- invasive and appears to be entirely without hazard. Images are produced by computer analysis of elec-tromagnetic signals from hydrogen nuclei, when they have been subjected

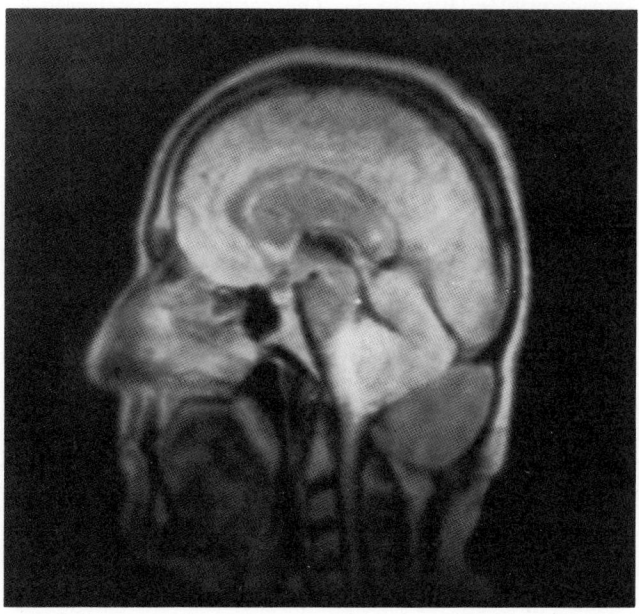

Fig. 15.1 Magnetic resonance imaging. This sagittal image shows an expanded, white area in the inferior brain stem signifying an intrinsic tumour. This tumour was not diagnosed on a new generation CT scanner or by positive contrast ventriculography. At surgery it proved to be a subependymoma and was removed using the surgical laser and leaving a small portion of its origin in the medulla.

to a powerful magnetic field. Images can be produced in any plain. MRI has the ability to reveal certain brain tumours that are not visualised by CT, particularly those in the posterior fossa and spinal cord (Fig. 15.1). Cystic components of spinal cord tumours can be easily seen, thus aiding surgical planning for these difficult lesions. Image enhancement with gadolinium-DTPA, a paramagnetic contrast agent, is a valuable new development.

BIOPSY TECHNIQUES

Brain tumour biopsy is accomplished by craniotomy or more frequently via a burr hole. Free hand burr hole biopsy using a suction cannula (designed over 40 years ago) remains adequate for large superficial lesions but for smaller, deeper lesions there is a perceptible incidence of negative biopsy and also complications such as haemorrhage. For this reason more precise techniques are now coming into practice.

CT directed stereotactic biopsy

A circular stereotactic frame is screwed to the patient's head under local anaesthesia and a CT scan is obtained. The three dimensional co-ordinates of the tumour relative to fixed points of the frame are then obtained from the scanner's computer (Fig. 15.2). The patient is transferred to the operating room where a burr hole is made and the co-ordinates for biopsy are transferred to the stereotactic device which is then fixed on to the frame.

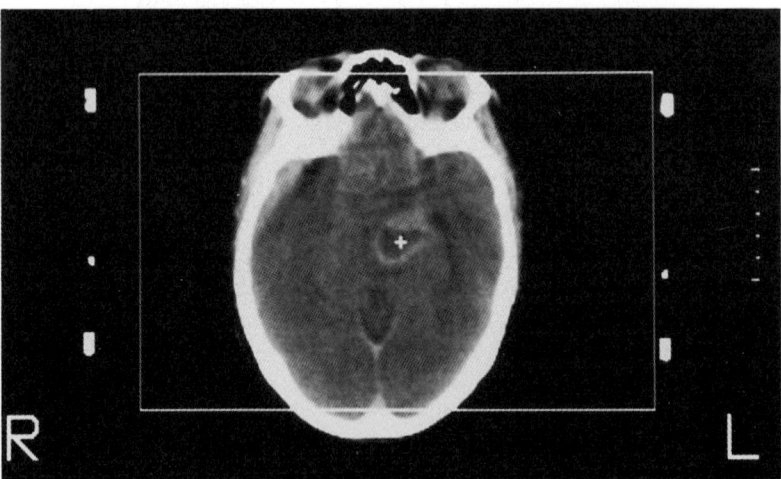

Fig. 15.2 The image obtained during CT scan directed stereotactic biopsy. The cursor has been placed in the centre of a deep tumour which proved to be an astrocytoma. The four posts of the frame are seen just outside the white oblong (courtesy of Professor E. Hitchcock).

This technique can be used to biopsy extremely small lesions in vital areas such as the brain stem and has also been employed to sample various parts of a tumour in order to correlate histology with the scan appearances (Thomas, 1984). It will soon be possible to use similar frames to achieve biopsies of magnetic resonance images in the same manner.

CT directed free hand biopsy

Stereotaxy is a little time consuming and for some lesions it is possible to use the alternative technique of free hand biopsy guided by CT. The biopsy is made via a previously placed burr hole, using a special cannula with the patient in the scanner. The computer measures the depth of the lesion and precise siting of the cannula can then be imaged by the scanner (Fig. 15.3).

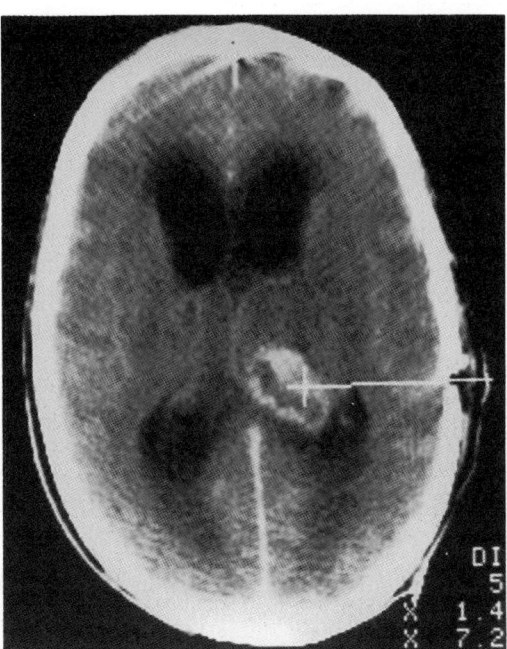

Fig. 15.3 CT directed free hand biopsy of a deep malignant glioma which is producing ventricular obstruction. A computer-generated line extends from the burr hole to a selected point in the lesion. The depth is measured and a special biopsy cannula is then passed along the same track and its position confirmed by repeat CT scan.

Endoscopic biopsy

This technique has not yet gained general usage although it is widely employed in the author's clinic (Griffith, 1975). It is useful in the manage-

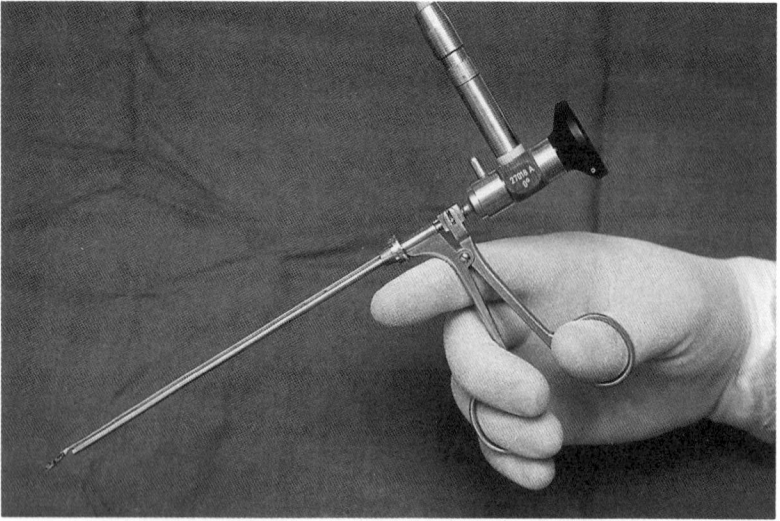

Fig. 15.4 The brain endoscope with biopsy device. Fine cup rongeurs can be seen at the end of the instrument.

ment of intraventricular tumours. The endoscope is a rigid 2 mm diameter end-viewing instrument. It has additional devices for biopsy, for irrigation and for fulguration (Fig. 15.4). A special trocar and cannula is used to make a trancortical track from a burr hole through which the instrument is passed and used to inspect dilated cerebral ventricles or cystic lesions. As in cystoscopy the lesions can be biopsied under direct vision and occasionally resected. This technique is particularly useful in the management of colloid cysts of the third ventricle and pineal tumours (Fig. 15.5).

ADVANCES IN NEUROPATHOLOGICAL TECHNIQUES

The diagnosis of brain tumour biopsies can present difficulties due to the nature of the tissue itself. Not uncommonly tumours consist of undifferentiated small round cells. Occasionally it is difficult to distinguish between a primary tumour, a metastasis and cerebral lymphoma. In addition the neurosurgeon may provide a biopsy fragment that is regarded as too small or is mechanically deformed by rongeurs. The pathologist will then need to resort to special techniques such as electromicroscopy and immunohistology. Immunohistology has progressed rapidly in the last 5 years due to an increase in available antibodies for various tissue components (Weller, 1985). The intermediate filament proteins which form part of the cytoskeleton of a tumour cell are particularly useful targets for identifying the tissue of origin. Examples of these are glial fibrillary acidic protein (astrocytes), cytokeratin (epithelium), and desmin (muscle derivatives). Vimentin, the fourth type of protein in this group, is less specific.

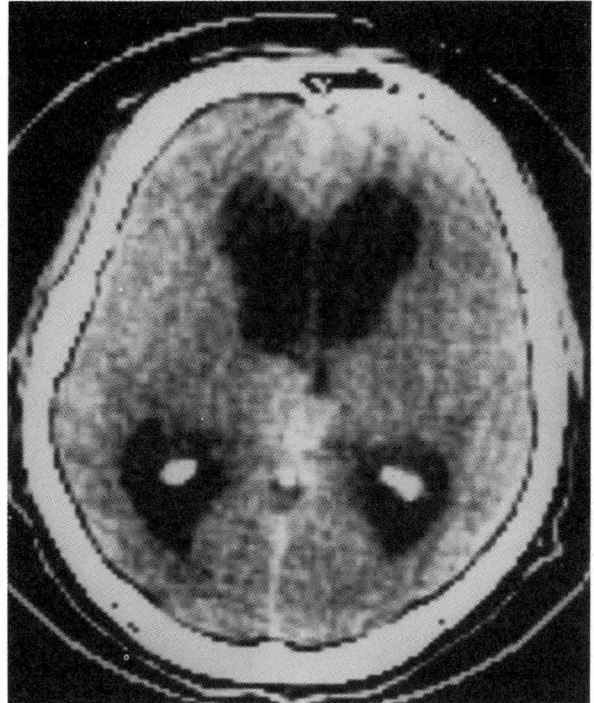

Fig. 15.5 CT scan showing a centrally placed white lesion which has obstructed the ventricles. Endoscopic biopsy was carried out via a right front burr hole, the instrument being passed across the dilated anterior horn. The tumour proved to be a pineoblastoma.

An ever increasing range of monoclonal antibodies directed against cytoplasmic and cell membrane antigens are now becoming available and should soon be widely used in both neuropathology and general pathology. Current evidence indicates that diagnostic accuracy is significantly increased and tumours are now being more fully characterised and understood (Coakham et al, 1985a).

Such antibody techniques are of even more value in cases of neoplastic meningitis and are extremely accurate in identifying and classifying the malignant cells within the cerebral spinal fluid (Coakham et al, 1985b).

ADVANCES IN SURGICAL TECHNIQUES

The basic techniques of craniotomy has changed little over the years. The strategy for dealing with various types of tumour also remains unchanged. Benign lesions are approached with the intent of total removal whenever possible whereas the intrinsic glial tumours are carefully de-bulked in the knowledge that total extirpation is not possible. If these malignant tumours are situated near a pole of a cerebral hemisphere then a formal lobectomy may be performed.

There is no doubt that operative morbidity and mortality has improved over the past decade.

A number of significant advances in technique are now available which enable tumour resection to be carried out more accurately and consequently more safely. For many years neurosurgeons have used microsurgical technique for brain tumour removal, employing either the operating microscope or optical loupes and headlight. The use of self-retaining retractors held by flexible metal 'snakes' and bipolar diathermy, greatly add to the accuracy of dissection.

Certain meningiomas arising from the skull base and the rarer haemangiopericytomas are extremely vascular. Using transfemoral catheter angiography these can be embolised in order to reduce operative blood loss and improve conditions (Fig. 15.6a, b).

Pituitary tumours

These lesions provide a good example of the successful application of microsurgical techniques. Pituitary tumours usually present as large suprasellar masses causing optic pathway compression or as small intrasellar tumours which cause endocrinopathy by over secretion of a specific hormone. Prolactinomas are the commonest example of this latter group and are a cause of female infertility. The endocrinologist will either opt for a course of bromocriptine to reduce serum prolactin levels or will refer the case for microadenomectomy. In the author's unit, these small tumours are approached microsurgically via the transnasal, transphenoidal route, using a speculum retractor passed up the right nostril. This technique is simpler and faster than the alternative sublabial route to the sphenoid sinus. The prolactinoma can be dissected from the anterior lobe of the pituitary with normalisation of prolactin level and retention of normal pituitary function. ACTH secreting adenomas can similarly be removed. Once conversant with this technique the surgeon can remove larger suprasellar tumours using imaging intensifier control. This will avoid the morbidity of craniotomy with includes a risk of post operative epilepsy and a mandatory ban on driving for six months regardless of whether seizures have occurred.

New instruments for tumour resection

Cerebral tumours are frequently firmer in consistency than the surrounding oedematous brain tissue. Routine techniques of removal with rongeurs and high vacuum sucker will inevitably transmit movement to the surrounding brain which may increase the risk of post operative deficit. Ultrasonic aspirators and surgical lasers allow more controlled and accurate removal of tumour tissue without disturbing adjacent brain.

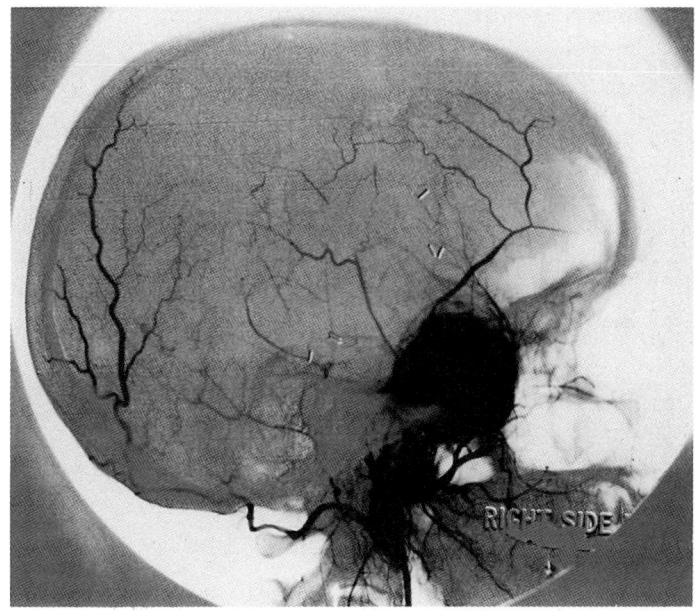

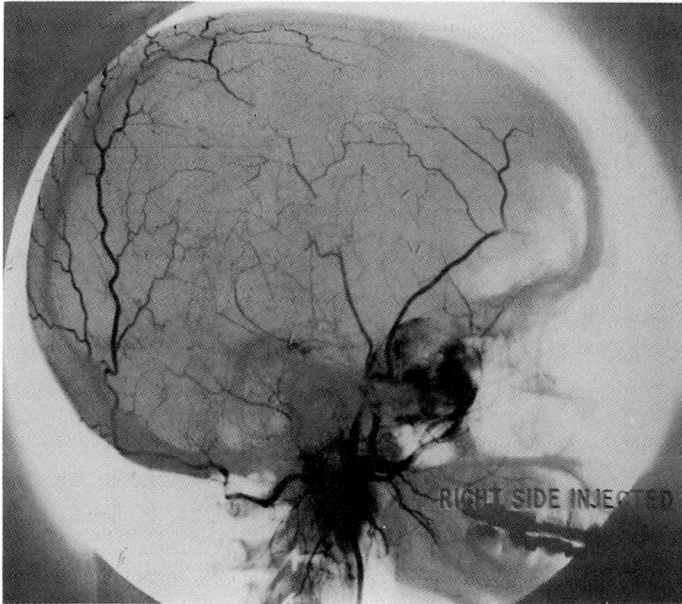

Fig. 15.6 An angiogram of a recurrent base of skull haemangiopericytoma before and after embolisation via a transfemoral catheter passed up the external carotid artery

Ultrasonic surgical aspirator

This device consists of a hand-held sucker with a sharp metal tip which vibrates ultrasonically to emulsify the tissue which it encounters. An irrigation channel is also present (Fig. 15.7). It is used for rapid and atraumatic de-bulking of many types of tumour but is at its most useful in the resection of large acoustic Schwannomas. Having exposed the tumour in the cerebello-pontine angle the ultrasonic aspirator will allow a relatively rapid de-bulking of the tumour thus greatly saving operating time and leaving the surgeon fresh for the more difficult task of dissecting the tumour from the brain stem and the facial nerve.

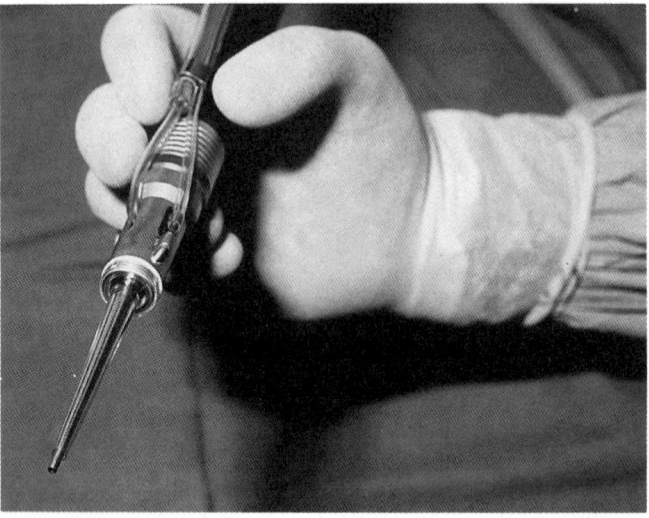

Fig. 15.7 The ultrasonic surgical aspirator. The metal suction tip vibrates ultrasonically. Irrigating saline passes down the outer plastic sheath.

Surgical lasers

(a) The *carbon dioxide laser* is used to accurately vaporise or cut tumour tissue (Fig. 15.8). It is the most commonly employed laser in neurosurgery, and will resect tissue regardless of its toughness without imparting any trauma to the surrounding brain. The laser beam is directed through the operating microscope field by a right angled mirror, using a helium neon target beam since the CO_2 energy is colourless. The beam is guided by a small joystick on the microscope. It is particularly useful for precise dissection of tumours from critical structures such as optic chiasm, parasellar region, brain stem and spinal cord. For the first time astrocytomas and ependymomas within the spinal cord can be safely approached using a combination of laser and ultrasonic aspirator. The CO_2 laser can also be used at high power (40–80 Watts) with the beam defocussed for de-bulking

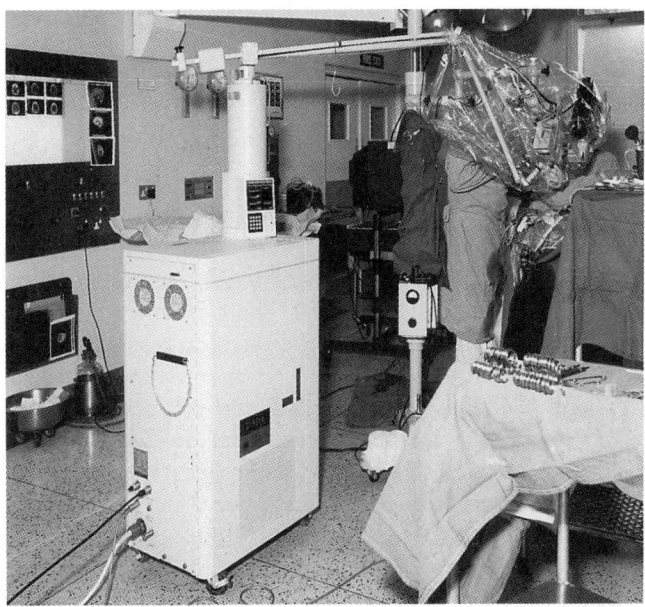

Fig. 15.8 The carbon dioxide laser used in neurosurgery. The laser beam passes through jointed pipes to the objective of the operating microscope which is covered with a sterile plastic bag.

large tough tumours such as meningiomas. The CO_2 laser beam is absorbed by water which limits its use within the ventricles but means that vital structures can be protected by saline soaked collonoid.

A few centres possess elaborate systems which allow small deep tumours to be approached down a narrow brain track via a narrow speculum retractor which is stereotactically guided by CT scan co-ordinates. A laser is then programmed to oblate the tumour having defined its margins on the CT scan image. It is not yet known whether this 'star wars' approach will have general application.

(b) The *Neodymium-YAG laser* is a hand-held unit. The energy produced is absorbed by tissues more deeply than the CO_2 beam and thus has a coagulating property. It can be used for hemastasis in deep-seated base of skull tumours, such as meningiomas and chordomas. The irradiation produced by this laser can be transmitted through cerebrospinal fluid thus allowing it to be used for intraventricular surgery via the endoscope.

(c) Photodynamic therapy requires the use of an argon pumped dye laser which emits red light of about 630 nm wavelengths. A photosensitive agent such as hematoporphyrin derivative is given intravenously about 48 hours previously and will be selectively taken up by tumour tissue. The argon laser is then applied and causes excitation of the photodynamic agent which releases cytotoxic free radicals with predominant damage to the tumour.

Human gliomas take up photodynamic agents as well and this modality shows promise but is still at the experimental stage.

ADJUNCTIVE THERAPY

Although accuracy of dissection and of pathological diagnosis has been markedly increased, the majority of malignant brain tumours are not curable by surgery and require post operative radiation therapy or chemotherapy. The role of external beam irradiation for supratentorial gliomas in adults remains somewhat controversial. There is now good evidence that radiotherapy will modestly increase the survival in cases of the more highly malignant gliomas (from a mean of about 6 months to a mean of about 12 months). Patient selection for further therapy is aided by the knowledge that advanced age and a marked neurological deficit at presentation are powerful indicants of a poor survival. Treatment is generally, therefore, reserved for young adults who are in good condition.

It is still not known whether radiotherapy influences the outcome in cases of low-grade astrocytoma although there is a clinical suspicion that it is beneficial. Multi-centre prospective trials are now underway to address this question.

Other malignant tumours in adults are generally treated with radiotherapy, especially the primary brain lymphomas which are extremely radiosensitive although tend to recur later. These lesions were originally classified as microgliomas. It is now known that they are non-Hodgkin B-cell lymphomas, and a proportion of cases go on to develop systemic deposits of lymphoma. This is one of the tumours associated with immunodeficiency states, and is being increasingly reported in cases of acquired immune deficiency syndrome (AIDS).

The cerebellar medulloblastomas of children are also radiosensitive and it is mandatory to treat these cases with a total neuraxis field to avoid early recurrences from seedlings within the CSF pathways. In addition to the benefit of radiotherapy it is now known that radical surgical resection confers an increase in survival. Germinomas are the commonest pineal tumours of children and young adults and can secrete antigenic markers which are of use in diagnosis (alphafoetoprotein, human chorionic gonadotrophin, carcinoembryonic antigen). This diagnosis is important to make since these tumours are extremely radiosensitive.

There is recent interest in the use of interstitial irradiation to treat gliomas that have recurred following conventional therapy. High energy beta emitting isotopes such as 192-Iridium or 125-Iodine are placed in the tumour, either by free hand technique or using stereotactic methods. At Frenchay Hospital we place small plastic tubes into the tumour bed following repeat craniotomy and de-bulking in younger patients with superficial tumours. Iridium wires are then inserted into the tubes for a period of time determined by dosimetry calculations (Fig. 15.9).

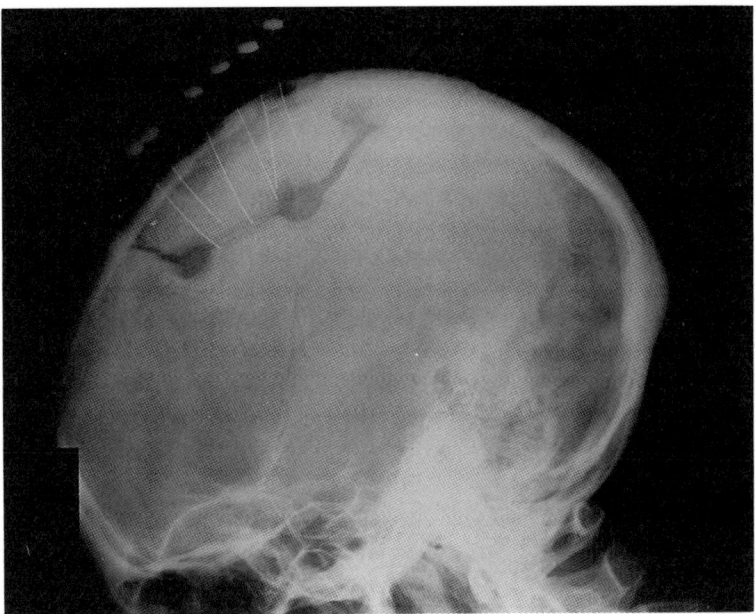

Fig. 15.9 Skull X-ray showing placement of Iridium wires for interstitial irradiation of a recurrent astrocytoma in the vertex region

All types of high dosage radiotherapy to the brain can be complicated by local radionecrosis which can mimic tumour recurrence, or by diffuse leukoencephalopathy which causes dementia. Dosimetry therefore requires careful judgement.

At present chemotherapy has a modest role in brain tumour treatment. Beneficial affects in supertentorial tumours of adults are marginal, although the nitrosourias (BCNU, CCNU) are sometimes given. Attempts to improve results by intracarotid delivery high concentrations of drugs by catheters are being evaluated. Other tumours such as brain lymphomas and germinomas may require chemotherapy regimes appropriate to the biology of the lesion.

Attempts are also being made to rationalise chemotherapy by in vitro sensitivity assays in which a panel of drugs are tested against cultured cells obtained from tumour biopsies of individual patients.

There is a more definite role for chemotherapy in some of the paediatric brain tumours. An example being 'high risk' medulloblastoma cases with residual tumour invading brain stem or the very young who cannot tolerate an adequate dose of irradiation. Combination chemotherapy regimes for other paediatic tumours are being vigorously assessed in a number of centres.

MANAGEMENT OF CEREBRAL METASTATIC DISEASE

Brain metastases represent an important cause of morbidity in cancer patients. Recent studies suggest that 15–20% of patients with cancer have intracranial metastases at autopsy, the majority of which produce symptoms during life. Some clinicians have noted an increase in frequency of brain metastases and have speculated that this may be the result of increasing longevity brought about by aggressive treatment of underlying lesion.

The current treatment of brain metastases is considered palliative, approximately 50% of patients with brain secondaries have multiple tumours demonstrated by CT scan. Even in patients with single brain lesions, there may be widespread systemic tumour deposits and these considerations preclude the possibility of curative treatment in most patients. Despite this, neurological improvement and increased survival can result from the removal of solitary cerebral secondaries in selected cases. Preoperative planning from CT scan along with the newer techniques of tumour resection have contributed to accurate removal of metastases with a very low surgical mortality. Postoperative whole brain irradiation is generally recommended in order to sterilise microscopic fragments of residual tumour and any existing micro-metastases which may be present. The survival will be determined by the nature of the primary tumour, the extent of underlying systemic disease and also the site of the cerebral deposit, a supratentorial metastasis being associated with a better survival than those in the posterior fossa. The incidence of various cancers metastasising to brain, and survivals following surgery and radiotherapy are shown in Table 15.2.

Table 15.2 Cerebral metastases, incidence and survival following surgery and radiotherapy*

Primary site		Median survival (months)	Percent survival at 2 years
Lung	40%	18	38
Skin (melanoma)	11.2%	6	14
Kidney	11.2%	6	31
Colon	8%	10	0
Sarcoma	8%	8	20
Breast	6.4%	12	25
Unknown	4.8%	5	17
Miscellaneous	10.4%	6	23
Overall survival		12	25

* from Sundaresan & Galicich (1985)

RECENT SCIENTIFIC ADVANCES

In recent years molecular biology has been advancing on two fronts. Monoclonal antibodies are now being used for both diagnosis and therapy of certain cancers. Recombinant DNA techniques have resulted in the detection of oncogenes which are related to various types of neoplasia. These genetic sequences which may also be found in tumour inducing viruses, are intimately associated with the malignant process and may masquerade as either cellular growth factors or growth factor receptors. The implications for this very new technology are exciting, for example, antibodies to oncogene peptide products would be highly specific markers for neoplastic cells.

Monoclonal antibodies have already been used to assist in the histological diagnosis of brain tumours but have a clear potential for use in vivo for targeted therapy. The attractive 'magic bullet' concept of employing specific antibody armed with lethal radio-isotope or toxin is at present being put to the test. Early results from clinical trials in Bristol suggest that 131-Iodine labelled monoclonal antibody is able to clean the CSF of neoplastic cells very effectively. The technique would be of value in treating all forms of neoplastic meningitis particularly when patients have already received maximal external beam irradiation.

ACKNOWLEDGMENTS

I am grateful to Mrs G. Wenczek for preparing the manuscript and also the Illustration Department, Frenchay Hospital, for photographs.

REFERENCES

Coakham H B, Garson J A, Allan P M, Harper E I, Brownell B, Kemshead J T, Lane E B 1985a Immunohistological diagnosis of cerebral nervous system tumours using a monoclonal antibody panel. Journal of Clinical Pathology 38: 165–173
Coakham H B, Garson J A, Brownell B, Allan P M, Harper E I, Lane E B, Kemshead J T 1985b Use of a monoclonal antibody panel to identify malignant cells in the cerebrospinal fluid. Lancet 1: 1095–1098
Griffith H B 1975 Technique of fontanelle and persutural ventriculoscopy and endoscopic ventricular surgery in infants. Childs Brain 1: 359–363
Thomas D G T, Anderson R E, DeBoulay G H 1984 CT guided stereotactic neurosurgery: experience in 24 cases with a new stereotactic system. Journal of Neurology, Neurosurgery and Psychiatry 47: 9–16
Weller R O 1985 The immunopathology of brain tumours. Bleehan N M (ed) Tumours of the Brain, Springer-Verlag, Berlin, ch 19
Bleehan N M 1985 Tumours of the Brain. Springer-Verlag, Berlin
Northfield D W C 1973 The Surgery of the Central Nervous System. J B Lippincott, Philadelphia
Punt J 1984 Intracranial tumours. In: Lumpley J S P, Craven J L (eds) Surgery, Vol. 1. Blackwell Scientific, Oxford, p 239–243
Rose F C, Fields W s 1985 Neuro-Oncology. Karger, Basel
Thomas D G T, Graham D I 1980 Brain Tumours. Scientific Basis, Clinical Investigation and Current Therapy. Butterworths, London

Index